Clinical Anatomy and Management of Cervical Spine Pain

CLINICAL ANATOMY AND MANAGEMENT OF CERVICAL SPINE PAIN

L. G. F. Giles MSc, DC(C), PhD

Reader
Department of Public Health and Tropical Medicine,
James Cook University of North Queensland, Townsville

Director
National Centre for Multidisciplinary Studies of Back Pain,
Townsville General Hospital

Honorary Clinical Scientist
Townsville General Hospital, Townsville, Queensland, Australia

and

K. P. Singer MSc, PT, PhD

Associate Professor
School of Physiotherapy,
Curtin University of Technology,
Shenton Park, Western Australia

Honorary Research Fellow
Departments of Radiology, Neuropathology and Bioengineering,
Royal Perth Hospital, Perth, Western Australia, Australia

With a Foreword by

Professor Jiri Dvorak MD

Head of Department of Neurology,
Spine Unit, Schulthess Clinic, Zurich, Switzerland

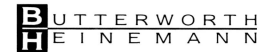

OXFORD AUCKLAND BOSTON JOHANNESBURG MELBOURNE NEW DELHI

Butterworth-Heinemann
Linacre House, Jordan Hill, Oxford OX2 8DP
225 Wildwood Avenue, Woburn, MA 01801-2041
A division of Reed Educational and Professional Publishing Ltd

A member of the Reed Elsevier plc group

First published 1998
Reprinted 2001

British Library Cataloguing in Publication Data
A catalogue record for this book is available from the British Library.

Library of Congress Cataloguing in Publication Data
A catalogue record for this book is available from the Library of Congress.

ISBN 0 7506 2397 7

For information on all Butterworth-Heinemann
publications visit our website at www.bh.com

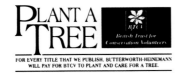

PLANT A TREE

British Trust for
Conservation Volunteers

FOR EVERY TITLE THAT WE PUBLISH, BUTTERWORTH-HEINEMANN
WILL PAY FOR BTCV TO PLANT AND CARE FOR A TREE.

Composition by Genesis Typesetting, Rochester, Kent
Printed in Great Britain by The Bath Press, Bath

Contents

Contributors

P. G. Baker
Associate Professor, Division of Community and Rural Health, University of Tasmania, Mersey Hospital, Latrobe, Tasmania, Australia

J. H. Bland
Professor of Medicine – Rheumatology, Emeritus, Rheumatology and Clinical Immunology Unit, University of Vermont, Burlington, USA

J. J. W. Boyle
School of Physiotherapy, Curtin University, Perth, Western Australia, Australia

R. Burtt
Spinal Research Unit, University of Huddersfield, Huddersfield, UK

R. Cailliet
Professor Emeritus, Department of Physical Medicine, University of Southern California, School of Medicine, Los Angeles, California, USA

R. Clarke
Spinal Research Unit, University of Huddersfield, Huddersfield, UK

M. I. Gatterman
Dean of Chiropractic and Clinical Sciences, Western States Chiropractic College, Portland, Oregon, USA

L. G. F. Giles
Reader, Department of Public Health and Tropical Medicine, James Cook University of North Queensland; Director, National Centre for Multidisciplinary Studies of Back Pain, Townsville General Hospital; Honorary Clinical Scientist, Townsville General Hospital, Queensland, Australia

N. R. Jones
Professor, Department of Neurosurgery, Royal Adelaide Hospital, South Australia, Australia

G. A. Jull
Associate Professor Physiotherapy Department, University of Queensland, St Lucia, Australia; Honorary Research Fellow, Department of Physiotherapy, University of Melbourne, Victoria, Australia

T. McClune
Spinal Research Unit, University of Huddersfield, Huddersfield, UK

N. Milne
Department of Anatomy and Human Biology, University of Western Australia, Perth, Western Australia, Australia

L. Penning
Emeritus Professor of Medical Imaging, Department of Neuroradiology, University Hospital, Groningen, The Netherlands

L. J. Rowe
Department of Medical Imaging, John Hunter Hospital, Newcastle, New South Wales, Australia

A. P. Shapiro
Department of Psychological Services, University Hospital, London, Ontario, Canada

K. P. Singer
Associate Professor, School of Physiotherapy, Curtin University of Technology, Shenton Park, Western Australia; Honorary Research Fellow, Departments of Radiology, Neuropathology and Bioengineering, Royal Perth Hospital, Perth, Western Australia, Australia

R. W. Teasell
Associate Professor and Acting Chairman,
Department of Physical Medicine and
Rehabilitation, London Health Sciences Center and
University of Western Ontario, London, Ontario,
Canada

A. G. J. Terrett
Associate Professor, School of Chiropractic,
Osteopathy and Complementary Medicine, Faculty
of Biomedical and Health Sciences, RMIT University,
Bundoora, Victoria, Australia

C. Walker
Spinal Research Unit, University of Huddersfield,
Huddersfield, UK

Foreword

The prevalence of neck pain is remarkably high, amounting to between 12 and 34% amongst the so-called normal population, depending on the age group. The aging population displays a higher incidence of neck pain, with or without radicular symptoms and signs, presenting with a decreased range of motion. One of the reasons for this might be the ongoing transformation of the bony structures, as observed by the German anatomist, Herbert von Luschka (1858) and scientifically studied by the Swiss anatomist, Gian Töndury (1947). Such a developmental transformation might be due to the upright position of the human body as well as the use and sometimes abuse of the cervical spine during daily working, leisure and sporting activities, leading to degenerative changes of the vertebral body and plates and the intervertebral and zygapophysial joints.

An understanding of these developmental changes, or – as pointed out by Töndury' – this 'ongoing transformation', is essential for the interpretation of altered motion patterns in relation to patient symptoms, clinical signs and radiological findings. The diagnosis will finally determine the appropriate therapeutic approach, mainly in deciding whether conservative or surgical treatment is indicated. Furthermore, an understanding of the underlying pathology will help the clinician to recognize the limits of the therapeutic procedure, especially when aggressive treatments might be counterproductive and simple 'wait and see' advice might be most beneficial for the patient in the long run.

Much too often we witness needlessly prolonged treatments of neck disorders from medical practitioners, chiropractors, osteopaths and other professional groups dealing with cervical spine disorders who do not always respect their limits and sometimes delude themselves concerning their therapeutic omnipotence.

The cervical spine is quite an unstable part of the spinal column where the equilibrium can easily be disturbed by minor trauma and sometimes even by aggressive treatment procedures. The most notable examples are the soft tissue injuries of the cervical spine as a result of car collisions.

The management of neck problems, due either to degenerative changes or trauma, is not an easy task, and requires a profound knowledge of the functional anatomy, the clinical biomechanics as well as the radiology and neurology of the cervical spine. This book impressively documents our current understanding of the above. The editors have invited world renowned authors to contribute to this book. The individual chapters are well balanced, reviewing the past development of our knowledge, combined with major new scientific advances.

The undersigned, in his own clinical life, regularly deals with cervical spine disorders, ranging from the easy-to-manage sprains to the more difficult problems such as narrowing of the spinal canal leading to severe cervical myelopathies which require extensive surgery. Based upon my own clinical experience and research work in the field of the cervical spine, I would highly recommend this book, not only to general practitioners, but also to specialists or to anybody who wishes to deal competently with cervical spine problems, bearing in mind that our major task is not to harm the patient (*primum non nocere* of Hippocrates). This is definitely important to recognize in the management of cervical spine disorders.

Zurich, September 1997
Professor Jiri Dvorak, MD
Head of Department of Neurology, Spine Unit,
Schulthess Clinic, Zurich, Switzerland

Preface

Our intention in compiling this new text series is to provide an international perspective on the rational approach to managing mechanical spinal pain. We present a comprehensive review and analysis of clinically relevant information on the basic sciences leading to diagnosis and treatment of mechanical neck disorders, with a chapter dedicated to contra-indications to spinal manipulation.

This text highlights the value of a team approach in appreciating the complexity of neck pain and a range of treatment approaches. Contemporary contributions from anatomy, pathology, clinical medicine, neurosurgery, chiropractic, osteopathy and physiotherapy are presented in this volume. Each part, written by experienced academic clinicians, provides a summary of pertinent material which will lead to an improved understanding of the causes of mechanical neck pain. Management strategies, based on routine assessment techniques, are proposed using clinical reasoning sequences. This text does not attempt to endorse a single therapy, rather to highlight the common approach to mechanical treatment which may be provided by chiropractic, osteopathy and physiotherapy practitioners.

Our goal is to present this information in a manner which will benefit both the undergraduate and postgraduate student of mechanical therapy, as well as all clinicians who seek a comprehensive review of mechanical neck pain. In the belief that quality illustrations facilitate the message, careful selection of material and detailed captions have been prepared to complement the text. A second objective is to encourage greater communication between the clinical schools interested in this important subject. Through this, we hope to contribute to a stronger scientific basis for cervical spine care.

The volume is organized so that it can be approached in several ways, according to the needs of the reader. The clinician who wishes a quick overview of clinical assessment concepts and techniques should consult Part 3: Diagnosis and management. This includes: imaging procedures for mechanical neck complaints, medical and surgical approaches to neck pain and separate chapters on the assessment and management strategies provided by chiropractors, osteopaths and physiotherapists.

Part 1 introduces the reasoning behind this text. Part 2 presents the clinical anatomy, pathology and biomechanics of the cervical spine.

Our general approach to both the clinical and scientific aspects of mechanical neck pain is to provide a contemporary review of the literature and to present logical examples of clinical reasoning behind three disciplines of mechanical therapy. Despite the need to validate theories behind mechanical intervention and to show the long-term efficacy of these therapies, this text also sets out our challenge, as clinician–scientists, to promote communication between all interested parties. Neck pain is multifaceted and it demands the sharing of ideas and knowledge to improve the management offered to our patients.

L. G. F. Giles
K. P. Singer

Section

I

Introduction

Introduction

L. G. F. Giles and P. G. Baker

Although many individuals (80–85%; Lewis *et al.,* 1993; Lahad *et al.,* 1994; Murtagh, 1994) will suffer from low back pain at some time during their lives, and only 35–40% will suffer from neck and arm pain (Bovim *et al.,* 1994; Day *et al.,* 1994), the latter can be a major source of mechanical spinal pain, and 30% of such patients will develop chronic symptoms (Shelokov, 1991). In addition, it has been known for many years that neck pain can be associated with referred pain to the head, the shoulders, upper extremities and anterior or posterior portions of the chest, between shoulders, and the mid and lower back (Jackson, 1977). Neck pain with or without cervicogenic headache uses an enormous volume of medical services and yet no clinical studies have addressed the validity of diagnostic or epidemiological factors associated with muscle lesions and disc lesions, but painful zygapophysial joints have been studied (Bogduk, 1995).

Many individuals suffer from cervicogenic headaches due to neck injuries and this is a major health problem in view of the increasing number of motor vehicle accidents which can cause a varied constellation of symptoms depending on which structures are injured in flexion–extension-type injuries of the cervical spine (Jackson, 1977; Chapter 5).

In order to appreciate the magnitude of suffering due to cervical spine injuries and degenerative changes, it is necessary to understand the anatomy and pathology of the cervical spine, including that of the cervicothoracic transitional junction (Bailey *et al.,* 1995), as briefly outlined here and in Chapters 2 and 3. In addition, serious psychosocial issues which can arise as a result of cervical spine injuries must also be considered (Merskey, 1993), as well as fibromyalgia syndrome (McCain, 1993) and myofascial pain syndrome (Fricton, 1993).

Motion (mobile) segment and its parts

The cervical spine has typical cervical vertebrae below the second spinal level (C2) whereas the vertebrae above the C3 vertebra are atypical (Chapter 2).

Lewin *et al.* (1961) and Hirsch *et al.* (1963) pointed out that the basic anatomical and functional unit of the vertebral column is the articular triad consisting of the fibrocartilaginous intervertebral joint and the two synovial zygapophysial joints. The motion (mobile) segment of Junghanns (Schmorl and Junghanns, 1971) is conveniently subdivided into anterior and posterior elements (Andersson, 1983) and consists of all the space between two vertebrae where movement occurs: the intervertebral disc with its cartilaginous plates, the anterior and posterior longitudinal ligaments, the zygapophysial joints with their fibrous joint capsules and the ligamenta flava, the contents of the spinal canal and the left and right intervertebral canals, and the ligamentum nuchae (Fig. 1.1).

The joints in the neck are responsible for first, flexibility, allowing a variety of movements such as flexion, extension, lateral bending and axial rotation, and second, load transmission and shock absorption for axial and torsional strains primarily as a result of the mechanical properties of the intervertebral disc (Shelokov, 1991). Furthermore, posture plays an important role in the cervical spine as it does in the thoracic and lumbosacral spines.

Posture

In normal posture, the line of weight is the perpendicular through the centre of gravity (Joseph, 1960).

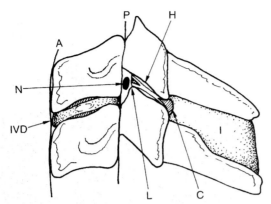

Fig. 1.1 The motion (mobile) segment of Junghanns. A and P = Anterior and posterior longitudinal ligament respectively; H = hyaline articular cartilage; I = interspinous ligaments; IVD = intervertebral disc with anulus fibrosus, nucleus pulposus and cartilage end-plates; C = joint capsule with associated synovial folds at the superior and inferior recesses; L = ligamentum flavum; N = neural structures. In addition, the space between the transverse processes and all corresponding muscular parts must be included. (Compare with histological section shown in Figure 1.10.)

The importance of this line lies in its relationship to the transverse axes of rotation of the joints of the vertebral column and the lower limbs since the body tends to fall forwards or backwards due to gravity according to whether the line of weight passes in front of, or behind, these axes, respectively (Joseph, 1960).

Posture and movement are related to the musculature of the back which has two functions: first, to hold the central supporting organ of the body (the spinal column) in its proper shape and position, and second, to supply the force for its movement. The muscles situated near the body's surface and far from the midline are highly effective motor agents, whereas the muscles situated adjacent to the spinal column are mainly concerned with maintenance of posture (Rickenbacher *et al.,* 1985).

Poor posture, in which the head is thrust forward with excessive spinal curves in the sagittal plane, sloping or hunched shoulders, protruding abdomen and hyperextended knees (Garlick, 1990; Fig. 1.2B) may be habitual or occupational (Mennell, 1960), and can be related to poor muscle tone. This can cause chronic postural strain which, in turn, can cause myofascial pain (Keim and Kirkaldy-Willis, 1987).

Thus it is important that good erect posture be maintained because poor posture can greatly increase the biomechanical stresses on the cervical spine (Chapter 7, Fig. 7.18). The human spine as a whole is a very complicated structure and it is considered by some to be a masterpiece of engineering (Keith, 1923; Farfan, 1978; Giles, 1991).

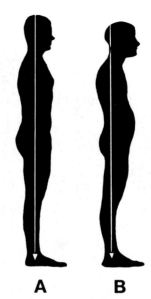

Fig. 1.2 A = Good posture due to proper muscle tone. B = Bad posture which develops when poor muscle tone is present. Note the hyperlordotic cervical and lumbar spines with the kyphotic thoracic spine. The line of weight in the neck, and the rest of the body, is no longer normal. From Giles (1991) with permission.

Although motion of the spine is under the control of active spinal musculature, further protective support is achieved from the complex ligamentous system (Farfan, 1978; Putz, 1992). Some ligaments have a dual role, for example the ligamenta flava are not only involved in resisting excess separation of adjacent vertebral laminae but also protect the neural elements from associated osseous structures, such as the laminae and zygapophysial joints, in parts of the spinal and intervertebral (foraminal) canals. Furthermore, under normal circumstances, the epidural and epiradicular adipose tissue affords an adequate reserve cushion for protection of neural and vascular structures within the spinal and intervertebral canals.

Three main factors make the cervical spine, including some of its neurovascular structures, vulnerable to abnormal mechanical stresses: first, apparent disregard for maintaining good posture; second, congenital or acquired anomalies of osseous and soft tissues; and third, our frequent inability to protect the spine from injuries, which may lead to joint dysfunction and degeneration.

Anomalies

Anomalies are varied and include first, osseous spinal anomalies such as unilaterally or bilaterally enlarged

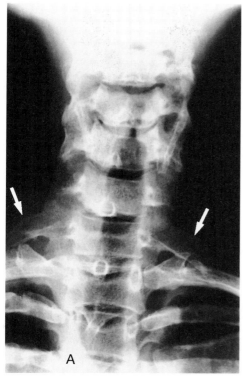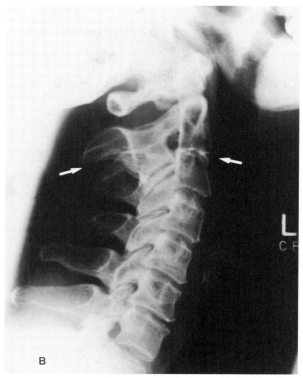

Fig. 1.3 Two congenital anomalies of the spine are shown as an example: A = bilaterally enlarged transverse processes, i.e. C7 rudimentary cervical ribs; B = blocked vertebrae.

C7 transverse processes or rudimentary cervical ribs (Fig. 1.3A), blocked vertebrae (Fig. 1.3B), which occur most commonly at C2–3 then at C5–6 (Brown *et al.*, 1964); and second, soft-tissue anomalies such as conjoined nerve roots, or fibrous bands in continuation with rudimentary cervical ribs (Adams and Hamblen, 1990). Enlarged transverse processes can affect the subclavian artery and the lowest trunk of the brachial plexus as they arch over this process due to mechanical pressure against it (Sunderland, 1968; Adams and Hamblen, 1990). In the case of congenitally blocked vertebrae, the freely movable articulations above and below the blocked segment are placed under additional mechanical stress, and this usually results in premature degenerative discogenic spondylosis and arthrosis at the fully articulated levels (Guebert *et al.*, 1996).

Spinal injuries

Our apparent inability to protect the neck from injury in many circumstances is an enormously complex issue which can be summarised as being due to unexpected trauma, or a poor understanding of spinal ergonomics and correct posture. The latter issue is beyond the scope of this volume but trauma is a serious problem in view of the ever-increasing number of motor vehicle accidents. This important issue will briefly be mentioned in this chapter but considered in detail in Chapter 5.

Innervation

A summary of the innervation of structures which may be injured in cervical spine trauma is briefly discussed here. In order to lay a foundation for understanding the possible clinical syndromes which may result from trauma to the cervical spine, reference should be made to original publications (Jackson, 1977) for a complete anatomical description.

The cervical zygapophysial joints are innervated by articular branches derived from the medial branches of the cervical dorsal rami; an ascending branch innervates the zygapophysial joint above and a descending branch innervates the joint below, resulting in a dual innervation for each zygapophysial joint (Lord *et al.*, 1993). Beyond the zygapophysial joint the medial branches of the cervical dorsal rami supply the

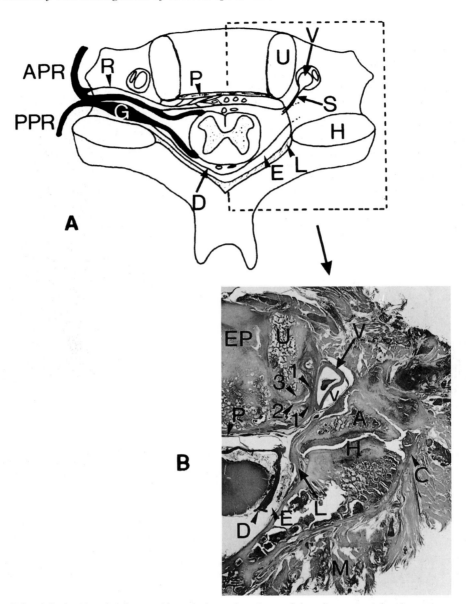

Fig. 1.4 A = Schematic drawing showing a mid cervical vertebra. Some of the adjacent peripheral nerve structures arising from the spinal cord are shown on the left side. On the right, the neural structures passing over the pedicle have not been illustrated but the spinal artery is shown arising from the vertebral artery. Note the anterior and posterior spinal arteries and veins, respectively and the small epidural vessels supplied by the recurrent meningeal nerve.

B = A 100 μm thick histological section cut in the horizontal plane through the right side of a cervical spine is shown (enlarged) for comparison with the overall view shown in A. Note the proximity of the vertebral artery to both the uncovertebral and zygapophysial joints. The sympathetic vertebral plexus located on the vertebral artery is not illustrated but is shown schematically in Figure 1.7.

A = Articular process (superior); APR = anterior primary ramus; C = capsule (fibrous) of zygapophysial joint; D = dural tube; E = epidural space; EP = end-plate on vertebral body; G = ganglion (spinal) on posterior nerve root; H = hyaline articular cartilage on the zygapophysial joint facets; L = ligamentum flavum; M = muscle; P = posterior longitudinal ligament; PPR = posterior primary ramus; R = recurrent meningeal nerve; S = spinal artery branch arising from the vertebral artery; U = uncinate process (raised lip) of the vertebral body showing part of the synovial joint of von Luschka with its (1) capsule, (2) synovial fold and (3) hyaline articular cartilage; V = vertebral artery and its adjacent thin-walled vein (v) within the foramen transversarium.

semispinalis and multifidus muscles (Lord *et al.,* 1993). An outline of the anterior and posterior nerve roots, the spinal ganglion, the spinal nerve dividing into anterior and posterior primary rami, and the recurrent meningeal nerve is shown in Figure 1.4A. In Figure 1.4B a histological section, cut in the horizontal plane through a mid cervical vertebra, is shown to illustrate some of the histological anatomy.

It should be remembered that Sunderland (1975) showed that two anatomical features in particular protect nerve roots from being overstretched: the arrangement of the dura at the entrance to the intervertebral canal (foramen), and the secure attachment of the C4–7 cervical spinal nerves to the gutter of the transverse processes (Fig. 1.5).

As each of the C4–7 spinal nerves leaves the intervertebral canal, it is immediately lodged in the gutter of the transverse process to which it is securely bound by

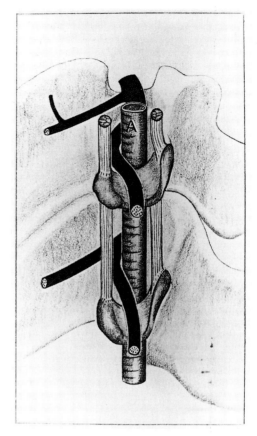

Fig. 1.6 Diagram to illustrate the manner in which the spinal nerve is forced against the posterior bony bar of the transverse process by the vertebral artery (A). From Sunderland (1975) with permission.

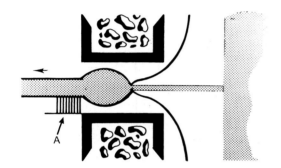

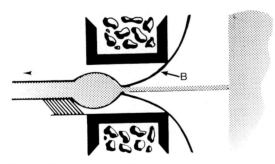

Fig. 1.5 Diagram showing the manner in which nerve roots are protected from being overstretched during lateral traction on the spinal nerve under normal circumstances. A = Attachment of the spinal nerve to the transverse process; B = plugging action of the dural sleeve as it is drawn into the foramen. Lateral displacement of the nerve complex is limited because of the attachments of the spinal nerve to the cervical transverse process and subsequently, and where no such attachments exist, by the plugging action of the dural funnel as it is drawn into the foramen. For simplification only one dorsal rootlet is shown. Abnormal forces may rupture the protective attachment at A and B. From Sunderland (1975) with permission.

its epineurial sheath, by reflections of the prevertebral fascia, by slips from the musculotendinous attachments to the transverse processes and by fibrous slips that descend from the transverse process above to blend with the epineurium of the nerve below (Sunderland, 1975). The nerve is also held backwards against the posterior bony bar of the transverse process by the vertebral artery whose adventitial coat blends with the sheath of the nerve (Sunderland, 1975). The artery usually lies within the foramen transversarium from C6 cephalad (Oh *et al.,* 1996; Fig. 1.6).

The autonomic nervous system

The autonomic nervous system includes parts of the central and peripheral nervous systems, the latter being concerned with the innervation of viscera, glands, blood vessels and non-striated muscle; it is the visceral (splanchnic) component of the nervous system (Williams and Warwick, 1980; Chusid, 1985). The autonomic nervous system is intimately responsive to changes in the somatic activities of the body, and while its connections with somatic elements are not always clear in anatomical terms, the physiological evidence of visceral reflex activities stimulated by somatic events is abundant (Williams and Warwick, 1980). The anatomy and physiology of the autonomic nervous system have been described over the years by several authors, such as Sheehan (1936), White *et al.* (1952), Kuntz (1953), Mitchell (1953, 1956), Pick (1970), and illustrated in detail by Netter (1962).

Anatomically, the autonomic nervous system is divided into two complementary divisions – the *sympathetic* and *parasympathetic nervous systems*. The preganglionic efferent fibres of the parasympathetic nervous system emerge through certain cranial and sacral spinal nerves and constitute the *craniosacral outflow*. The cell bodies of the postganglionic neurons in the parasympathetic system are situated peripherally, either as discrete collections forming ganglia nearer to the structures innervated than to the central nervous system, or sometimes dispersed in the walls of the viscera themselves (Williams and Warwick, 1980). The cell bodies of the postganglionic neurons in the sympathetic system are generally situated in ganglia of the sympathetic trunk or as ganglia in more peripheral plexuses, almost always nearer to the spinal cord than to the effectors which they innervate.

The sympathetic nervous system (thoracolumbar outflow), which is the larger division of the autonomic nervous system, includes the two ganglionated sympathetic trunks, their branches, plexuses and subsidiary ganglia, and innervates sweat glands and arrector pili muscles of the skin, the muscular walls of blood vessels everywhere, the heart, lungs and abdominopelvic viscera (Williams and Warwick, 1980; Barr and Kiernan, 1983). The preganglionic fibres, which are myelinated, are the axons of nerve cells in the lateral column of the grey matter of all the thoracic and upper two to three lumbar segments of the spinal cord; they emerge from the spinal cord through the ventral roots of the corresponding spinal nerves and pass into the spinal nerve trunks and the commencement of their ventral rami, which they leave in the white rami communicantes, to join either the corresponding ganglia on the sympathetic trunks or their interganglionic parts (Williams and Warwick, 1980). The possibility of a limited outflow of preganglionic fibres in other spinal nerves has been suggested and it is certain that nerve cells of the same type as those in the lateral grey column also exist at levels above and below the thoracolumbar outflow (Mitchell, 1953) and that small numbers of their fibres issue in corresponding ventral roots.

The cervical portion of the sympathetic trunk lies in the posterior wall of the carotid sheath and includes the superior, middle and inferior sympathetic ganglia (Fig. 1.7); the inferior cervical ganglion (located on the anterior aspect of the first rib head) is frequently fused with the first thoracic ganglion to form the stellate, or cervicothoracic, ganglion and it is joined by the white communicating ramus of the first thoracic nerve and is sometimes connected with the C6, C7, C8 and T1 nerves by sympathetic roots (Kuntz, 1964). Figure 1.7 has been simplified from Jackson's (1977) textbook and gives an overview of the extent of the cervical sympathetics.

Jackson (1977) has documented possible sympathetic responses to injury of the cervical sympathetics and other authors have written on this topic (von Torklus and Gehle, 1972; Chapters 2 and 5). According to Shelokov (1991), bizarre vasomotor symptoms can be explained when one considers that spondylosis (specifically involving the joints of Luschka) can irritate the vertebral artery sympathetic nerves.

With respect to the sympathetic supply of structures in the head and thorax, the preganglionic fibres terminate in ganglia of the sympathetic trunk: for smooth muscles and glands in the head, the synapses between pre- and postganglionic neurons are mainly in the superior cervical ganglion of the sympathetic trunk (Barr and Kiernan, 1983); for thoracic viscera, the synapses are in the three cervical sympathetic ganglia (superior, middle and inferior) and in the upper five ganglia of the thoracic portion of the sympathetic trunk (Barr and Kiernan, 1983).

Autonomic innervation includes the muscles of the iris and ciliary body in the eye, smooth muscles in the orbit, the lacrimal, salivary glands and sweat glands, and all blood vessels (Barr and Kiernan, 1983; Fig. 1.7).

The superior cervical sympathetic ganglion is located on the ventral aspect of the transverse processes of the C2–4 vertebrae and receives preganglionic fibres through the sympathetic trunk from the first four or more thoracic nerves; sympathetic roots arising from this ganglion join the C1 and C2 (and sometimes C3 and C4) nerves and fibres derived from this ganglion make up the major portion of the *internal* and *external carotid plexuses* (Kuntz, 1964). The latter branches of the superior cervical ganglion consist of grey rami communicantes to the C1–4 nerves and to some of the cranial nerves (Williams and Warwick, 1980). The *vertebral artery plexus* arises from the middle, intermediate and inferior sympathetic trunk ganglia (Kuntz, 1964) but is derived mainly from a thick branch of the cervicothoracic ganglion (Williams and Warwick, 1980). From the vertebral artery plexus, deep rami communicantes pass to the anterior rami of the C1 to C5–6 spinal nerves and the plexus continues into the skull via the basilar arteries and their branches as far as the posterior cerebral artery where it meets with the plexus derived from that on the internal carotid artery (Williams and Warwick, 1980). Lazorthes

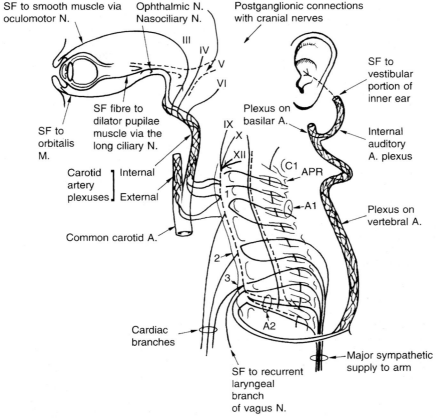

Fig. 1.7 The cervical sympathetic nerves. The preganglionic fibres are indicated by broken lines and the postganglionic fibres by solid lines. C1 = First cervical nerve roots, spinal ganglion and spinal nerve; APR = anterior primary ramus of the spinal nerve (its adjacent posterior primary ramus is not marked). Irritation of postganglionic fibres at A1 may cause reflex stimulation of the cervical sympathetic nerves. Interruption of preganglionic fibres at A2 will give paralysis of the cervical sympathetic supply. Postganglionic connections with cranial nerves III–VI, IX, X and XII are illustrated. 1 = Superior cervical sympathetic ganglion; 2 = middle cervical sympathetic ganglion; 3 = inferior cervical sympathetic ganglion (stellate ganglion). SF = sympathetic fibres. Simplified from Jackson (1977).

(1949) and Mitchell (1952) consider that the vertebral artery plexus represents the main intracranial extension of the sympathetic system.

Pain

Neck pain may be associated with anomalous cervical vertebrae such as agenesis of the anterior and/or posterior arches of the atlas vertebra, hemivertebra(e), congenital block vertebrae or rudimentary or cervical rib(s) (Sunderland, 1968; Jackson, 1977; Adams and Hamblen, 1990). Agenesis of the anterior or posterior arches of the atlas, and hemivertebra(e), are rare (Guebert *et al.,* 1996). The percentage of congenital block

vertebrae is 0.7 (Brown *et al.,* 1964); the percentage of rudimentary cervical ribs in the population is 0.5–1.00 (Haven, 1939; Steiner, 1943; Jones *et al.,* 1984) and can be clinically significant or asymptomatic. It appears that precipitating factors such as injury, faulty posture or unaccustomed hard labour are a few of the factors which can convert a latent condition into one causing trouble (Sunderland, 1968).

Joint injury often results from motor vehicle accidents which can result in well-documented lesions, such as illustrated in Figure 1.8.

The soft tissues of the cervical zygapophysial vertebral joints are poorly seen with plain film radiographs, computed tomography (CT) and magnetic resonance imaging (MRI). Nevertheless, joint capsule tears have been shown at surgery (Jeffreys,

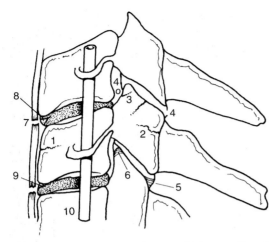

Fig. 1.8 The more common lesions which may affect the cervical spine following whiplash. 1 = Vertebral body fracture; 2 = articular pillar fracture; 3 = fractures involving the articular facet subchondral bone plate; 4 = tears of the zygapophysial joint capsule; 5 = haemarthrosis in the zygapophysial joint; 6 = synovial fold trauma with possible nipping; 7 = tear of the anterior longitudinal ligament; 8 = tear of the anulus fibrosus of the intervertebral disc; 9 = end-plate avulsion; 10 = vertebral artery which has an extensive sympathetic nerve plexus, both of which can be traumatized.

1980) and other injuries have been found during postmortem examination such as intervertebral disc and soft-tissue injuries of the zygapophysial joints (Taylor and Kakulas, 1991; Taylor and Twomey, 1993). Other injuries from postmortem material have shown injuries of the ligamentum flavum, uncovertebral joints and cartilaginous end-plate avulsions (Jonsson *et al.*, 1991).

Cervical spine joint dysfunction due to injury can often be shown by cervical spine flexion and extension stress (functional) views. An example of a cervical spine extension stress view in a 29-year-old female, who sustained a neck injury in a rear-end motor vehicle accident 16 months prior to radiography, highlights this issue (Fig. 1.9). There is joint hypermobility and instability between vertebrae at the C3–4 and C4–5 levels, as indicated by backward displacement of the vertebral bodies upon each other and 'gapping' between some paired zygapophysial joint facet surfaces.

Because soft tissues which could be injured are not visible on plain X-ray images such as shown in Figure 1.9, nor in any detail on CT or MRI, Figures 1.10 and 1.11 show some of the soft tissues which could be injured and which should be borne in mind when examining a patient.

Most soft-tissue structures of the cervical spine have a good nociceptive nerve supply so that pain

will warn of incorrect spinal movements and strains. This pain is a main cause of disability and expense from work-related injuries accounting for approximately 4% of workers' compensation injuries, and is the eighth most common cause of injuries (Workers' Compensation Board of Queensland Annual Report, 1995). In spite of this, cervical spine basic science studies received very little attention until relatively recently with the studies of Giles (1986), Jonsson *et al.* (1991), Taylor and Kakulas (1991) and the clinical studies by Jackson (1977), Barnsley *et al.* (1993) and Lord *et al.* (1993), in spite of the possibly serious implications of cervical spine injury. Central cord syndrome is now a well-established entity in spinal cord injury which is most often seen in hyperextension injuries in patients with cervical spondylosis or narrow spinal canals (Chang, 1995). The syndrome is characterized by greater involvement of

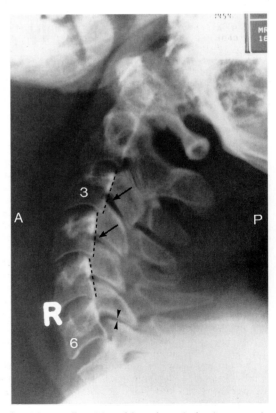

Fig. 1.9 A well-positioned lateral cervical spine extension (stress) view. Note: (1) backward displacement of C3 vertebral body on C4 (as shown by the dotted line on the posterior aspect of the vertebral bodies); (2) backward displacement of C4 vertebral body on C5; (3) the facet joint planes are parallel, except at the C3–4 and C4–5 levels where the joints 'gap' anteriorly (arrows). A = Anterior; P = posterior.

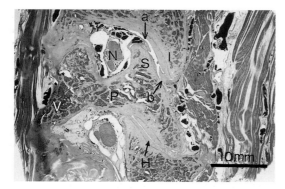

Fig. 1.10 Parasagittal section from a cervical spine showing part of the anterolateral aspect of the vertebral body (V) and the superior (S) and inferior (I) articular processes of the zygapophysial joint. Note the superior (a) and inferior (b) highly vascular synovial folds which can be nipped between joint surfaces during injury. H = Hyaline articular cartilage on the lower joint's facet surfaces, which is essentially normal. Note that the cartilage on the upper joint facets one level above has almost worn away on the superior articular process (S). N = Neural structures in the intervertebral foramen which are surrounded by fatty tissue and many blood vessels. P = Pedicle joining the vertebral body and the posterior spinal elements, i.e. superior and inferior articular processes, etc. The darkly stained muscle groups anteriorly and posteriorly are illustrated. From Giles (1986) with permission.

upper-extremity motor function compared with that of the lower extremities, and sensory symptoms most typically consisting of a burning sensation or hyperpathia in the upper extremities (Hopkins and Rudge, 1973; Maroon, 1977; Wilberger *et al.,* 1986). The pathophysiology of this syndrome is believed to be an oedematous type of process in the central part of the spinal cord (Chang, 1995).

Refractory neck and head pain is a serious problem which is difficult to treat (Carpenter and Rauck, 1996). New surgical techniques have been established in order to combat the problem of cervical disc herniation with radiculopathy (Jho, 1996) as well as for craniovertebral junction surgery (Al-Mefty *et al.,* 1996) and some cases requiring cervical spine surgical intervention are illustrated in Chapter 8.

The clinical entity of cervical spondylotic myelopathy became well-recognized in the 1950s through the work of Brain and associates (Brain *et al.,* 1952; Brain and Wilkinson, 1967) as well as that of Clarke and Robinson (1956), who identified cervical spondylotic myelopathy as resulting from the spondylotic process, although the pathophysiology of cervical myelopathy is probably multifactorial (Bohlman, 1995).

Law *et al.* (1995) schematically illustrated the various structures that can contribute to the patho-

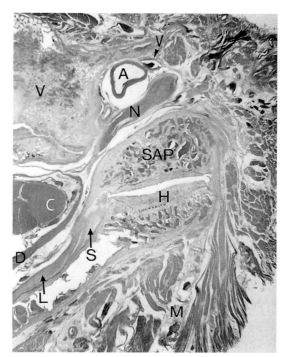

Fig. 1.11 Further soft tissues which could be injured in the mid cervical spine by trauma.

Partial horizontal section cut through the mid cervical spine showing part of the vertebral body (V) and the superior (SAP) and inferior articular processes with their zygapophysial joint facet and a synovial fold (S) which can be nipped between joint surfaces during injury. A = Vertebral artery within the foramen transversarium with its adjacent vein (V arrow); C = spinal cord; D = dural tube; H = hyaline articular cartilage on the facet surfaces, which is essentially normal; L = ligamentum flavum; N = neural structures in the intervertebral foramen, including the ganglion which are surrounded by fatty tissue and blood vessels. The darkly stained muscle groups (M) anteriorly and posteriorly are illustrated.

logical anatomy of cervical spondylotic myelopathy and these can be summarised as protruding intervertebral disc, ossification of the posterior longitudinal ligament, hypertrophy of the ligamentum flavum, osteoarthrosis of the zygapophysial or uncovertebral joints, or any combination of these.

An example of some osseous degenerative changes which can occur in the cervical spine is given in Figure 1.12 which shows the superior and inferior aspects of the sixth vertebra.

The medial margin of a normal uncovertebral joint to the medial margin of the foramen transversarium which contains the vertebral artery ranges from approximately 4.0 to 6.3 mm (Oh *et al.,* 1996). Therefore, relatively minor osteophytic

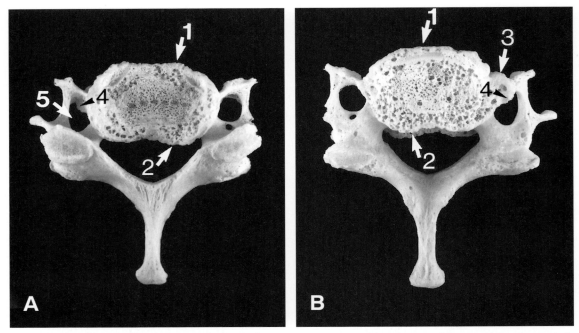

Fig. 1.12 Superior (A) and inferior (B) views of the C6 vertebra showing spondylotic lipping of the vertebral body anteriorly (1), posteriorly into the spinal canal (2), and at the lateral margins of the uncovertebral joint (3). Osteophytic encroachment by the C6–7 uncovertebral joint (4) of particularly the left transverse foramen (5) through which the vertebral artery passes indicates how vulnerable the vertebral artery can be. The left superior articular facet slightly encroaches upon the adjacent transverse foramen in this specimen.

development at the lateral margins of the uncovertebral joint can encroach upon the foramen transversarium and its contents.

Despite the spine's excellent design (Keith, 1923; Farfan, 1978; Giles, 1991), with its normal cervical and lumbar lordoses and its thoracic kyphosis being well-adapted to the function of the vertebral column, any major aberrations in these spinal curves are mechanically unsound (Rickenbacher *et al.,* 1985). It is well-known that radiologically normal but painful spines (Benson, 1983; El-Khoury and Renfrew, 1991) may have pathological changes which cannot be demonstrated radiologically (Dixon, 1980). It is suggested that pain in these cases may be due to mechanical irritation of various pain-sensitive soft-tissue structures which cannot be visualized by imaging procedures but can be found at postmortem, as shown by macroscopic studies (Jonsson *et al.,* 1991; Taylor and Kakulas, 1991; Taylor and Twomey, 1993), although it is not possible to correlate pathological findings in cadavers with pain. Many spinal structures probably play a role in pain production, as all innervated structures in the motion segment are possible sources of pain (Haldeman, 1977; Nachemson, 1985).

Magnitude of the problem of neck pain

Acute injury of the cervical spine presents the treating clinician with numerous diagnostic and management issues, and successful long-term treatment is contingent on early recognition of the injury (Slucky and Eismont, 1994). Acute and chronic neck pain, although sometimes due to frank pathological causes, can result from alterations from the normal in the vertebral column and constitutes a major health problem (National Health and Medical Research Council, 1988; Spitzer *et al.,* 1995).

Two important factors compound the problem of spinal pain mechanisms (Haldeman, 1977): pain may have a multifactorial aetiology, and there may be several types of pain which closely mimic each other. Part of the problem relates to the fact that the neck region is extremely complex, both anatomically and functionally (Chapter 2). We await further elucidation of the pathophysiology of spinal pain since the pathologic aetiology of many varieties of spinal pain remains undiscovered (Pearcy *et al.,* 1985; Tajima and Kawano, 1986).

In spite of many attempts to provide a rationale for clinicians to order diagnostic examinations properly and prescribe treatments that maximize the quality and efficiency of patient care (Spitzer *et al.,* 1995), the complex problem of neck pain continues unabated. Many psychological factors are believed to contribute to the development, exacerbation and/or maintenance of chronic spinal pain (Kinney *et al.,* 1991) and, when evaluating patients with chronic neck pain (Chapters 5–12), it is necessary to understand clinical findings in relation to issues of everyday functioning, such as employment, social adjustment and activities of daily living (Millard and Jones, 1991; James and McDonald, 1996; Chapter 7).

In general, the answer to the complex issue of spinal pain may well depend upon multidisciplinary cooperation and, as Frymoyer *et al.* (1991) state, centres for spinal care will emerge as part of larger health care systems. This principle is as important in cervical spine pain syndromes as it is in thoracic and lumbosacral spine syndromes.

Degenerative processes

Degeneration of the intervertebral disc and associated osteoarthrosis of the synovial zygapophysial joints and joints of von Luschka (uncovertebral joints; Compere *et al.,* 1959; Williams and Warwick, 1980) can cause neck pain resulting from a synovitis, in all probability due to an increase of synovial fluid causing pressure on the richly innervated capsular structures and adjacent nerve root (Jackson, 1977). According to Butler *et al.* (1990), disc degeneration occurs before zygapophysial joint osteoarthrosis which may be secondary to mechanical changes in the loading of the zygapophysial joints. It has also been suggested that intervertebral disc herniation is associated with vertebrogenic pain and the autonomic syndrome (Jinkins *et al.,* 1989; Giles, 1992). Jackson (1977) clearly illustrated the possible role of the cervical sympathetics in the cervical syndrome in the presence of irritation of the vertebral arteries and the internal and external carotid arteries and their sympathetic plexuses (Fig. 1.7), as well as injuries to the cervical nerve roots and the spinal cord.

In addition, pain of vascular origin, due to deformation of blood vessels and venous stasis within blood vessels of the lumbar spinal and intervertebral canals, has been suggested by Giles (1973), Hoyland *et al.* (1989), Giles and Kaveri (1990) and Jayson (1997). Degenerative joint changes in the cervical spine would most likely result in similar changes to cervical spine blood vessels. Pain may be experienced in the absence of radiologically obvious degenerative joint disease, or other pathological changes, as a result of traction on normal pain-sensitive structures, for

example, the innervated joint capsules, or pinching and tractioning of the highly vascular and innervated intra-articular synovial folds within the zygapophysial joints (Giles, 1989; Fig. 1.10). Because diagnostic imaging procedures may well not provide a diagnosis in cases where pain is due to mechanical dysfunction of joints, some authors stress psychological factors (Hoehler and Tobis, 1983).

Diagnostic problems

Neck pain may originate from many different innervated spinal tissues making it difficult to evaluate a patient with neck pain of mechanical origin, with or without referred pain; the painful structure or structures are not amenable to direct scrutiny, so a tentative diagnosis is usually arrived at for an individual by taking a case history and employing a format similar to the examination procedures indicated in Chapters 7–12.

However, in spite of following routine examination procedures, one often merely eliminates demonstrable pathologies and the cause of spinal pain of mechanical origin often remains obscure (Margo, 1994), especially when dysfunction and degenerative pathology of spinal joints occur. In severe cases of neck pain, injections of anaesthetic, with or without steroid suspension, are sometimes used to augment the clinical evaluation (Lord *et al.,* 1993), for example to determine whether pain originates in the zygapophysial joint(s). Imaging procedures such as plain film radiography, CT, MRI, myelography, and bone scans (Chapter 6) have diagnostic limitations, and even three-dimensional MRI techniques (Ross, 1995) have limitations. Specifically, diagnostic problems relate first to, inadequacies in the precise knowledge of the anatomy of the cervical spine and its related soft-tissue structures; second, there are multifactorial causes of pain at a given level of the spine in some cases, and third, many diagnostic procedures have limitations. Also, there is often disagreement on which imaging procedures have diagnostic validity for neck pain of mechanical origin. Certainly, the use of flexion and extension plain film radiography, with measurement of segmental motion in the sagittal plane, is a valuable method for determining pathological conditions such as hypo- and hypermobility (Dvorak *et al.,* 1988) and can demonstrate instability secondary to ligamentous laxity (Gibson, 1991). As shown in Figure 1.9, stress views of the cervical spine can demonstrate regions of anatomical hypermobility and instability. Such views can also demonstrate hypomobility.

Furthermore, some diagnostic and therapeutic chemical agents may be harmful, for example when such agents injected into intervertebral discs extravasate into the epidural space (Weitz, 1984; Adams *et al.,* 1986; MacMillan *et al.,* 1991) during discography, causing complications due to contact between these chemical agents and neural structures (Eguro, 1983; Dyck, 1985; Merz, 1986; Watts and Dickhaus, 1986). Therefore, such diagnostic tests should only be performed to provide reliable information about a patient's condition and if the result is likely to influence the patient's management (Modic and Herzog, 1994).

In many cases of neck pain with radiculopathy, intervertebral disc prolapse has been described as being the pathological cause (Mixter and Ayer, 1935), although radicular arm pain can be due to irritation or compression of a cervical nerve root due to other causes (Chapter 8). Herniated nucleus pulposus does not necessarily produce radiculopathy and may only cause vague referred pain. Therefore, caution must always be exercised prior to manipulation of the cervical spine as radiculopathy may not necessarily be the first symptom of cervical disc prolapse. An example to highlight such a case is that of a 52-year-old man who only experienced mild paraesthesiae in the lateral border of the left little finger, even though he had significant right-sided C5–6 intervertebral disc prolapse on CT (Fig. 1.13).

Based on lumbar spine studies, many authorities believe that disc herniation has been overemphasized as the principal source of spinal pain and that advocating early surgery, even for patients with appropriate pathology such as herniated nucleus pulposus, is not recommended given the favourable history of natural recovery for the majority of these patients (Lehmann *et al.,* 1993). Spontaneous recovery from pain thought to be associated with lumbar intervertebral disc herniation is well-known and it is reasonable to suspect that such neck pain may also have a favourable history of natural recovery.

It is likely that cervical zygapophysial joint pain is a common condition which is frequently overlooked (Wedel and Wilson, 1985; Lord *et al.,* 1993) and the alleviation of the pain by injection of local anaesthetic, with or without steroid suspension, into the joints, under fluoroscopic control, supports this diagnosis (Lord *et al.,* 1993).

Limitations of investigative methods

All imaging procedures only provide a shadow of the truth (Giles and Crawford, 1997) as detailed anatomy and early histopathology cannot be perceived (Fig. 1.10). CT, MRI and bone scans, although able to give additional and different types of information to that provided by plain film radiographs, still have limitations. For example, although MRI has proved to be a valuable diagnostic tool in the initial evaluation of the patient with discogenic pain, Schellhas *et al.* (1996)

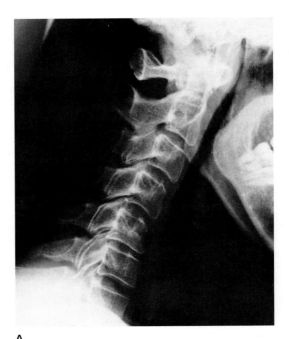

A

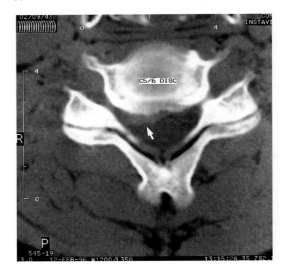

B

Fig. 1.13 (A) The C5–6 intervertebral disc has thinned by approximately 40% as seen on the cervical spine flexion view. (B) The computed tomographic scan view shows the right-sided C5–6 intervertebral disc herniation, but the left intervertebral canal is stenotic.

showed that significant cervical disc anular tears often escape MRI detection when compared with discography. It should be noted that, although MRI is useful for nuclear anatomy, it is not helpful for symptomatology (Buirski and Silberstein, 1993). The anatomical basis of primary cervical discogenic pain provoked with discography has been described by Bogduk *et al.* (1988).

MRI is useful for assessing spinal cord anatomy and pathology, ligamentous integrity (Brightman *et al.,* 1992), particularly the integrity of the anterior and posterior longitudinal ligaments (McArdle *et al.,*

1986), epidural fat, cerebrospinal fluid and marrow space (Lauterbur, 1973) and, used in conjunction with CT and plain film radiography, it can also aid in the evaluation of bony injuries (Brightman *et al.,* 1992). Therefore, although spinal imaging can be informative (Chapter 6) it has limitations (Carroll, 1987), and there is often a discrepancy between the degree of pain and the severity of radiographic changes (Stockwell, 1985). For example, disabling zygapophysial joint syndromes can be associated with normal or nearly normal plain film radiographs (Eisenstein and Parry, 1987).

Table 1.1 *Some possible causes of mechanical neck pain with or without arm pain*

Nerve root conditions
Adhesions between dural sleeves and (a) the joint capsule with nerve root fibrosis (Wilkinson, 1967; Sunderland, 1968; Jackson, 1977) and (b) intervertebral disc herniation (Wilkinson, 1967)

Intervertebral disc degeneration and fragmentation (Schiotz and Cyriax, 1975), or nucleus pulposus extrusion (Mixter and Ayer, 1935) causing nerve root compression or nerve root chemical radiculitis (Marshall and Trethewie, 1973)

Zygapophysial joint conditions
Joint derangement (subluxation) due to ligamentous and capsular instability (Hadley, 1964; Cailliet, 1968; Jackson, 1977; Macnab, 1977; van Norel and Verhagen, 1996)

Joint capsule tension, encroachment of the intervertebral foramen lumen (Jackson, 1977)

Joint degenerative changes, e.g. meniscal incarceration (Schmorl and Junghanns, 1971), traumatic synovitis due to pinching of synovial folds (Giles, 1986), synovial fold tractioning against the pain-sensitive joint capsule (Hadley, 1964) and osteoarthrosis (Jackson, 1977)

Joint effusion with capsular distension which may (a) exert pressure on a nerve root (Jackson, 1977); (b) cause capsular pain (Jackson, 1966) or (c) cause nerve root pain by direct diffusion (Haldeman, 1977)

Joint capsule adhesions (Jackson, 1977; Farfan, 1980; Giles, 1989)

Intervertebral disc conditions
Significant disc herniation into the spinal and intervertebral canals

Spondylosis (Young, 1967; Jackson, 1977)

Miscellaneous conditions
Spinal and intervertebral canal (foramen) stenosis (Young, 1967; Jackson, 1977; Epstein and Epstein, 1987; Rauschning, 1992)

Intervertebral canal (foramen) venous stasis (Sunderland, 1975)

Myofascial genesis of pain (trigger areas); Travell and Rinzler, 1952; Bonica, 1957; Simons and Travell, 1983)

Baastrup's syndrome (Bland, 1987)

Osseous spinal anomalies, e.g. bilateral cervical ribs, block vertebra (Jackson, 1977)

Possible causes of mechanical neck pain with or without upper limb pain

Table 1.1 briefly summarizes some possible causes of neck pain of mechanical origin, with or without arm pain, and provides a summary of some literature references over the years in order to provide a historical background to this complex issue.

Many other causes of neck pain, with or without progressive radiculopathy, should be considered, and Table 1.2 summarizes some well-established disorders of the neck and cervical spine.

Table 1.2 *Classification of disorders of the neck and cervical spine*

Deformities
Infantile torticollis
Congenital short neck
Congenital high scapula

Arthritis of the spinal joints
Rheumatoid arthritis
Ankylosing spondylitis
Osteoarthritis of the cervical spine (cervical spondylosis)

Infections of bone
Tuberculosis of the cervical spine
Pyogenic infection of the cervical spine

Mechanical derangements
Prolapsed intervertebral disc
Cervical rib
Cervical spondylolisthesis
Joint dysfunction

Tumours
Benign and malignant tumours in relation to the cervical
   spine, spinal cord and nerve roots

Modified from Adams and Hamblen (1990).

Summary

It is not our intention to list all the possible causes of neck pain in this chapter summarising some anatomy and pathology which may have a bearing on cervical spine pain of mechanical origin but rather to provide an overview of this complex issue as an introduction to following chapters. In order to appreciate a neck pain sufferer's signs and symptoms, it is necessary to understand normal erect posture and the complex anatomy and possible subtle or overt pathology of the cervical spine and the cervicothoracic junction (see Chapters 2 and 3). The following chapters review the basic anatomy and pathology of the cervical spine, followed by kinematics, the clinical picture of whiplash-type injuries, radiology and clinical management.

References

Adams, J.C., Hamblen, D.L. (1990) *Outline of Orthopaedics,* 11th edn.. Edinburgh: Churchill Livingstone, p. 154.

Adams, M.A., Dolan, P., Hutton, W.C. (1986) The stages of disc degeneration as revealed by discogram. *J. Bone Joint Surg.* **68B:** 36.

Al-Mefty, O., Borba, A.B., Aoki, N., Angtuaco, E., Pait, T.G. (1996) The transcondylar approach to extradural non-neoplastic lesions of the craniovertebral junction. *J. Neurosurg.* **84:** 1-6.

Andersson, G.B.J. (1983) The biomechanics of the posterior elements of the lumbar spine. *Spine* **8:** 326.

Bailey, A.S., Stanescu, S., Yesting, R.A. *et al.* (1995) Anatomic relationships of the cervicothoracic junction. *Spine* **20:** 1431-1439.

Barnsley, L., Lord, S., Bogduk, N. (1993) The pathophysiology of whiplash. In: *Cervical Flexion-Extensions/Whiplash Injuries* (R.W. Teasell, A.P. Shapiro, eds). Spine: State of the Art Review, vol. 7. Philadelphia: Hanley and Belfus, pp. 329-354.

Barr, M.L., Kiernan, J.A. (1983) *The Human Nervous System,* 4th edn. Philadelphia: Harper & Row.

Benson, D.R. (1983) The spine and neck. In: *Musculoskeletal Diseases of Children* (Gershwin M.E., Robbins D.L., eds). New York: Grune & Stratton, p. 469.

Bland, J.H. (1987) *Disorders of the Cervical Spine. Diagnosis and Medical Management.* Philadelphia: WB Saunders.

Bogduk, N. (1995) Editorial. Scientific monograph of the Quebec task force on whiplash associated supplementary disorders. *Spine* **20:** 8S-9S.

Bogduk, N., Windsor, M., Inglis, A. (1988) The innervation of cervical intervertebral discs. *Spine* **13:** 2-8.

Bohlman, H.H. (1995) Cervical spondylosis and myelopathy. In: *Instructional Course Lectures* (Jackson D.W., ed.). Illinois: Academy of Orthopaedic Surgeons, pp. 81-97.

Bonica, J.J. (1957) Management of myofascial pain syndromes in general practice. *J.A.M.A.* **164:** 732-738.

Bovim, G., Schrader, H., Sand, T. (1994) Neck pain in the general population. *Spine* **19:** 1307-1309.

Brain, L., Wilkinson, M. (eds) (1967) *Cervical Spondylosis and Other Disorders of the Cervical Spine.* Philadelphia: WB Saunders.

Brain, W.R., Northfield, D., Wilkinson, M. (1952) The neurological manifestations of cervical spondylosis. *Brain* **75:** 187-225.

Brightman, R.P., Miller, C.A., Rea, G.L. *et al.* (1992) Magnetic resonance imaging of trauma to the thoracic and lumbar spine. *Spine* **17:** 541-550.

Brown, M.W., Templeton, A.W., Hodges, F.J. (1964) The incidence of acquired and congenital fusions in the cervical spine. *A.J.R.* **92:** 1255-1259.

Buirski, G., Silberstein, M. (1993) The symptomatic lumbar disc in patients with low-back pain. *Spine* **18:** 1808-1811.

Butler, D., Trafimow, J.H., Andersson, G.B.J. *et al.* (1990) Discs degenerate before facets. *Spine* **15:** 111-113.

Cailliet, R. (1968) *Low Back Pain Syndrome,* 2nd edn. Philadelphia: F.A. Davis.

Carpenter, R.L., Rauck, R.L. (1996) Refractory head and neck pain. A difficult problem and a new alternative therapy. *Anesthesiology* **84:** 249-252.

Carroll, G. J. (1987) Spectrophotometric measurement of proteoglycans in osteoarthritic synovial fluid. *Ann. Rheum. Dis.* **46:** 375-379.

Chang, H.S. (1995) Cervical central cord syndrome involving the spinal trigeminal nucleus: a case report. *Surg. Neurol.* **44:** 236-240.

Chusid, J.G. (1985) *Correlative Neuroanatomy and Functional Neurology,* 19th edn. California: Lange Medical Publications, p. 162.

Clarke, E., Robinson, P.K. (1956) Cervical myelopathy: a complication of cervical spondylosis. *Brain* **79:** 483-510.

Compere, E.L., Tachdjian, M.O., Kernahan, W.T. (1959) The Luschka joints. Their anatomy, physiology and pathology. *Am. J. Orthop. Surg.* **1:** 159-168.

Day, L.J., Bovill, E.G., Trafton, P.G. *et al.* (1994) Orthopedics. In: *Current Surgical Diagnosis and Treatment* (Way L.W., ed.) Connecticut: Appleton Lange, pp. 1011-1104.

Dixon, A. St. (1980) Diagnosis of low back pain - sorting the complainers. In: *The Lumbar Spine and Back Pain* (Jayson M., ed.), 2nd edn. Kent: Pitman Medical, pp. 135-156.

Dvorak, J., Froehlich, D., Penning, L. *et al.* (1988) Functional radiographic diagnosis of the cervical spine: flexion/extension. *Spine* **13:** 748-755.

Dyck, P. (1985) Paraplegia following chemonucleolysis. *Spine* **10:** 359.

Eguro, H. (1983) Transverse myelitis following chemonucleolysis. *J. Bone Joint Surg.* **65A:** 1328.

Eisenstein, S.M., Parry, C.R. (1987) The lumbar facet arthrosis syndrome. Clinical presentation and articular surface changes. *J. Bone Joint Surg.* **69B:** 3-7.

El-Khoury, G.Y., Renfrew, D.L. (1991) Percutaneous procedures for the diagnosis and treatment of lower back pain: diskography. Facet joint injection, and epidural injection. *A.J.R.* **157:** 685-691.

Epstein, N.E., Epstein, J.A. (1987) Individual and coexistant lumbar and cervical spinal stenosis. In: *Spinal Stenosis* (Hopp E., ed.) Spine: State of the Art Reviews **1:** 401-420.

Farfan, H.F. (1978) The biomechanical advantage of lordosis and hip extension for upright man as compared with other anthropoids. *Spine* **3:** 336-345.

Farfan, H.F. (1980) The scientific basis of manipulative procedures. *Clin. Rheum. Dis.* **6:** 159-178.

Fricton, J.R. (1993) Myofascial pain and whiplash. In: *Cervical Flexion-Extension/Whiplash Injuries* (Teasell R.W., and Shapiro A.P., eds). Spine: State of the Art Reviews **7**: 403-422.

Frymoyer, J.W., Ducker, T.B., Hadler, N.M. *et al.* (1991) The future of spinal treatment. In: *The Adult Spine: Principles and Practice* (Frymoyer J.W., ed.). New York: Raven Press, pp. 43-52.

Garlick, D. (1990) *The Lost Sixth Sense. A Medical Scientist looks at the Alexander Technique*. Kensington, NSW: Biological and Behavioural Sciences Printing Unit, The University of NSW.

Gibson, G. (1991) Radiographic evaluation of the cervical spine. In: *Cervical Spine Disease* (Regan J.J., ed.) Spine: State of the Art Reviews **5**, 177-187.

Giles, L. G. F. (1973) Spinal fixation and viscera. *J. Clin. Chiropract. Arch.* **3**: 144-165.

Giles, L.G.F. (1986) Lumbo-sacral and cervical zygapophyseal joint inclusions. *Man. Med.* **2**: 89-92.

Giles, L.G.F. (1989) *Anatomical Basis of Low Back Pain*. Baltimore: Williams & Wilkins.

Giles, L.G.F. (1991) A review and description of some possible causes of low back pain of mechanical origin *Homo sapiens*. *Proc. Aust. Soc. Human Biol.* **4**: 193-212.

Giles, L.G.F. (1992) Paraspinal autonomic ganglion distortion due to vertebral body osteophytosis: a cause of vertebrogenic autonomic syndromes? *J. Manipul. Physiol. Ther.* **15**: 551-555.

Giles, L.G.F., Crawford, C.M. (1997) Shadows of the truth in patients with spinal pain: a review. *Can. J. Psychiatry*, **42**: 44-48.

Giles, L.G.F., Kaveri, M.J.P. (1990) Some osseous and soft tissue causes of human intervertebral canal (foramen) stenosis. *J. Rheumatol.* **17**: 1471-1481.

Guebert, G.M., Yochum, T.R., Rowe, L.J. (1996) Congenital anomalies and normal skeletal variants. In: *Essentials of Skeletal Radiology*, 2nd edn. (Yochum T.R., Rowe L.J., eds). Baltimore: Williams & Wilkins, pp. 197-306.

Hadley, L.A. (1964) *Anatomico-Roentgenographic Studies of the Spine*. Springfield, IL: Charles C. Thomas.

Haldeman, S. (1977) Why one cause of back pain? In: *Approaches to the Validation of Manipulation Therapy* (Buerger A.A., Tobis T.S., eds). Springfield, IL: Charles C. Thomas, pp. 187-197.

Haven, H. (1939) Neurocirculatory scalenus anticus syndrome in presence of developmental defects of first rib. *Yale J. Biol. Med.* **11**: 443.

Hirsch, C., Ingelmark, B.E., Miller, M. (1963) The anatomical basis for low back pain. *Acta Orthop. Scand.* **33**: 1-17.

Hoehler, F.K. and Tobis, J.S. (1983) Psychological factors in the treatment of back pain by spinal manipulation. *Br. J. Rheumatol.* **22**: 206-212.

Hopkins, A., Rudge, P. (1973) Hyperpathia in the central cervical cord syndrome. *J. Neurol. Neurosurg. Psychiatry* **36**: 637-642.

Hoyland, J.A., Freemont, A.J., Jayson, M.I.V. (1989) Intervertebral foramen venous obstruction. A cause of periradicular fibrosis? *Spine* **14**: 558-568.

Jackson, R. (1966) *The Cervical Syndrome*, 3rd edn. Springfield, IL: Charles C. Thomas.

Jackson, R. (1977) *The Cervical Syndrome*, 4th edn. Spingfield, IL: Charles C. Thomas.

James, B., McDonald, F. (1997) Psychosocial aspects of back pain. In: *Clinical Anatomy and Management of Low Back Pain* (Giles L.G.F., Singer K.P., eds). Oxford: Butterworth-Heinemann.

Jayson, M.I.V. (1997) Why does acute back pain become chronic? *Spine*, **22**: 1053-1056.

Jeffreys, E. (1980) Soft tissue injuries of the cervical spine. In: *Disorders of the Cervical Spine*. Oxford: Butterworth, pp. 81-89.

Jho, H-D. (1996) Microsurgical anterior cervical foraminotomy for radiculopathy: a new approach to cervical disc herniation. *J. Neurosurg.* **84**: 155-160.

Jinkins, J.R., Whittemore, A.R., Bradley, W.G. (1989) The anatomic basis of vertebrogenic pain and the autonomic syndrome associated with lumbar disk extrustion. *A.J.N.R.* **10**: 219-231.

Jones, M.D., Edwards, K.C. and Ong, E. (1984) The cervicothoracic junction on chest radiograph. *Radiol. Clin. North Am.* **22**: 487-496.

Jónsson, H., Bring, G., Rauschning, W., Sahlstedt, B. (1991) Hidden cervical spine injuries in traffic accident victims with skull fractures. *J. Spinal Disorders* **4**: 251-263.

Joseph, J. (1960) *Man's Posture: Electromyographic Studies*. Springfield, IL: Charles C Thomas, p. 14.

Keim, H.A., Kirkaldy-Willis, W.H. (1987) *Clinical Symposia. Low Back Pain*, vol. 39. New Jersey: Ciba-Geigy.

Keith, A. (1923) Man's posture: its evolution and disorders. *Br. Med. J.* **3247**: 499-502.

Kinney, R.K., Gatchel, R.J., Mayer, D.G. (1991) The SCL-90R evaluated as an alternative to the MMPI for psychological screening of chronic low-back pain patients. *Spine* **16**: 940-942.

Kuntz, A. (1953) *The Autonomic Nervous System*, 4th edn. Philadelphia: Lea & Febiger.

Kuntz, A. (1964) The autonomic nervous system. In: *Nervous System*, vol. 1. The Ciba Collection of Medical Illustrations. New York: Ciba Pharmaceutical Company.

Lahad, A., Malter, A.D., Berg, A.O., Deyo, R.A. (1994) The effectiveness of four interventions for the prevention of low back pain. *J.A.M.A.* **272**: 1286-1291.

Lauterbur, P. C. (1973) Image formation by induced local interactions: examples employing nuclear magnetic resonance. *Nature* **242**: 190-191.

Law, M.D., Bernhardt, M., White, A.A. (1995) Evaluation and management of cervical spondylotic myelopathy. In: *Instructional Course Lectures* (Jackson D.W., ed.). Illinois: Academy of Orthopaedic Surgeons, pp. 99-110.

Lazorthes, G. (1949) *Le Système Neurovasculaire*. Paris: Masson.

Lehmann, T.R., Spratt, K.F., Lehmann, K.K. (1993) Predicting long-term disability in low back injured workers presenting to a spine consultant. *Spine* **18**: 1103-1112.

Lewin, T., Moffett, B., Viidik, A. (1961) The morphology of the lumbar synovial intervertebral arches. *Acta Morphol. Neerlando-Scand.* **4**: 299-319.

Lewis, D.J., Frain, K.A., Donnelly, M.H. (1993) Chronic pain management support group: a program designed to facilitate coping. *Rehabil-Nurs.* **18**: 318-320.

Lord, S., Barnsley, L., Bogduk, N. (1993) Cervical zygapophyseal joint pain in whiplash. In: *Cervical Flexion-Extension/Whiplash Injuries* (Teasell R.W., Shapiro A.P., eds). Spine: State of the Art Reviews **7**, 355-372.

MacMillan, J., Schaffer, J.L., Kambin, P. (1991) Routes and incidence of communication of lumbar discs with surrounding neural structures. *Spine* **16**: 167-171.

Macnab, I. (1977) *Backache*. Baltimore: Williams & Wilkins.

Margo, K. (1994) Diagnosis, treatment and prognosis in patients with low back pain. *Am. Fam. Physician* **49:** 171-179.

Maroon, J.C. (1977) Burning hands in football spinal cord injuries. *J.A.M.A.* **238:** 2049-2051.

Marshall, L.L., Trethewie, E.R. (1973) Chemical irritation of nerve root in disc prolapse. *Lancet* **2:** 320.

McArdle, C.B., Crofford, M.J., Mirfakhraee, M. *et al.* (1986) Surface coil MR of spinal trauma: preliminary experience. *A.J.N.R.* **7:** 885-893.

McCain, G.A. (1993) Diagnosis and treatment of fibromyalgia. In: *Cervical Flexion-Extension/Whiplash Injuries* (Teasell R.W., Shapiro A.P., eds). Spine: State of the Art Reviews **7,** 423-441.

Mennell, J. McM. (1960) *Back Pain. Diagnosis and Treatment using Manipulative Techniques.* Boston: Little, Brown.

Merskey, H. (1993) Psychological consequences of whiplash. In: *Cervical Flexion-Extension/Whiplash Injuries* (Teasell R.W., Shapiro A.P., eds). Spine: State of the Art Reviews **7,** 471-480.

Merz, B. (1986) The honeymoon is over: spinal surgeons begin to divorce themselves from chemonucleolysis. *J.A.M.A.* **256:** 317.

Millard, R.W., Jones, R.H. (1991) Construct validity of practical questionnaires for assessing disability of low-back pain. *Spine* **16:** 835-838.

Mitchell, G.A.G. (1952) Rostral extremities of sympathetic trunks. *Nature* **129:** 533-534.

Mitchell, G.A.G. (1953) *Anatomy of the Autonomic Nervous System.* Edinburgh: Livingstone.

Mitchell, G.A.G. (1956) *Cardiovascular Innervation.* Edinburgh: Livingstone.

Mixter, W.J., Ayer, J.B. (1935) Herniation or rupture of the intervertebral disc into the spinal canal. *N. Engl. J. Med.* **213:** 385-.

Modic, M.T., Herzog, R.J. (1994) Imaging corner. Spinal imaging modalities. What's available and who should order them? *Spine* **19:** 1764-1765.

Murtagh, J.E. (1994) The non pharmacological treatment of back pain. *Aust. Prescriber* **17:** 9-12.

Nachemson, A.L. (1985) Advances in low-back pain. *Clin. Orthop.* **200:** 266-278.

National Health and Medical Research Council (1988) *Management of Severe Pain.* Canberra: Australian Government Publishing Service.

Netter, F.H. (1962) *Nervous System.* Ciba Collection of Medical Illustrations, vol. 1. New York: Ciba Pharmaceutical Company.

Oh, S-H., Perin, N.I., Cooper, P.R. (1996) Quantitative three-dimensional anatomy of the subaxial cervical spine: implication for anterior spinal surgery. *Neurosurgery* **38:** 1139-1144.

Pearcy, M., Portek, I., Shepherd, J. (1985) The effect of low back pain on lumbar spinal movements measured by three-dimensional x-ray analysis. *Spine* **10:** 150-153.

Pick, J. (1970) *The Autonomic Nervous System.* Philadelphia: Lippincott.

Putz, R. (1992) The detailed functional anatomy of the ligaments of the vertebral column. *Ann. Anat.* **174:** 40-47.

Rauschning, W. (1992) Spinal anatomy: the relationship of structures. In: *Principles and Practice of Chiropractic* (Haldeman S., ed.), 2nd edn. Norwalk: Appleton and Lange, pp. 63-72.

Rickenbacher, J., Landolt, A.M. Theiler, K. (1985) *Applied Anatomy of the Back.* Berlin: Springer-Verlag, pp. 93, 184-186.

Ross, J.S. (1995) Imaging corner. Three-dimensional magnetic resonance techniques for evaluating the cervical spine. *Spine* **20:** 1099-1102.

Schellhas, K.P., Smith, M.D., Gundry, C.R., Pollei, S.R. (1996) Cervical discogenic pain. Prospective correlation of magnetic resonance imaging and discography in asymptomatic subjects and pain sufferers. *Spine* **21:** 300-312.

Schiotz, E.H., Cyriax, J. (1975) *Manipulation Past and Present.* London: Heinemann Medical.

Schmorl, G., Junghanns, H. (1971) *The Human Spine in Health and Disease,* 2nd edn. New York: Grune & Stratton, pp. 22, 37, 148, 197.

Sheehan, D. (1936) Discovery of the autonomic nervous system. *Arch. Neurol. Psychiatry* **35:** 1081-1115.

Shelokov, A.P. (1991) Evaluation, diagnosis, and initial treatment of cervical disc disease. In: Cervical Spine Disease (Regan J.J., ed.). *Spine: State of the Art Reviews* **5**(2), pp. 167-176.

Simons, D.G., Travell, J. (1983) Common myofascial origins of low back pain. *Postgrad. Med.* **73:** 55-108.

Slucky, A.V., Eismont, F.J. (1994) Treatment of acute injury of the cervical spine. *J. Bone Joint Surg.* **76:** 1882-1896.

Spitzer, W.O., Skovron, M.L., Salmi, L.R. *et al.* (1995) Scientific monograph of the Quebec Task Force on whiplash-associated disorders: redefining "whiplash" and its management. *Spine* **20:** (8S).

Steiner, H.A. (1943) Roentgenologic manifestations and clinical symptoms of rib abnormalities. *Radiology* **40:** 175.

Stockwell, R.A. (1985) *A Pre-clinical View of Osteoarthritis.* A Sir John Struthers Lecture. Teviot Place, Edinburgh: The Medical School.

Sunderland, S. (1968) *Nerves and Nerve Injuries.* Edinburgh: E.S. Livingstone.

Sunderland, S. (1975) Anatomical perivertebral influences on the intervertebral foramen. In: *The Research Status of Spinal Manipulative Therapy* (Goldstein M., ed.) NINCDS Monograph no. 15. Bethesda, Maryland: US Department of Health, Education, and Welfare, Public Health Service, National Institutes of Health, National Institute of Neurological and Communicative Disorders and Stroke, pp. 129-140.

Tajima, N., Kawano, K. (1986) Cryomicrotomy of the lumbar spine. *Spine* **11,** 376-379.

Taylor, J. R., Kakulas, B.A. (1991) Neck injuries. *Lancet* **338:** 1343.

Taylor, J.R., Twomey, L.T. (1993) Acute injuries to cervical joints. An autopsy study of neck sprain. *Spine* **18:** 1115-1122.

Travell, J., Rinzler, S.H. (1952) Myofascial genesis of pain. *Postgrad. Med.* **11:** 425-434.

van Norel, G.J., Verhagen, W.I.M. (1996) Drop attacks and instability of the degenerate cervical spine. *J. Bone Joint Surg.* **78B:** 495-496.

von Torklus, D., Gehle, W (1972) *The Upper Cervical Spine. Regional Anatomy, Pathology and Traumatology. A Systematic Radiological Atlas and Textbook.* London: Butterworths.

Watts, C., Dickhaus, E. (1986) Chemonucleolysis: a note of caution. *Surg. Neurol.* **26:** 236.

Wedel, D.J., Wilson, P.R. (1985) Cervical facet arthrography. *Reg. Anaesth.* **10:** 7-11.

Weitz, E.M. (1984) Paraplegia following chymopapain injection. *J. Bone Joint Surg.* **66A:** 1131.

White, J.C., Smithwick, R.H., Simeone, F.A. (1952) *The Autonomic Nervous System*, 3rd edn. London: Kimpton.

Wilberger, J.E., Abla, A., Maroon, J.C. (1986) Burning hands syndrome revisited. *Neurosurgery* **19:** 1038-1040.

Wilkinson, M. (1967) Pathology. In: *Cervical Spondylosis and other Disorders of the Cervical Spine* (Brain L., Wilkinson M., eds). London: Heinemann, pp. 98-123.

Williams, P.L., Warwick, R. (1980) *Gray's Anatomy*, 36th edn. Edinburgh: Churchill Livingstone.

Workers' Compensation Board of Queensland Annual Report (1995) Brisbane, Australia.

Young, A.C. (1967) Radiology and cervical spondylosis. In: *Cervical Spondylosis and other Disorders of the Cervical Spine* (Brain L., Wilkinson M., eds). London: William Heinemann, pp. 133-196.

Section

II

Anatomy, Pathology and Biomechanics

2

Anatomy and pathology of the cervical spine

J. H. Bland

Introduction

The cervical spine is surely the most complicated articular system in the body: there are 37 separate joints whose function it is to carry out the myriad movements of the head and neck in relation to the trunk, and subserve all special sense organs, e.g. eyes, ears, nose, taste, touch and proprioception. The seven small cervical vertebrae with their ligamentous, capsular, tendinous and muscle attachments appear poorly designed to protect their contents, compared to the skull above and the thorax below. The contents of this anatomical cylinder interposed between skull and thorax include carotid and vertebral arteries, the spinal cord, and all anterior and posterior nerve roots and, in its uppermost portion, the brainstem. The extremely flexible cervical spine balances a 4.5–5.5 kg (10–12 lb) 'ball', the head, on the lateral masses (zygapophysial joints) of the atlas. The head acts as a cantilever on top of the highly mobile neck.

Normally the neck moves over 600 times an hour, awake or asleep; no other part of the musculoskeletal system is in such constant motion. The cervical spine is subject to stress and strain in ordinary everyday activities - speaking, gesturing, rising, sitting, walking, turning about, even at rest lying down (Kapandji, 1977). The position of the cervical spine discloses mood, attitude, how you feel about yourself and the world about you. The cervical spine in flexion suggests depression, withdrawal, sadness, mourning - sometimes prayer, as in bowing the head in prayer and supplication, while chin-up extension of the cervical spine reflects optimism, confidence, *savoir faire*, 'all's right with the world'. This section of the spine is constantly communicating, with a myriad of subliminal gestures, poses, questions and answers. A 'pain in the neck' is such an unpleasant experience that it is used as an invective for any annoying event or person. How about the verb 'to neck,' i.e. kissing and caressing - a terminology currently out of style! Normal function requires that all movement be made without damage to the spinal cord, the entire vascular supply to the head and neck, many millions - or perhaps billions - of receptors and nerve fibres, passing through it and the intervertebral foramina.

Anatomy and physiology of the cervical spine

Clinical symptoms and signs, subjective and/or objective, generally reflect discomfort or disease and result from abnormal function of a tissue or an organ system which, as Rudolph Virchow taught over 130 years ago, must originate in cellular disturbances. Disease in most instances has a visible component and the study of morbid anatomy has been the classic approach to its understanding. The scientific fashion today is for molecular and cell biology; gross anatomical studies are thought by many to be outmoded, old-fashioned, even irrelevant. On the other hand, as William Blake has written, one need not be limited to the 'Vegetated Mortal Eye's perverted and single, flat vision' (Blake, 1925).

Enormous advances have been made in the last 100 years, mainly from intensive study of biochemistry and immunology which, along with evolution and maturation of cell biology, have illuminated morbid anatomy - but only because morbid anatomy had been studied in great detail for it to be illuminated! For example, immunofluorescent studies in renal pathology allowed us to see, disclosing the detailed cellular and molecular understanding of these complex diseases.

Too seldom perceived in medical research is that morbid anatomy remains, and always will be, key to our understanding of clinical disease.

Once something has been observed, what was previously invisible is obvious. The discovery of perspective in painting is an example, and so seemingly simple now! Anatomical abnormality, or normality for that matter, once well-comprehended, becomes a diagnostic tool in the hands of the radiologist, the clinician, the surgical pathologist and at the autopsy table (Bullough, 1987).

In the case of the cervical spine, relatively little morbid and microscopic anatomy has been done compared to the lumbar spine, presumably because of difficulty in obtaining whole specimens of human cervical spines to study. Major works describing the pathology of the cervical spine have been reported by Payne and Spillane (1957), Schmorl and Junghanns (1971), Ten Have and Eulderink (1980), Penning (1988) and Bland (1994). This chapter reflects a deep enduring interest in cervical spine anatomy and pathology dating back to a single clinical experience in 1955. During this period, a total of over 191 whole human cervical spines have been removed at post-mortem or obtained from anatomical laboratories and the coroner's office (Bland, 1991, 1994).

Phylogenetic anatomy of clinical importance

1. The nerve supply to this area is from C1, C2 and C3, and clinical disease is reflected in referral patterns of those roots; the myotomal and sclerotomal derived structures, when abnormal, are perceived in the forehead and retro-orbital areas.
2. The intervertebral foramina carry the anterior and posterior nerve roots, the respective posterior root ganglia and the recurrent meningeal nerve (see Fig. 1.4). The nerves occupy about 25% of the available space. The remainder of the space is taken up by lymphatics, blood vessels, areolar and fatty tissue, which constitute a compressible safety cushion space, allowing physiological encroachment without damage to nerve roots. The bony prominence, the uncus or uncinate process on the lateral and posterolateral aspect of the cervical vertebrae from C3 through C7 (see Fig. 1.4), constitutes the phylogenetic remainder of the costovertebral joint. The clinical significance is that this bony elevation enlarges from age 9 to 14 years such that, beyond the age of 40 years, it constitutes a bony bulwark acting to prevent herniation laterally or postero-laterally (Bland, 1994).
3. The free rotary movement of the head became possible with the eccentrically located axle of the axis, the odontoid, allowing relatively enormous mobility at that level, particularly in rotation.
4. The neural traffic from the extremities requires an increase in the diameter of the spinal cord and the nerve roots, particularly the sensory roots, are larger in the cervical spine than in the thoracic and lumbar spines.
5. The nucleus pulposus, present at birth and up until 9–14 years, is made up of remnants of the primitive notochord, that is, collagen and proteoglycan material. However, in the cervical spine, in contrast to events in the lumbar spine, this nucleus pulposus gradually disappears. In 191 whole human cervical spines we have found no evidence of a gel-like nucleus pulposus in adults. The intervertebral disc in the cervical spine is dry and is very much more like a ligament than a disc. It was found to be fibrous and gradually breaking up in various-sized pieces, seemingly a universal, probably physiological, development. This is consistent with the early observations of Töndury (1959).

Clinical surface anatomy

Familiarity with surface anatomy is important to the clinician since the main structures of the neck can be seen and felt easily in the thin patient; they are more difficult to see and feel in the obese, pyknic body type with a short neck. The sternocleidomastoid muscle runs from one corner to the other of a quadrilateral area formed by the anterior midline, the clavicle and the leading edge of the trapezius muscle; the mastoid–mandibular line divides the side of the neck into anterior and posterior triangles (Fig. 2.1).

There is little to be seen in the posterior triangle, which is really a pyramid (Fig. 2.2). The first rib is palpable at the base of the triangle where it is crossed by the subclavian artery and the lower trunks of the brachial plexus. A cervical rib (see Fig. 1.3), or its fibrous extension, may be felt here. The spinal accessory nerve runs forward to the sternomastoid muscle, dividing the triangle into an upper 'safe' and lower 'dangerous' area. The upper area of the transverse processes of cervical vertebrae can be felt, though they are deep. The external jugular vein and the platysma muscle cross the sternomastoid muscle in the anterior triangles; both are prominent in breath-holding. The pulsation of the carotid artery is easily seen.

The hyoid bone, a horseshoe-shaped structure, is felt at the level of C3 on a horizontal plane just above the thyroid cartilage (Fig. 2.3). The anterior body of the bone and its two stems are readily felt by a pincer-like action of the finger and thumb. With swallowing, the movement of the hyoid bone is easily palpable.

Moving down with the fingers, the upper edge of the thyroid cartilage is felt at the level of C4–5; the lower border of the thyroid cartilage is at the level of C5–6. The thyroid cartilage also moves with swallow-

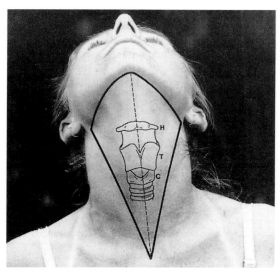

Fig. 2.1 Anterior and right/left triangles are bounded by the anterior edge of the sternocleidomastoid muscle, the midline, the lower border of the mandible. Some anatomists describe a large upside-down triangle bounded by the two anterior borders of the sternocleidomastoid muscle and the two lower borders of the mandible, with its apex at the sternal notch and its base at the mandible.

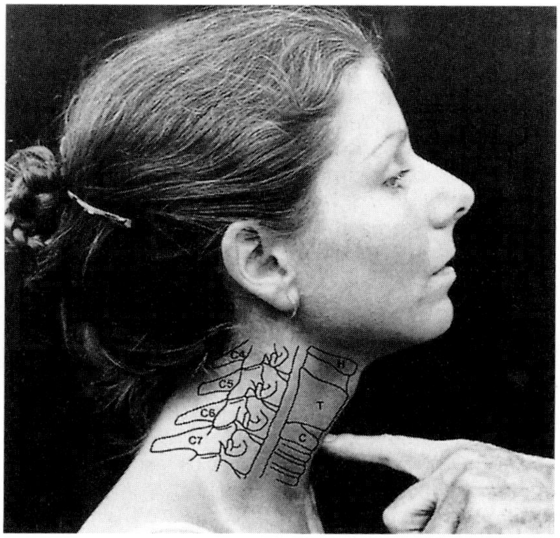

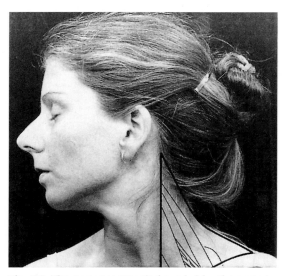

Fig. 2.2 The posterior triangle bounded by the posterior border of the sternocleidomastoid muscle, the clavicle, and the leading edge of the trapezius muscle.

Fig. 2.3 Lateral view of the four main landmarks to cervical spine level: the hyoid bone (C3–4), the upper (C4–5) and lower (C5–6) margins of the thyroid cartilage (T), the cricoid ring (C6), the first of the tracheal rings (C6–7). The examiner's finger is at the lower margin of the thyroid cartilage.

ing and is, of course, the Adam's apple. The first bite of the forbidden apple was said to have stuck in Adam's throat, hence the name.

Progressing downward, the first tracheal ring is felt immediately below the sharp lower border of the thyroid cartilage and at the level of the C6 vertebra. It is the only complete ring of the cricoid series and is an integral part of the trachea. The first ring is immediately above the site for emergency tracheostomy. Applying gentle pressure upon palpation prevents initiating the gag reflex. With swallowing, the cricoid ring moves, but does so less obviously than the thyroid cartilage.

Moving laterally 2.5 cm from the first cricoid ring, one palpates the carotid tubercle, the anterior tubercle of the C6 transverse process. Although the carotid tubercle is small, located about 2.5 cm from the midline and deep beneath overlying muscles, it is still clearly palpable. It is especially well-detected by pressing posteriorly from the lateral position.

Carotid tubercles should be palpated separately because simultaneous palpation of these tubercles and other structures of the neck may occlude flow in both carotid arteries, resulting in the carotid reflex, a drop in blood pressure and fainting. The carotid tubercle is the anatomical landmark for an anterior surgical approach to C5–6 and the site for injection of the cervical stellate ganglion (see Fig. 1.7). The neurovascular bundle can be compressed against the carotid tubercle (level of C6 vertebra). At the apex of the triangle, the transverse process of the atlas can be felt as a small hard lump, just posterior to the internal carotid artery. It lies between the angle of the jaw and the mastoid process of the skull just behind the ear. The examining fingertip rolls over the tip of the styloid process and the stylohyoid ligament.

The transverse processes of the atlas are the broadest in the cervical spine and are readily palpable – an easily identifiable anatomical point of orientation. The anterior arch of the hyoid bone, the notch of the thyroid cartilage, the cricoid and the upper rings of the trachea are readily felt in the anterior midline.

The vertebra prominens, the spinous process of the seventh cervical vertebra, just above the first thoracic vertebra, marks the lower end of the midline sulcus formed by the ligamentum nuchae, which extends from the spinous process to the occiput.

The splenius capitis muscle forms a rounded ridge on either side of the sulcus; the trapezius muscle origin is tendinous without muscle and extends from the inion to the T12 spinous process (Fig. 2.4). The 'dowager hump' is the upper part of the vertebra prominens, always more obvious in obese people or in those with cervical osteoarthritis.

The posterior landmarks of the cervical spine include the occiput, the inion, the superior nuchal line and the mastoid process. The occiput is the posterior portion of the skull including the floor. The inion (bump of knowledge) is a dome-shaped bump in the middle of the occipital region and is the centre of the nuchal line. The superior nuchal line is felt by moving laterally from the inion and is a small transverse bony ridge extending out on both sides of the inion. Palpating laterally from the lateral edge of

the superior nuchal line is found the rounded mastoid process of the skull (Fig. 2.4).

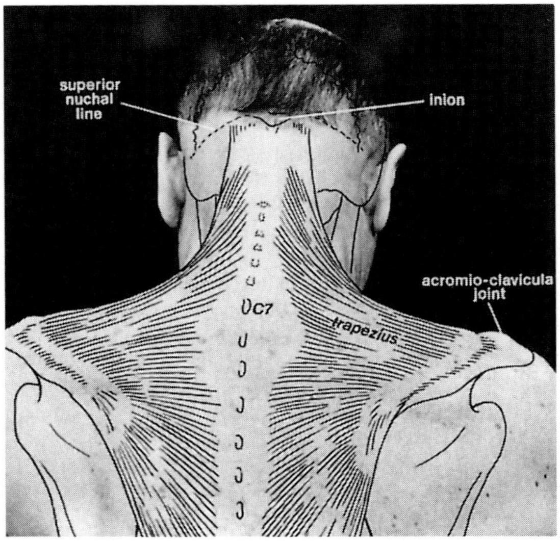

The spinous processes of the cervical vertebrae are in the posterior midline of the cervical spine. No muscle crosses the midline, so there is an indentation there. The lateral soft tissue bulges outlining the indentation are made up of the deep paraspinal muscles and the superficial trapezius.

The C1 posterior arch of the atlas lies deep and has a small tubercle. The C2 spinous process, the axis, is large and easy to feel. The neck normally is in lordosis, but each spinous process can be felt. The cervical spinous processes are often bifid, having two small excrescences of bone. The C7 and T1 spinous processes are larger than those above them. Normally, the spinous processes are in line with each other unless they have developed asymmetrically. Misalignment can result from unilateral dislocation of a zygapophysial joint or fracture of a spinous process due to trauma (Fig. 2.5).

The zygapophysial joints are palpable about 25 mm lateral to the respective spinous processes (Fig. 2.6). They are often tender if abnormal and they feel like little domes lying deep below the trapezius muscle. The patient should be completely relaxed for palpable perception of these joints. The vertebral level of any one of the posterior joints can be ascertained by lining up the joint level with the anterior structures of the neck: hyoid bone, thyroid cartilage and the first cricoid ring at C6 (Fig. 2.3).

The cervical spine is a superb example of the biological principle of adaptation of structure to function. It supplies support for the head, a flexible and buffered tube for the transmission and protection

Fig. 2.4 Posterior aspect of the head and neck with landmarks drawn in. The trapezius muscle originates from the inion, extends through all the thoracic vertebral processes to T12, is inserted into the clavicle and scapula, and overlies all superficial structures in the posterior cervical spine.

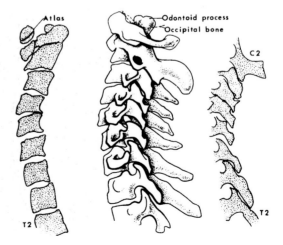

Fig. 2.5 A drawing of a whole cervical spine specimen illustrating the large C2 spinous process, the vertebra prominens (C7), the atlas–axis relationship, the zygapophysial joints and the exiting intervertebral foramina.

of the upper spinal cord, provision for the entry and exit of spinal nerves, and extremely serviceable mobility. Viewed from the front it appears as a truncated pyramid, widening from the axis downwards; laterally in the neutral position, there is a mild lordosis with an anterior convexity (Fig. 2.7). Slight scoliosis to the left is normal at the cervicothoracic junction in 80% of people and to the right in 20%.

Head and neck mobility

Erect posture, binocular vision and cervical spine mobility allow human beings to look quickly behind themselves, over their shoulders, to gaze up at the stars or peer down at their feet, far more efficiently than most animals. Many head and neck movements are social signals; non-verbal communication is indicative of mood, attitude of the moment and emotion. We are not even aware of many of these signals. The cervical spine moves in flexion, extension, lateral flexion and rotation (Penning and Wilmink, 1987; Dvorak, 1988; Dvorak *et al.,* 1991). The latter two movements are always combined to some extent. Nodding occurs primarily at the atlanto-occipital joint with the atlantoaxial joints participating to some degree. Rotation mainly occurs at the atlantoaxial joints, particularly the atlanto-odontoid rotation. The atlanto-occipital joints allow movement only in flexion and extension, not in rotation. Thus, the atlas and skull move in rotation as a unit and the position of the

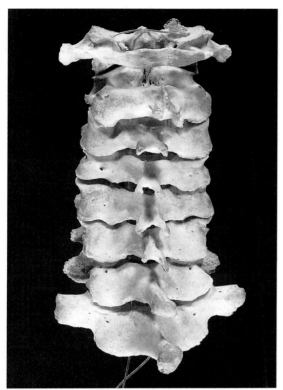

Fig. 2.6 Posterior view of the whole cervical spine. Note the bilateral zygapophysial joints and the bifid spinous processes.

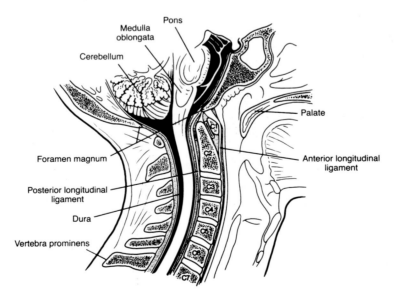

Fig. 2.7 Drawing of a sagittal view of the cervical spine showing the relationships of the brainstem, the medulla oblongata, the foramen magnum and the spinal canal. The lower portion of the medulla is really outside and below the foramen. Thus, with subluxation of the atlas on the axis, compression of the brainstem can occur by pressure of the odontoid against the upper spinal cord and the medulla. Note that the anterior arch of the atlas is only millimetres from the pharynx.

skull is a clear indication of the position of the atlas in rotation. The limiting factor in extension is the trapping of the posterior arch of the atlas between the occiput and the spinous process of the axis; lateral flexion is likewise limited. Further extension is allowed by participation of the lower elements. Bony impingement limits further extension at the atlanto-occipital joint. Flexion is arrested when the posterior ligaments are taut and when the tip of the odontoid process abuts against the bony anterior lip of the foramen magnum (the atlas is tightly bound to it by the transverse ligament). In these movements the atlas does not move appreciably on the axis. With fusion of the atlas and axis, flexion and extension are unchanged. All three atlantoaxial joints constitute the most complex joints in the body. Four distinct movements occur here: rotation, flexion, extension and vertical approximation/lateral glide of the atlas on the axis.

The normal cervical spine can rotate as much as 160° and, rarely, up to 180°. Approximately 50% of the rotation occurs at the atlantoaxial articulation; the remainder occurs in joints below that level, with joints rotating in decreasing magnitude from above down. The atlas, like a wheel with an eccentrically placed axle, pivots around the laterally central, but anteriorly eccentric, odontoid process. The odontoid process is tightly bound to the occiput by the apical and alar ligaments which, together with the capsule of the atlantoaxial zygapophysial joints, limit rotation each way to 45° (Figs 2.8 and 2.9).

Figure 2.10 illustrates a lateral view of the cervical spine's atlas and axis. In rotation, the wall of the spinal canal at the atlas level swings laterally across the spinal canal at the axis level, narrowing the area of the canal at this level by about one-third. Fortunately, the canal is at its most capacious here and accommodates such rotation. The diameter of the canal at C1 level is equally occupied by the odontoid process, free space and the cord (Figs 2.11 and 2.12). The free space allows for safe rotation and an accommodation to the spinal cord. Ligamentous structures, remarkably enough, are sufficiently lax to allow this wide range, but are inelastic with high tensile strength and can limit further motion without impingement on vital structures. Lateral flexion of the head produces as much, or more, associated rotation of the axis than does simple rotation of the head. With head tilt, the spinous process of the axis, and of those vertebrae below, rotates to the opposite side to a greater degree in the upper than in the lower portion of the cervical spine. Lateral glide occurs in

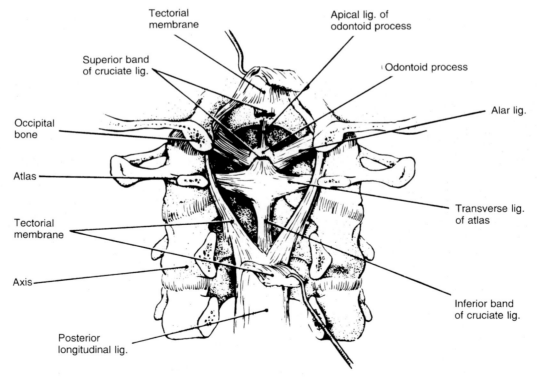

Fig. 2.8 Coronal view of the upper cervical spine showing the critical transverse/cruciate ligaments and the apical and alar (checkrein) ligaments of the odontoid.

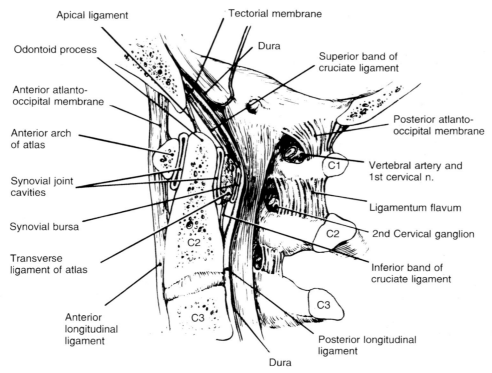

Apical ligament
Tectorial membrane
Odontoid process
Dura
Superior band of
cruciate ligament
Anterior atlanto-
occipital membrane
Anterior arch
of atlas
Posterior atlanto-
occipital membrane
Synovial joint
cavities
C1
Vertebral artery and
1st cervical n.
Ligamentum flavum
Synovial bursa
C2
2nd Cervical ganglion
Transverse
ligament of atlas
C2
Inferior band of
cruciate ligament
Anterior
longitudinal
ligament
C3
C3
Posterior longitudinal
ligament
Dura

Fig. 2.9 Sagittal view of the upper cervical spine showing the atlanto-odontoid joint with synovial joint cavities located anteriorly and posteriorly to the odontoid process. The cervical spinal canal is at its widest at the level of the foramen magnum.

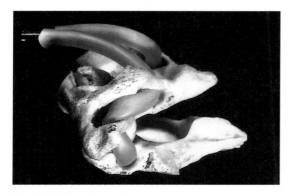

Fig. 2.10 The atlas and axis are shown as the vertebral artery winds its way through the foramina transversaria of the two vertebrae. The odontoid process and the anterior arch of the atlas are visible just below the two arteries. Note the sharp deviation outwards and upwards that the artery must make from axis to atlas, followed by a complete return about the posterior aspect of the lateral mass of the atlas before proceeding to the clivus to join the other vertebral artery as the basilar artery. This is a normal specimen; consider the implications of this situation with atherosclerotic plaques, narrow joint spaces, loss of intervertebral disc height and extensive osteophytosis.

normal people, with the atlas shifting to the side of the tilt. It is observable on radiographic film as a narrowing of the space between the odontoid process and the lateral mass of the atlas on the side of the tilt, and a widening of the other side.

The vertebral artery normally enters the transverse foramen at the transverse process of the sixth cervical vertebra and ascends through the foramina transversaria to enter the skull (see Figs 1.4, 1.11 and 1.12). It is protected in the foramen except between the axis and the atlas, where there is about 1.5–2.0 cm of artery lying outside the canal. In addition, the artery is normally subject to the stress and stretch between atlas and axis, since it is situated at the periphery of the marked rotation. The artery is pulled forwards and backwards by the rotary action. The clinical consequences must be considered in any rotary dislocation, fracture or malalignment of the atlas and axis (Fig. 2.10; see Chapter 12).

Below the axis, rotation, flexion–extension and lateral flexion occur in decreasing magnitude from the top down. Normally, the cervical spine is in slight lordosis but a linear pattern is not necessarily abnormal. There is even reversal of the standard

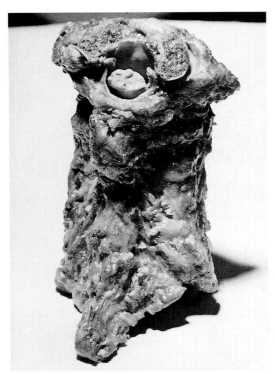

Fig. 2.11 Specimen of a whole human cervical spine, vertically positioned and viewed from the posterior aspect. The upper third of the picture shows the spinal cord in the capacious spinal canal at the foramen magnum level; the occipital condyles were cut off the skull with a sharp chisel (laterally situated) and the edges of the atlanto-occipital joint are visible; the anterior and posterior arches of the atlas can be identified.

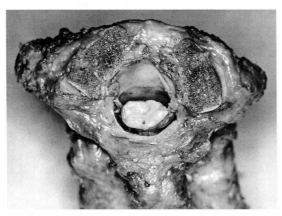

Fig. 2.12 A close-up view of Figure 2.11 showing the odontoid 'peeking' through.

lordosis in a few normal people. During flexion, the cervical spine appears to lengthen. This seems to be attributable to straightening of the lordosis rather than to actual lengthening of the cervical spine (Fineman, 1963; Ball and Meijers, 1964).

Specific structural anatomical characteristics correlated with age

Nucleus pulposus

The nucleus pulposus of the cervical intervertebral discs, present at birth, is less and less evident in adolescence and above age 40 it mainly disappears. The adult disc is ligamentous, dry, composed of fibrocartilage, islands of hyaline cartilage, even some tendon-like material, and certainly with very little proteoglycan. Thus, after age 40 years, it is generally impossible to herniate the nucleus pulposus clinically, since there is none there! Figure 2.13 is a coronal section of the cervical spine of a 4-year-old boy, which shows that the nucleus pulposus is clearly present in the mid-disc region.

By ages 9–14 years, the nucleus pulposus is far less evident and bilateral clefts have developed in the posterolateral anulus fibrosus; medial to the growing uncinate processes of the vertebra, and posterolaterally situated. This cleft is the site of the joints of Luschka (uncovertebral or neurocentral joints; Fig. 2.14; Cave *et al.*, 1955; Boreadis and Gershon-Cohen, 1956; Hadley, 1964; Hall, 1965; Töndury, 1974; Bland and Boushey, 1987; Bland, 1994). At age 20–35, the clefts have gradually enlarged and are dissecting tissue planes toward the midline, where each finally meets its counterpart from the opposite side (Figs 2.15 and 2.16). This phenomenon proved to be universal in our spine studies, therefore it is believed to be a physiological event, peculiar to the human cervical spine's biomechanics. Meanwhile, the disc is changing overall tissue characteristics with gradual disappearance of the nucleus pulposus and acquisition of ligamentous, fibrocartilage-like gross characteristics (Figs 2.15 and 2.16). An example of the uncinate processes is shown in Figure 2.17.

In cervical spines of people aged 60 and above, the anular dissection has reached the midline, suggesting a bisected disc from uncinate process to uncinate process. The overall material in the disc has become dry with little proteoglycan, acquiring dense ligamentous character and marked loss of volume of disc tissue. It is formulated that these events are a physiological consequence of shearing planes of tissue – a biophysical, biomechanical consequence of the relatively extreme repetitions of motion that the cervical spine enjoys, especially rotation (Milne, 1991).

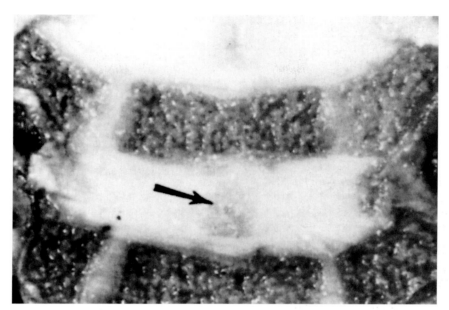

Fig. 2.13 This specimen is a close-up of a coronal section of the cervical spine of a 4-year-old boy. The nucleus pulposus is obvious in the centre of the disc (arrow). The uncinate processes are well-developed. From Hall (1965) with permission.

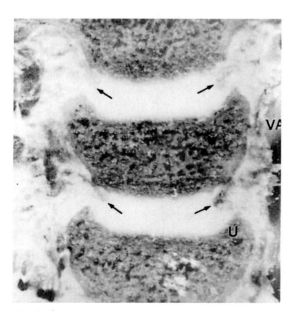

Fig. 2.14 Coronal section of a cervical spine from a 3-year-old child. Note VA (vertebral artery) and U (uncinate process). Arrows point to developing clefts in the postero-lateral anulus fibrosus. From Hall (1965) with permission.

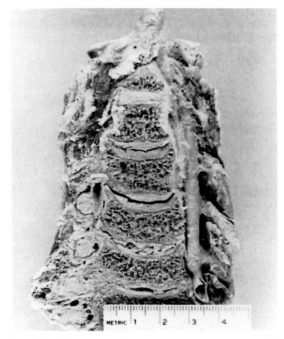

Fig. 2.15 Whole cervical spine specimen (cut coronally) from an 80-year-old woman. Note the striking decrease in overall disc substance, marked narrowing of all discs and completely bisected disc surfaces facing one another.

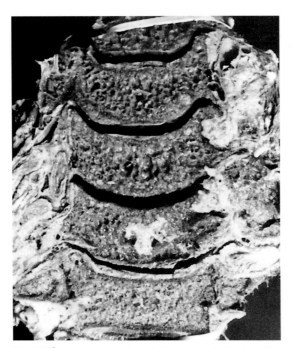

Fig. 2.16 A coronal section of a lower cervical spine taken from a 92-year-old man. Note the spaces between all of the intervertebral discs with most of the material gone, except in the lowest intervertebral disc. In life this is clearly only a potential space and has a pressure below that of the atmosphere, the two surfaces are normally in close and well-moulded apposition.

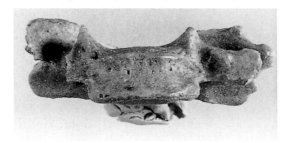

Fig. 2.17 An anterior view of the C4 vertebra illustrating a sharp remodelled uncinate process on the viewer's left and blunt remodelling uncinate process on the right.

Pieces of disc tissue are frequently found as separate hard marginally elastic fragments free within the disc which conceivably could herniate.

Uncinate processes

The uncinate processes (*uncus* = a small hook) are normal bony developments of cervical vertebrae,

laterally and posterolaterally from C3 to C7 (Figs 2.16 and 2.17).

With increasing age the uncinate processes enlarge and often flatten, losing their sharp bony edge. This osteogenic phenomenon forms a bulwark of bone laterally, and to some degree posterolaterally which, it is believed, prevents disc herniation in this area. Figure 2.15 is an anterior view of an articulated cervical spine from an 80-year-old woman which illustrates this principle. Figure 2.18 shows a coronal section of the uncinate process from a 28-year-old man, while Figure 2.19 is an illustration of the same uncinate process viewed from within the disc.

The normal physiological sequence of events and anatomical structures here constitutes an accurate description of normal cervical intervertebral disc physiology and pathology. These findings are virtually universal.

At age 9–14 years a cleft appears in the lateral and posterolateral anulus fibrosus, a function of the unusual ability in obligate bipeds to rotate the cervical spine. This cleft, or fissure, gradually dissects toward the midline to meet its counterpart coming

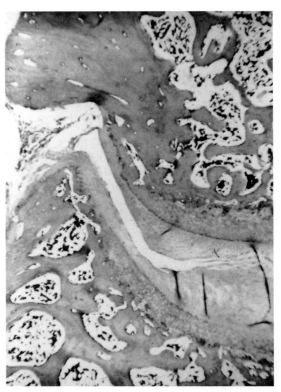

Fig. 2.18 Coronal section of the uncinate process from a 28-year-old man. The cleft or fissure medial to the uncinate process shows disc fibrocartilage fibrillation.

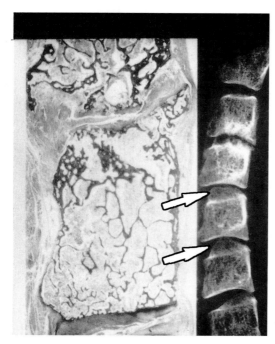

Fig. 2.19 On the viewer's right is a parasagittal section seen on X-ray. Arrows point to the uncinate process as seen from within the disc, looking from inside out. On the left is a parasagittal section of the same anatomical specimen showing C5 vertebra in the middle and the lower half of C4 above. Note the through-and-through clefts above and below C5. From Ball (1964) with permission.

from the other direction. In this space there are patches of synovium. With increasing age, the disc is finally bisected in a transverse plane and the two surfaces are made up of a peculiar mix of connective tissues, anulus-like tissue, fibrocartilage, hyaline cartilage, even some tendon-like tissues as well as bony islands. Thus, there are caudal and cephalad portions of the normal transected cervical intervertebral discs. The disc overall becomes narrower with the passage of time, sometimes nearly disappearing. We dubbed this 'the grin of Luschka' when the process is complete, as per the smile of the Cheshire cat (Fig. 2.15).

Nerve root exit sites

At the C3–C4 level the anterior and posterior nerve root exit sites through the dural root sleeves are below the level of the intervertebral discs by approximately 4 mm. This is as a consequence of the formation of the nervous system, being followed later by rapid growth of the spine. With growth and extension of the cervical spine, physiological traction is exerted on the cord and nerve roots and the dural root sleeve exit sites are at the level of vertebral bodies rather than at the disc level; the root exit zone is generally below the level of the disc (Bland, 1994; Fig. 2.20). Incidentally, virtually all dural root sleeves become fibrotic, rigid and stiff after the age of 45–50 years.

Anatomy of the anterior (motor) nerve root

The anterior nerve root is normally situated low in the intervertebral foramen and hence is very unlikely to be compressed (Fig. 2.21). The posterior nerve root is well-protected from the point of any disc herniation. However, the zygapophysial joints could become enlarged due to osteophytosis, and the posterior root could become compressed, resulting in radiculopathy (though radiculopathy itself is unusual in the author's experience).

Spinal cord volume vs the measured transverse diameter of spinal cords and the bony spinal canal

There is normally a considerable individual disparity between the spinal cord volume and space available in the bony canal. This seems a constitutional, or genetic, characteristic. Thus, clinically, if one inherited a wide spinal cord and a relatively small bony canal, the development of osteoarthritis compromise cord function. The ideal is clearly a narrow cord and a capacious spinal canal – the luck of the draw (Fig. 2.22)!

Anatomy of anterior and posterior spinal canal

In people over age 45–50, the anterior spinal canal is characterized by bars of osteophytes at the level of the intervertebral discs (Fig. 2.23). These osteophytes commonly compress the cord to varying degrees (Fig. 2.24), not always resulting in symptoms. The ligamentum flavum (Fig. 2.25) is hypertrophied and hyperplastic, projecting into the spinal canal, and may compress the spinal cord posteriorly, with varying symptomatic consequences.

The posterior longitudinal ligament in the cervical spine is three- to fivefold thicker and more developed than in either the thoracic or lumbar spines, where it tends strongly towards attenuation. Since

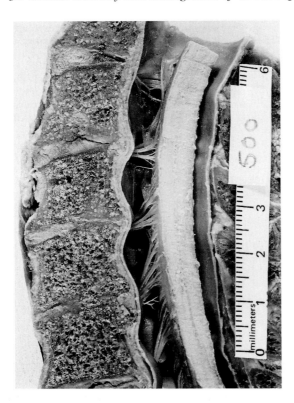

Fig. 2.20 A sagittal section of a whole cervical spine showing nerve exit sites (dural root sleeves) and that they are at the upper level of the vertebrae rather than at the level of the discs.

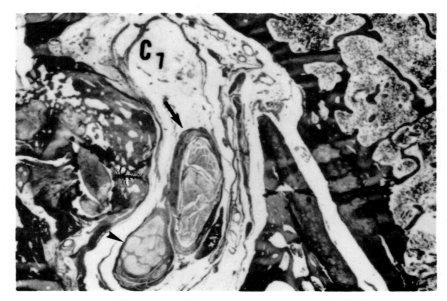

Fig. 2.21 Coronal section through the intervertebral foramen at C7–T1. The upper arrow points to the posterior (sensory) root and the arrowhead to the anterior (motor) root. The level in the foramen is proximal to the posterior root ganglion. The motor root is anatomically situated low in the foramen, well-protected from any osteophytic compression throughout its course from the spinal cord.

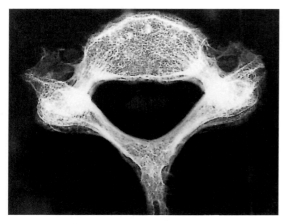

Fig. 2.22 A transverse view of C6 vertebra illustrating the very spacious spinal canal and the relatively small spinal cord – there is a great tolerance for extensive osteoarthritis without cord compression and myelopathy.

the posterior longitudinal ligament is in a position to prevent herniation posterolaterally and posteriorly, this may be a partial explanation for the unusual occurrence of disc herniation in the cervical spine.

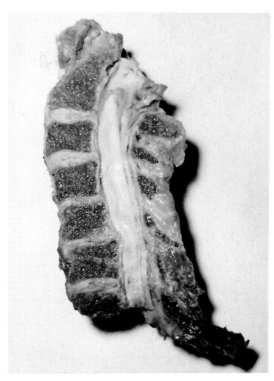

Fig. 2.24 This specimen is a gross midline section of a cervical spine. Note anterior arch of the atlas at the top; the odontoid is eroded and the anterior atlanto-occipital joint is filled with granulomatous tissue; the spinal cord is cut in the sagittal plane and compressed by intensive intervertebral disc granuloma and osteophytes at the C5-6 level; the C2-3 and C3-4 discs are of normal height.

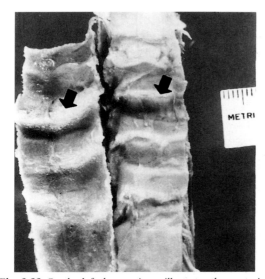

Fig. 2.23 On the left the specimen illustrates the posterior surface of cervical vertebrae seen from inside the spinal canal, showing massive posterior vertebral body osteophytes at the margins of the intervertebral discs, protruding into the anterior cervical spine canal (arrow). The posterior longitudinal ligament is greatly thickened. On the right is a section illustrating the posterior surface of the spinal canal with immensely thickened and protruding ligamenta flava (arrow).

The anterior longitudinal ligament is attached firmly to the vertebral bodies, but only loosely at the disc area. Conversely, posterior longitudinal ligament is firmly attached to the disc but loosely to the vertebral body surface. This anatomical fact may explain why osteophytes (following the path of least resistance) are larger and more common anteriorly than posteriorly. In the cervical region only, the posterior longitudinal ligament is very broad throughout, while in the thoracic and lumbar regions it narrows strikingly behind each vertebral body.

A strange and poorly understood cervical spine characteristic is that of marked remodelling hypertrophy and hyperplasia of cervical vertebrae with increasing chronological age.

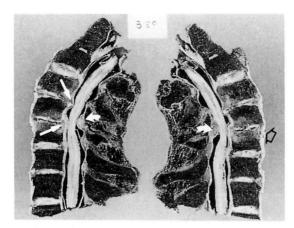

Fig. 2.25 A whole cervical spine cut sagittally down the midline, dividing the spine and spinal cord into two facing halves. The white spinal cord is in mid-section. The left and right bisected specimens show a greatly hypertrophied and hyperplastic anterior longitudinal ligament (arrowhead) and a very narrow disc and an extremely thickened posterior longitudinal ligament and large osteophytes compress the spinal cord anteriorly (white arrow). A severely thickened ligamentum flavum compressing the spinal cord posteriorly (curved arrow).

We are thrust into this world by smooth muscle, which is under the control of the autonomic nervous system. From moment to moment we are dependent for our conscious existence on the moderate contraction of blood vessels, routinely kept in this state by autonomic impulses. Most of the complicated processes of digestion, from the initial outpouring to the final riddance of waste, require the participation of autonomic nerves. Any vigorous exercise in which we may engage depends on cooperation of autonomic government of appropriate effectors, thus throughout eons of past time the physical struggle for existence has been made possible by that 'government' which preserves the stable states of the fluid matrix that are required for steady response to every call to action.

Once the great importance of the involuntary or vegetative nervous system was established and proven to be absolutely requisite to efficient func-

Synovial folds (menisci) of zygapophysial joints

All zygapophysial joints have synovial folds (menisci) in a circular arrangement about the periphery of the joint with varying degrees of projection into the joint (Fig. 2.26; see Fig. 1.10). These have a propensity to proliferate in a fibrous-like pannus in disease of the zygapophysial joints (Bland, 1994). There is evidence that if the hyaline cartilage surface is damaged, fibrillation of the surface and chondrocyte clone formation occur. The proliferation may be related to immobilization, relative or absolute. There is no secure knowledge of physiological function of the menisci other than that of lubrication.

The autonomic nervous system and the cervical spine

Pertinent to the cervical spine is the fact that a very large part of our nervous system (and that of all other animals) is concerned with activities and vital functions of which we are totally unaware and over which we have no voluntary control. Claude Bernard (1957) proposed that a divine providence considered these autonomic activities far too important to entrust to a capricious will.

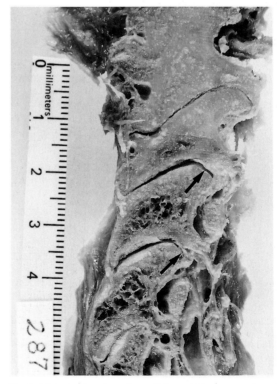

Fig. 2.26 Sagittal section through four of the zygapophysial joints. Note the menisci which are reasonably normal (black arrows). The menisci are capable of proliferation and may result in a fibrous-like pannus proliferating over the hyaline cartilage surface.

tioning of the human organism, physiologists the world over, led by Walter B. Cannon, have worked long and hard to elucidate the functions of the autonomic nervous system in maintenance of *le milieu interne*, necessary to health, the continuation of the race, and the myriad natural reflex mechanisms of controlling glands and smooth muscles. However, only in the last two decades has research attention been paid to the manner in which the autonomic nervous system participates in neurological diseases, or how the sympathetic–parasympathetic nervous system may be selectively deranged by pathological processes. Only recently have clinical investigators made significant advances in the neurology of the autonomic nervous system. The pathology of the sympathetic nervous system has been, for the first time, surveyed in many important medical and neurological diseases. Neuropathological experiments are today, with the use of modern neuroimmunological methods, done on the autonomic nervous system in the hope of clarifying human diseases.

Pertinent to the human cervical spine and its clinical syndromes is the fact that there are no preganglionic sympathetic fibres in the neck, all coming from T1, T2 and T3 levels, having their first synapse in one of the three cervical sympathetic ganglia, stellate, middle and superior. Variations of this have been demonstrated in preganglionic fibres from the C7 and as low as the L4 cord segments (Appenzeller, 1994). The postganglionic fibres then go in three directions: first, out into the upper extremities, providing all autonomic functions, circulatory vasomotion, sweating, proprioception, etc.; second, re-entering the spinal cord through the intervertebral foramen and having synaptic connections in the vestibular apparatus, the cerebellum, the thalamus and the hypothalamus; third, large segments of postganglionic fibres accompany the vertebral and carotid arteries following their distribution in the brain (see Fig. 1.7).

The earliest description of sympathetic nervous system syndromes was by Barre in 1926 and further described by his student Lieou in 1928. So diverse, bizarre and widespread were the symptoms and signs that some authors did not regard it as a disorder associated with the cervical spine (Lieou, 1928; Rotes-Queral *et al.*, 1949; Kovaks, 1955).

My current view is that the apparently nebulous, bizarre and atypical complaints are well-within clinical experience and are explicable on the basis of known autonomic neurological and pathophysiological events (Hines *et al.*, 1981; deJong and Bles, 1986; see Chapter 1). Clinical appreciation recognizes the interplay between the cervical sympathetic system, the vertebral arteries, the brain and spinal cord, the zygapophysial joints, the scalene muscle system, a pre-existing degree of arteriosclerosis and collateral circulation – all related to mechanical derangements of the cervical spine (Rotes-Queral *et al.*, 1949; Stewart, 1980; Bland and Boushey, 1987; Bland, 1994). In addition, subluxations and deformations of the zygapophysial joint importantly contribute to the aetiology of headache (Kovaks, 1955).

Though it was already known by the ancient Egyptians by the 16th and possibly the 30th century BC that spinal cord injury involved more than just motor and sensory loss (Breasted, 1930), we still don't have a full grasp of the physical and physiological complexities of autonomic functional alteration in general, and of cervical spine generated clinical syndromes in particular. Our understanding of the physiology and pathophysiology of autonomic function is limited (Stewart, 1980). Nevertheless, we do have valid clinical, physiological explanations for such common cervical spine occurrences as cervical dizziness and ataxia, nystagmus, various puzzling syndromes such as loss

Table 2.1 *Symptoms and signs of dysfunction arising from pathophysiological changes in the cervical spine*

Symptoms	Signs
Pain	Falling
Headache	Tender scalp
Dizziness	Tender bones
Vertigo	Anaesthesia
Paraesthesia	Hyperaesthesia
Fatigue	Dysaesthesia
Insomnia	Atrophy
Restless arms and legs	Hypertrophy
Cough	Hyperplasia
Sneeze	Weakness in the upper extremity
Diarrhoea	Sweating, or lack of
Syncope	Nystagmus
Visual disturbances	Tender muscle
Auditory disturbance	Fasciculation
Drop attack	Pathological gait
Arm and leg ache/pain	Transient hearing loss
Stiff neck	Fainting
Torticollis	Spastic gait
Gait abnormality	Reflex changes (deep tendon
Balance poor	superficial and autonomic
Proprioceptive loss	reflexes)
Speech disturbance	Carotid sinus sensitivity
Muscle twitch	Benign paroxysmal positional
Mood depression	nystagmus
Tinnitus	Vertebrobasilar insufficiency
Diplopia	Sensory ataxia
	Physiological head extension
	vertigo
	Cervicocollic reflex
	Cervico-ocular reflex
	Vestibulo-ocular reflex

Adapted from Bland (1994).

of proprioception, and reproducible reflexes such as the cervical ocular reflex, vestibulo-ocular reflex, pupillary dilation on extension of the neck, postural and pathological gaits induced by cervical spine disease and ataxia during the Romberg test (Hines *et al.*, 1981; deJong and Bles, 1986).

The goal of this part is simply to call attention to, and broadly review, the subject of the cervical spine's specific and peculiar relationship to the autonomic nervous system. Table 2.1 lists symptoms and signs arising from pathophysiological changes in the cervical spine.

In summary, from a postmortem examination of 191 cervical spines, the following observations are made:

1. Although present at birth, the nucleus pulposus is absent in the adult.
2. The uncinate processes, present from early life, gradually enlarge superiorly, forming a lateral and posterolateral bulwark of bone which constrains the cervical disc.
3. The posterior longitudinal ligament is four to five times thicker in the cervical spine than in the thoracic and lumbar regions, probably preventing posterior disc herniation.
4. From C3 to C4, the nerve root exit sites are below the disc level. Together with the uncovertebral joints, these nerve roots are protected from the disc.
5. Normally, anterior nerve roots are too low in the intervertebral foramen to be subject to compression. Except for zygapophysial joint osteoarthritis, the posterior roots are also normally well-protected.
6. A cleft appears in the lateral anulus fibrosus from an early age and progressively disects medially from both sides, eventually bisecting the disc.
7. There are no preganglionic autonomic fibres in the cervical spine; all arise from T1–3 levels before synapsing in the cervical ganglia.

References

Appenzeller, O. (1994) The autonomic nervous system in cervical spine disorders. In: *Disorders of the Cervical Spine*, 2nd edn (Bland, J.H., ed.). Philadelphia: Saunders, pp. 313–327.

Ball, J. (1964) The articular pathology of rheumatoid arthritis. International Study Center for Rheumatic Diseases (ISRA), International Congress Series 61. Radiological aspects of rheumatoid arthritis **61**: 25–39.

Ball, J., Meijers, K.A. (1964) On cervical mobility. *Ann. Rheum. Dis.* **23**: 429–436.

Barre, J. (1926) Le Syndrome sympathique cervicale posterieur et sa cause frequent l'Arthritie Cervicale. *Rev. Neurol.* **33**: 1246-1254.

Bernard, C. (1957) *An Introduction to the Study of Experimental Medicine* (translated by Greene, H.C.). New York: Dover Press.

Blake, W. (1925) Jerusalem. In: *The Writings of William Blake,* vol. 3 (Keynes, G., ed.) London: Nonesuch Press.

Bland, J.H. (1991) Cervical and thoracic pain. *Curr. Opin. Rheumatol.* **3**: 218–225.

Bland, J.H. (1994) *Disorders of the Cervical Spine,* 2nd edn. Philadelphia: Saunders.

Bland, J.H., Boushey, D.R. (1987) *Disorders of the Cervical Spine*, pp. 182–224. Philadelphia: Saunders.

Boreadis, A., Gershon-Cohen, J. (1956) Luschka joints of the cervical spine. *Clin. Orthop. Rel. Res.* **66**: 181–186.

Breasted, J.H. (1930) *The Edwin Smith Surgical Papyrus*, cited in: Brain, L.. (1967) *Cervical Spondylosis*. Philadelphia: Saunders.

Bullough, P.C. (1987) Understanding osteoarthritis, the value of anatomical studies. *J. Rheumatol.* **14**: 189–190.

Cave, A.J.E., Griffith, J.D., Whitley, M.M. (1955) Osteoarthritis deformans of the Luschka joints. *Lancet* **1**: 176–178.

deJong, J.N.B.V., Bles, W. (1986) Cervical dizziness and ataxia. In: *Disorders of Posture and Gait*. Elsevier Science.

Dvorak, J. (1988) Functional radiographic diagnosis of the cervical spine; flexion/extension. *Spine* **13**: 748–755.

Dvorak, J., Panjabi, M.M., Novotny, J.E., Antinnes. J.A. (1991) *In vivo* flexion/extension of the normal cervical spine. *J. Orthop. Res.* **9**: 828–834.

Fineman, S. (1963) The cervical spine: transformation of the normal lordotic pattern into a linear pattern in the neutral posture. *J. Bone Joint Surg.* **45A**: 1179–1183.

Hadley, L. (1964) *Anatomico-roentgenographic Studies of the Spine*. Springfield, IL: Charles C. Thomas.

Hall, M.C. (1965) *Luschka's Joint*. Springfield, Illinois

Hines, S., Houston, M., Robertson, D. (1981) The clinical spectrum of autonomic dysfunction. *Am. J. Med.* **70**: 2091–2096.

Kapandji, I. (1977) *The Trunk and Vertebral Column,* 2nd edn. Edinburgh: Churchill.

Kovaks, A. (1955) Subluxation and deformation of the apophyseal joints: a contribution to etiology of headache. *Acta Radiol.* **43**: 1–6.

Lieou, Y.C. (1928) *Syndrome sympathique cervical posterieur et arthritie cervicace chronique. Etude Clinique et Radiologique*. Strasbourg: Schuler & Minh.

Milne, N. (1991) The role of zygapophysial joint orientation and uncinate processes in controlling motion in the cervical spine. *J. Anat.* **178**: 189–201.

Payne, E.E., Spillane, J.D. (1957) The cervical spine: an anatomico-pathological study of 70 specimens (using a special technique) with particular reference to the problem of cervical spondylosis. *Brain* **80**: 571–596.

Penning, L. (1988) Differences in anatomy, motion, development and aging of the upper and lower cervical disk segments. *Clin. Biomechanics* **3**: 37–47.

Penning, L., Wilmink, J. (1987) Rotation of the cervical spine. *Spine* **12**: 732–738.

Rotes-Queral, J., Crespi, P.B., Pariggros, A.C. (1949) Studies on locomotor syndromes of possible psychogenic origin. II. The so-called Barre-Lieou syndrome. *Med. Clin. (Barc)* **33**: 235–246.

Schmorl, G., Junghanns, H. (1971) *The Human Spine in Health and Disease,* 2nd edn. New York: Grune & Stratton.

Stewart, D.Y. (1980) Current concepts of the Barre syndrome or the posterior cervical sympathetic syndrome. *Clin. Orthop.* **24:** 4048.

Ten Have, H. A. M. J. and Eulderink, F. (1980) Degenerative changes in the cervical spine and their relationship to its mobility. *J. Pathol.* **132:** 133–159.

Töndury, G. (1974) Morphology of the cervical spine. In: *The Cervical Spine* (Jung A., Kahn P., Matert F. *et al.*, eds). Bern: Hans Huber.

Töndury, G. (1959) La colonne cervicale, son développement et ses modifications durant la vie. *Acta Orthop. Belg.* **25:** 602–627.

Veleanu, C. (1975) Contributions to the anatomy of the cervical spine. *Acta Anat.* **92:** 467–480.

3

Clinical anatomy of the cervicothoracic junction

J. J. W. Boyle, K. P. Singer and N. Milne

Introduction

The head balances precariously on the slender chain of seven cervical vertebrae. By means of their zygapophysial and uncovertebral joints, intervertebral discs and a complex system of ligaments and muscles, this configuration allows considerable motion in all planes. The mobile cervical spine in turn rests upon the relatively rigid thorax which consists of the thoracic vertebrae and ribcage. The intersection of these two regions defines the human cervicothoracic transition. This chapter reviews the anatomy, mechanics, injuries and pathologies of this transitional region which, according to Kazarian (1981), remains one of the least described junctions within the human spine.

Normal anatomy

In contrast to typical cervical segments, the thoracic vertebrae are distinguished by the presence of the ribs and their articulations. The rib tubercles articulate with the transverse processes (costotransverse joint) and the rib heads typically articulate with the vertebrae at the intervertebral disc and the adjacent demifacets above and below the disc (costovertebral joint). The exception to this rule in the upper thoracic spine is the first rib, which frequently articulates with a single costal facet on the lateral aspect of the first thoracic vertebra. The rigidity of the thoracic spine is increased markedly by the presence of the ribcage and this plays a significant role in regulating thoracic spine motion (Stokes, 1997).

The transition from the thoracic to the cervical spine in humans is unusual compared to other mammals (Milne, 1990; Bland 1994). With respect to the orientation of the articular facets as seen in the transverse plane, there is a well-described transition between the lumbar and thoracic regions (Singer, 1996), but the cervicothoracic transition is not as clear. In non-human mammals there is a distinct transition at the second thoracic vertebra from the thoracic-type (or tangentially oriented articular facets) to the lumbar type (or radially oriented facets) found in the cervical spine (Milne, 1990). Measurements of the interfacet angles (posterior angle between the left and right superior articular facets) in humans show that the thoracic pattern (interfacet angles greater than 180°) continues into the cervical spine. There is a more subtle transition at C4 to interfacet angles slightly less than 180° in the upper two typical cervical motion segments (Milne, 1990). Med (1973) reported a similar change from his subjective study of the orientation of these joints. Others have observed this change in the upper cervical spine and attributed it to a transition between the typical cervical vertebrae and the suboccipital segments (Overton and Grossman, 1952; Mestdagh, 1976). Interfacet angles less than 180° provide a much more stable configuration and it is possible that this provides a more stable platform for the highly mobile atlantoaxial and atlanto-occipital motion segments.

Considering the orientation of the articular facets of the zygapophysial joints, as seen in the sagittal plane, there is a gradual transition in humans between the vertically oriented facets in the lumbar and thoracic regions to the obliquely oriented facets in the cervical spine (Milne, 1990, 1991). This transition occurs between about the C5–6 and T2–3 segments.

There are other morphological features which help to define this transitional zone (Fig. 3.1). Panjabi *et al.* (1991a) stated that the transition from the cervical to

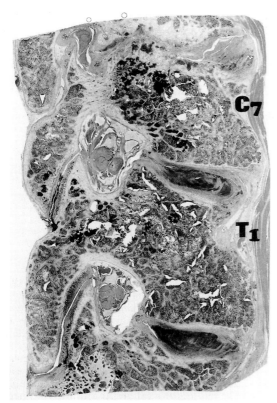

Fig. 3.1 Parasagittal 150 μm thick histological section through the cervicothoracic junction, immediately medial to the uncovertebral joints. Note the biplanar pattern for the zygapophysial joint of the T1-2 level; the tip of the inferior articular process forming an articulation with the lamina of T2. Uncovertebral joints are apparent at C7-T1 and T1-2. The larger sensory branch of the spinal nerve is clearly shown compared to the motor branch. The intervertebral discs show the greatest vertical height anteriorly.

the thoracic region is readily apparent from the vertebral body dimensions. In the cervical spine the upper end-plate dimensions at C6 and C7 are significantly greater than those of the more superior cervical vertebrae. There is a trend towards increasing values from C3 to T1 for the transverse dimensions of both the vertebral body and the superior articular facets (Milne, 1991). Uncinate processes are best developed at C3-6, but they are still evident down to T2 or T3 (Fig. 3.1). This would infer that the upper boundary of the cervicothoracic transition probably begins at the level of the sixth cervical vertebra.

As for the lower boundary of this transitional zone, Panjabi *et al.* (1991b) state that the thoracic spine can be divided into three distinct regions. The upper region is characterized by a narrowing of the end-plate and spinal canal width from T1 to T4, while the

depths remained relatively constant. As a result, the width to depth radio decreases from T1 to T4, suggesting that the fourth thoracic vertebra represents the lower boundary of the cervicothoracic transition.

The transitional zones of the human spinal column frequently show variations in their morphology as the vertebrae and zygapophysial joints assume the features of the adjacent region (Schmorl and Junghanns, 1971; Fig. 3.2). In the cervicothoracic region this was thought to involve more commonly the vertebral arch. There are, however, additional variations in the anatomy of this transition which will be discussed in this chapter.

Of all the spinal literature the thoracic region has not received the same attention as the other regions. There are numerous studies describing the cervical morphology using cadaveric (Veleanu, 1971; Med, 1973; Panjabi *et al.*, 1991a), dry specimens (Francis, 1955a, 1995b, 1956, Milne, 1991; Stanescu *et al.*, 1994) or radiological techniques (Gilad and Nissan, 1986; Liguoro *et al.*, 1994) as a basis for measurement. Logically these studies include the cervical vertebrae to the level of the seventh cervical and on rare occasions have included the first thoracic vertebra. There is a smaller body of literature describing the morphological characteristics of the thoracic vertebrae (Med, 1972; Veleanu *et al.*, 1972; Taylor and Twomey, 1984; Scoles *et al.*, 1988; An *et al.*, 1991; Panjabi *et al.*, 1991b). However within these studies a strong bias exists towards describing the lower thoracic region and its interrelationship with the lumbar spine. In addition, recent literature on the upper thoracic region has focused predominantly on pedicular anatomy relative to surgical stabilization techniques (An *et al.*, 1991; Stanescu *et al.*, 1994). Both of these studies report very small margins for error in inserting pedicle screws due to the high degree of variability in the angle of attachment of the pedicle to the vertebral body. Stanescu *et al.* (1994) reported a 7° difference in pedicle angulation between C7 and T1 and a total of 38° variation from C5 to T5. The angle between the pedicle and the lamina in the sagittal plane was more consistent, with only a 10° change between C5 and T5. However, 7° of change occurred at the C7-T1 junction.

There are very few data available on the upper thoracic vertebrae, focusing specifically on vertebral body and zygapophysial joint morphology. Panjabi *et al.* (1991b) provided a three-dimensional anatomical description of all thoracic segments, and lower cervical segments (Panjabi *et al.*, 1991a), from only 12 cases. This metric analysis provides linear and angular measures on the anatomical morphology of this transition. In recent work, we have disclosed gender differences from analysing cervicothoracic vertebral morphology. Using mean data, female vertebrae were consistently smaller than in males for the C6-T4 vertebral levels based on all vertebral body

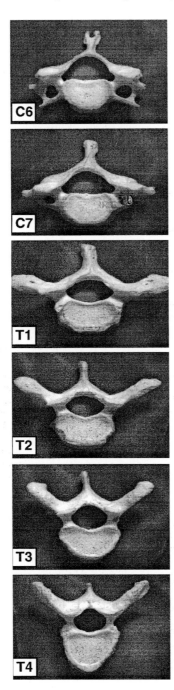

Fig. 3.2 Morphological changes through the cervicothoracic transitional region (C6–T4 vertebrae). Note the change in width of the vertebral body, widest at T1, and the progressive increase caudally in depth of the thoracic vertebral bodies. The transverse process is widest at T1 with a progressive posterior change in direction from T1 to T4 as the rib angle increases.

heights and end-plate surface area measures (Boyle *et al.*, 1966).

Taylor and Twomey (1984), in their morphological study of the thoracolumbar spine, reported that gender differences in spinal growth produce a more slender thoracolumbar spine in females than in males, as seen in the coronal plane. They postulated that the relatively thinner and taller vertebrae of females were potentially more unstable and may be related to the greater prevalence of progressive scoliosis in adolescent females. A vertebral index (the superior end-plate surface area divided by the posterior vertebral body height) was calculated (Boyle *et al.*, 1996) and indicated a non-significant trend for a smaller index in females. However, for both sexes, the upper thoracic vertebrae are narrower and more slender than their lower cervical counterparts.

In the transitional zone at the thoracolumbar junction, differences in the pattern of transition from coronal to sagittal joint orientation have been well-described. Singer *et al.* (1989), in a prospective study of 630 routine thoracolumbar CT scans (T10–L2), confirmed previous reports of a higher incidence of asymmetry between zygapophysial joints at these transitional segments and indicated the variability in the level at which the transition occurred. The morphology of the cervicothoracic transition was examined by Boyle *et al.* (1996), with particular reference to the orientation of the zygapophysial joint pairs relative to the plane of the superior end-plate (disc–facet angle) and the sagittal midline (facet angle; Fig. 3.3). Measures were recorded from 51 disarticulated skeletons, totalling 306 vertebrae. There was a marked change in the disc–facet angle from C6 to T1 with a significantly larger disc–facet transition in females (16° variation) than in males (14° variation). The incidence of asymmetry (>10°) between the left and right disc–facet angles was highest at the T1 level (8%). Similarly, there was a high freqency of right versus left facet angle asymmetry (>10°) through the lower cervical (24% at C6 and 18% at C7) and first thoracic (16%) vertebrae; however, no gender differences were evident.

Motion characteristics at the cervicothoracic junction

There have been many studies on the motion characteristics of the cervical spine (Lysell, 1969; Penning and Wilmink, 1987), but motion in the thoracic region is less well-studied (White, 1969). Recent studies performed by Milne (1993a,b) examined the motion characteristics between the second cervical and the third thoracic vertebra. The cervical spine was highly mobile compared with the thoracic spine and this is reflected in the results where a

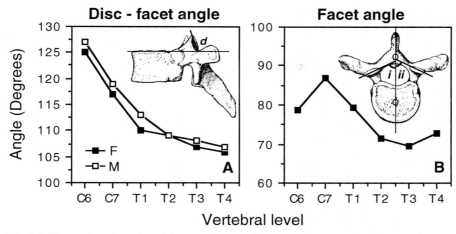

Fig. 3.3 Changes in orientation of the superior articular processes (zygapophysial joints) through the cervicothoracic junction (C6–T4) using mean data from 51 cases (Boyle *et al.*, 1996). Data for the disc–facet angle is given for males (M) and females (F) separately, while both male and female data are combined for the mean facet angle results. A schematic representation of the angles is included (*d* = disc–facet angle, *i,ii* = right and left facet angles).

steady decline from the C5–6 motion segment to the upper thoracic segments was found, as depicted in Figure 3.4.

Due to the oblique orientation of the cervical articular facets, motion in the sagittal plane incorporates some sliding as well as tilting within the cervical discs during flexion and extension. The centre of rotation in the cervical region is situated well below the disc, within the subjacent vertebral body. As you move into the lower cervical and the thoracic motion segments the position of this centre of motion moves close to the intervertebral disc, indicating that the

motion has relatively more tilting and less sliding within the disc (Lysell, 1969; Penning, 1988; Milne, 1993b).

Again, due to the oblique orientation of the cervical articular facets, the movements of rotation and lateral flexion are coupled within the cervical spine so that rotation is accompanied by ipsilateral lateral flexion. This motion can be considered to occur about a single axis which is perpendicular to the plane of the zygapophysial joints, as seen in the lateral projection (Penning and Wilmink, 1987; Milne, 1993b). As the lower cervical and thoracic

Segmental ranges of motion and trauma patterns

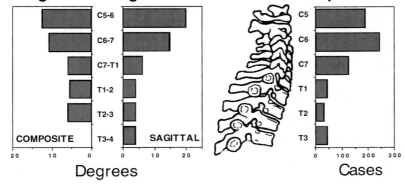

Fig. 3.4 Comparison of segmental composite rotation (Milne, 1993b) and combined flexion–extension range of motion (White and Panjabi, 1990) for the vertebral segments of the cervicothoracic transition. The reduction in mobility from C5 to T3 corresponds with representative data for cervical trauma (Jefferson, 1927).

articular facets become more vertical (Fig. 3.3), the axis of coupled motion could be expected to become more horizontal (involving more lateral flexion). However, the interfacet angles have been shown to have a bearing on the axis of coupled motion (Milne, 1993b; Fig. 3.5). At C3 and C4 the interfacet angles are less than 180° and the orientation of the axis of coupled motion is constrained to a narrow band perpendicular to the facets. In the lower cervical and thoracic regions where the interfacet angles are greater than 180° (Fig. 3.3) the orientation of the axis of coupled motion can vary greatly depending on whether the applied force was axial rotation or lateral flexion.

Axes of motion in the cervicothoracic spine

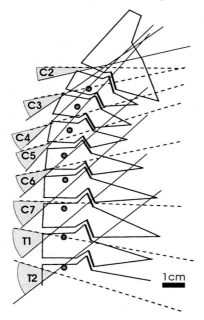

Fig. 3.5 The axes of coupled lateral flexion and axial rotation in the cervicothoracic spine (C2–T2). The solid lines indicate the axes of coupled motion when the applied force was rotary, and the interrupted lines indicate the axes when the applied force was lateral bending. The shaded sectors indicate the range of possible orientations that the axes can take. The axes in the upper two motion segments are constrained to a very narrow band. The axes in the lower three segments shown can take on a wide range of orientation, but the range of motion here is quite limited. However in the middle three motion segments where disc degeneration is most frequent there is the greatest range of motion and the axes have an intermediate range of possible orientations. The small circles represent the centres of rotation for sagittal motion in the cervicothoracic spine. Adapted from Milne (1993b).

Spinal curvature and weight transmission

The thoracic kyphosis has been shown to be highly variable in normal individuals (Fon *et al.*, 1980; Bernhardt and Bridwell, 1984; Singer *et al.*, 1990b). Bernhardt and Bridwell (1984) state that the kyphosis in the thoracic spine usually starts at T1–2 (averaging about 1° at that segment) and incrementally increases at each segment caudally until the apex of the kyphosis, centred around the T6–7 disc, is reached. Fon *et al.* (1980) reported that females have a slightly greater kyphosis and that the kyphosis, in both sexes, tended to increase slightly with age, with the upper limits of normal in elderly adults being as high as 56°. In addition to soft-tissue ageing, Fon *et al.* (1980) speculated that the increased kyphosis in females was due to relative physical inactivity, probably related to occupation, and that dependent breasts may further accentuate the kyphotic curvature.

The articular surfaces of the cervical vertebrae not only regulate the direction and type of movement but, because of their oblique inclination, in a ventrodorsal direction, they also transmit the weight of the head (Med, 1973). In investigating weight transmission in the cervical and upper thoracic regions of the vertebral column, compressive forces are thought to be transmitted through three parallel columns in the cervical spine and through two columns in the thoracic spine (Pal and Routal, 1986). Their study proposed that the transfer of load from the cervical to the upper thoracic spine occurs at the transition of the cervical and thoracic curvatures. They postulate three reasons for this: first, that there is a sharp decline in the zygapophysial joint surface area in the upper thoracic region as compared to the cervical region; second, that the pedicles at T1 and T2 are large compared to those above and are inclined downwards and forwards from the lamina to the bodies, and finally, that the posterior column becomes more closely placed to the anterior column. Thus, putatively there is a transfer of weight transmission from the posterior column in the cervical region to the anterior column in the thoracic region.

However, to facilitate weight transmission in this region a proportionate increase in the surface area of the vertebral bodies in the upper thoracic spine would be expected, yet this is not the case (Boyle *et al.*, 1996). This may indicate why this could be an area where stress is concentrated. Similarly, one would postulate that there should be an increase in bone mineral density at the cervicothoracic junction. However, the bone mineral density of the seventh cervical vertebra (approximately 0.6 g/cm²) is significantly lower than the levels above (Curylo *et al.*, 1996). The bone mineral density further decreases at the first thoracic vertebra, approximately 0.45 g/cm², and approximately 0.35 g/cm² were recorded for the second and third thoracic vertebrae (Singer *et al.*, 1995).

Based on these findings any added stress, due to the putative transfer of weight to the anterior thoracic column, would be applied to a narrower and more slender thoracic vertebra with a lower bone mineral density. It is proposed that, in combination, these findings may, in part, contribute to the higher incidence of degenerative changes in the zygapophysial joints reported at C7–T1, and to the continuing high incidence of discal degenerative changes reported in the upper thoracic region (Boyle *et al.*, 1997).

Transitional anomalies

The incidence of cervical ribs is thought to be about 1% of the population (Jones *et al.*, 1984), with approximately one-half of these cases being bilateral. Jones *et al.* (1984) report that these ribs vary from remnants emanating from the seventh cervical vertebra to complete ribs articulating with the manubrium or first rib. Gladstone and Wakeley (1932) described 10 cases of cervical ribs and rudimentary first thoracic ribs. Coupled with a review of the literature, they indicated that these anomalies were developmental defects probably occurring in the early stage of embryonic life. Anomalies in the nervous and vascular systems were frequently associated.

Variations in the morphology of the first rib may have a causative role in thoracic outlet syndrome. A thick or abnormally curved first rib may compromise the neurovascular bundle in its passage about this region and is often associated with changes in the muscular attachments to the first rib, scalenus anterior and medius. Similarly, an anomaly of the clavicle can lead to a pincerlike action between it and the first rib (Jones *et al.*, 1984).

Vertebral degenerative changes

There is limited literature on degenerative changes of the vertebrae of the cervicothoracic junctional region. Shore (1935) considered osteoarthritis (OA) of the zygapophysial joints of the vertebral column and reported an increased incidence of disease in the cervicothoracic junction – a finding he termed the cervicodorsal peak. Shore speculated that the explanation for this finding may lie in the alteration of the column in order to maintain the position of the head in the upright posture on a changing thoracic kyphosis. The change in direction (inflexion) of curve coupled with different functional demands might tend to localize stress on the cervicothoracic zygapophysial joints. Certainly there has been support for an increasing thoracic kyphosis in the aged female

population (Fon *et al.*, 1980; Dalton, 1989; Singer *et al.*, 1990b). Griegel-Morris *et al.* (1992) also studied altered head position, suggesting that there is a relationship between the presence of some postural variations and the incidence of pain. They investigated 88 healthy subjects, aged 20–50 years, and reported that subjects with increased kyphosis and rounded shoulders had an increased incidence of interscapular pain. Additionally those subjects with a forward head posture had an increased incidence of cervical and intrascapular pains and headache. There was no relationship, however, between the severity of the postural abnormality and the severity and frequency of pain.

Oegema and Bradford (1991) posed the hypothesis that a decrease in disc space may lead to altered mechanics of the zygapophysial joints and that the changes in motion and/or pressure on these joints may lead to degenerative change. However, Malmivaara *et al.* (1987), in investigating the thoracolumbar region, reported that anular disruption of the disc was not related to zygapophysial joint asymmetry, nor was there an increase in zygapophysial joint osteoarthrosis, although, at T11–12, facet joint asymmetry was associated with more OA on the side with the more sagitally oriented facet. This finding was consistent with a report by Giles (1987), who noted anecdotal histological evidence of zygapophysial joint degeneration affecting the more sagitally oriented joint as compared to the joint oriented to the coronal plane, from an examination of the lumbosacral transition. Similarly, Farfan and Sullivan (1967) reported a high correlation between asymmetrical orientation of the zygapophysial joints and the level of disc pathology, and between the side of disc prolapse and the side of the more oblique oriented joint in patients with low back pain with sciatica. By comparison, Hägg and Wallner (1990), in a study of 47 cases of lumbar disc protrusion, were of the opinion that there was no relationship between facet asymmetry and intervertebral disc protrusion. At the thoracolumbar junction, the variability in zygapophysial joint orientation was not shown to influence the degenerative patterns, recorded histologically, of these joints (Singer *et al.*, 1990a). With no data as yet recorded for the cervicothoracic junction the debate on the relationship between zygopophysial joint orientation and vertebral degenerative patterns remains inconclusive.

In addition, the analysis of association between zygapophysial joint degeneration and zygapophysial joint asymmetry must be approached with some degree of caution. There appear to be limited normative data on aged zygapophysial joint appearance and in particular what constitutes degenerated joint appearance. Fletcher *et al.* (1990), in a small series of 20 cadavers, demonstrated that the majority of cervical zygapophysial joints do not have a normal appearance. They reported that, in cadaveric specimens, 37 years of age or older, articular cartilage is reduced to a thin, discoloured or microscopic layer and that menisci are non-existent. In contrast, Bland (1994) showed synovial folds (menisci) with cervical facet joints to be a common occurrence across the age span. Fletcher *et al.* (1990) indicated that about half of the cervical joints in adults have thickening of subchondral bone or osteophytes, as well as cartilage loss. In particular, the lower and mid cervical levels were usually more severely affected. These data are supported by Friedenberg and Miller (1963), who reported that 25% of their asymptomatic patients demonstrated degenerative changes on radiographic examination by their fifth decade and by the seventh decade, 75% showed roentgenographic degenerative changes.

Similarly, analysis of degenerative changes of the intervertebral discs must be approached with some caution. Ten Have and Eulderink (1980) rated cervical discs on the presence or absence of discal splits. The limitation with the Ten Have and Eulderink (1980) disc analysis is that clefts may be found in the middle of healthy cervical discs on coronal inspection (Töndury, 1959, 1972; Bland, 1994). These clefts may start to appear in the uncovertebral joint region as early as 9 years of age. Töndury (1959) and Ecklin (1960) both deny that the formation of uncovertebral fissures in the cervical intervertebral discs should be regarded as a degenerative process.

Of particular interest, given the proposed effects of the uncovertebral joints in the development of discal clefts, is the influence of the ribs in their articulation with the thoracic discs. Luschka (1858) suggested that the uncinate processes are homologous with the rib heads. This postulation has gained some support in the literature (Bull, 1948; Hall, 1965; Bland, 1994). It has been speculated that the contact of the rib head with the fibrocartilage of the anulus may produce the same kind of changes as seen in uncovertebral joints (Milne, 1993). Figure 3.6 demonstrates the similarity between

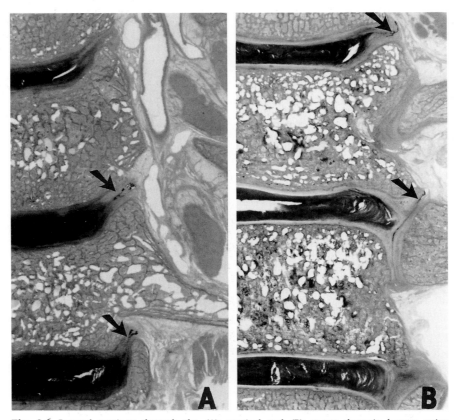

Fig. 3.6 Coronal sections through the (A) cervical and (B) upper thoracic human spine demonstrating carbon particles in the uncovertebral joints and the costovertebral joint of the second rib (arrows) following injection of suspended carbon into the centre of the intervertebral discs. The migration of carbon within these joints demonstrates fissures within the disc tissue and communication with the costovertebral and uncovertebral joints.

the uncovertebral and costovertebral joints with leakage of radiopaque dye from upper thoracic discograms into the costovertebral joints.

Given the scarcity of literature on degenerative patterns of the intervertebral disc through the cervicothoracic transition, 96 vertebral columns from the sixth cervical to the fourth thoracic vertebra were studied (Boyle *et al.*, 1997). The disc-grading scale of Ten Have and Eulderink (1980) was used, complemented by the categories of discal changes of Nachemson (1960) which has previously been used to rate lumbar discs. Comparison with other studies was limited to previous cervical investigations. However, data from this study compared favourably with the findings of Ten Have and Eulderink (1980). Analysis of these cases revealed that there was a decline in the incidence of degenerative changes in the intervertebral discs from the C6-7 to the T1-2 segments. However, there was increased incidence recorded at the T2-3 segment and comparable results at the segment below, which were more consistent with the lower cervical findings (Fig. 3.7). This increasing incidence is surprising given the presumed stabilizing effect of the thoracic cage and increased stiffness of the thoracic spine (Panjabi *et al.*, 1976).

The high frequency of degenerative findings in the mid cervical spine is well-documented (Fletcher *et al.*, 1990; Milne, 1991). This finding relates to the combination of disc-facet and interfacet angles seen in the mid cervical vertebrae which allows for larger anteroposterior translation during sagittal motion and a greater freedom in combined lateral flexion and axial rotation (Milne, 1991; Milne, 1993a,b; Fig. 3.5).

This pattern of movement is thought to result in greater shearing forces in the intervertebral discs (Töndury, 1959). The variations in orientation of the zygapophysial joints through the cervicothoracic transition may in part account for the discal degeneration in the upper thoracic spine. Unfortunately a causal link between the angular asymmetries and the pattern of discal degeneration in the cervicothoracic junctional region could not be measured in our study (Boyle *et al.*, 1997) due to prior autopsy procedures rendering measurement of zygapophysial configuration impossible.

In inspecting degenerative changes in the cervicothoracic transition, significant trends with respect to age were identified (Boyle *et al.*, 1997), consistent with the view that there is an increasing frequency of degenerative lesions with ageing of the human spine. In the youngest age group (11-29 years), 75% of all discs were graded normal, with the majority of the remainder demonstrating minor lesions. Ratings of normal declined steadily through the age categories, with the 30-49-year group recording 62% of all discs as having no degenerative lesions and the 50-69-year group scoring 57%. In the oldest age group (greater than 70 years), only 42% of all discs were graded normal and, of the remainder, over half were moderately to severely degenerated.

The frequency of osteophytic lipping decreased dramatically from the C6-7 vertebral segment and thereafter remained constant in frequency into the upper thoracic region (Boyle *et al.*, 1997). The lowest incidence of marginal vertebral osteophyte formation occurred at the C7-T1 vertebral segment. The report

Segmental patterns of degenerative changes

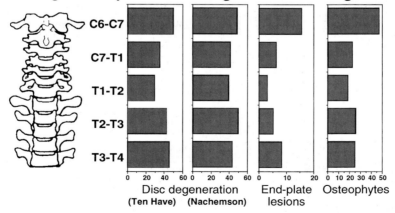

	Disc degeneration (Ten Have)	Disc degeneration (Nachemson)	End-plate lesions	Osteophytes

Fig. 3.7 Graphical summary of the incidence of degenerative changes for the vertebral segments of the transition from sagittal midline inspection of 96 vertebral columns, based on two reported scales of discal degeneration (Nachemson, 1960; Ten Have and Eulderink, 1980). Patterns of end-plate lesions and marginal osteophyte formation are also presented. In general, the last cervical (mobile) segment tends to be affected most. Modified from Boyle *et al.* (1997).

by Nathan (1962) showed a similar trend, suggesting that T1 and T2 were least likely to develop anterior vertebral body osteophytes in the whole vertebral column. In contrast, Nathan added that C6 had the highest frequency of osteophyte formation in the cervical spine. The comparison of discal degenerative changes, as defined by Nachemson's grading, with the incidence of osteophyte presence, indicates that if the disc is normal then osteophyte formation is not common. However, in this series of 96 cases, one-third of the degenerated intervertebral discs were not associated with evidence of osteophyte formation on sagittal midline inspection.

The relationship between the presence of cervical degenerative lesions and patients' complaints of symptoms was studied by Friedenberg and Miller (1963) in 160 asymptomatic patients and compared 92 of them to age- and gender-matched patients with cervical pain. Using radiographic examination they reported no difference between these two groups in the incidence of changes at the posterolateral margins of the vertebral bodies, the intervertebral foramina or the zygapophysial joints. The association, by these authors, between postmortem observations and clinical pain syndromes was considered tenuous.

Spinal trauma

Transitional regions of the human spinal column are considered to be vulnerable to injury due to the abrupt changes in vertebral morphology which alter spinal mechanics and load transmission (Kazarian, 1981). The biomechanics of the cervicothoracic junction are considered somewhat unique due to the transition from a very mobile cervical spine to the relatively rigid thoracic spine. Rogers *et al.* (1980), reviewing 35 cases of upper thoracic spinal trauma, searched for patterns of resultant bony lesions. They reported a basic pattern of injury occurring in 22 cases with a fracture involving two contiguous vertebrae with the superior vertebrae dislocated anteriorly. Additionally, associated secondary spinal injuries were common (17% incidence) and usually represented a hyperextension injury of the upper cervical spine.

Dislocation or fracture dislocation at the C7–T1 levels is a rare injury. Evans (1983) reported 14 cases from 27 years of spinal injury management at his centre, out of a series of 587 cervical traumas. A similar incidence rate is reported by Allen *et al.* (1982), who recorded 10 cases from 165 lower cervical injuries over 15 years. In an ongoing review of spinal injury cases from the Sir George Bedbrook Spinal Unit at the Royal Perth Rehabilitation Hospital, Western Australia (Boyle, unpublished), 6 cases have been identified. This series represents an 11-year review (1985–1995) out of a total of 865 spinal injury cases. Five of the 6 cases reflect the basic pattern described by Rogers *et al.* (1980), and would be classified under the distractive-flexion category (Allen *et al.*, 1982; Fig. 3.8), although a rotary component appears to be an additional features in two cases. The final case is consistent with the vertical compression category using this classification (represented in Fig. 3.9).

There appears to be general consensus in the literature that, although these lesions are uncommon, they are easily missed and closer scrutiny is required when examining trauma in this region. Evans (1983) reported that nearly two-thirds of all cases reviewed were not properly diagnosed on admission and that

Mechanisms of cervicothoracic junction trauma

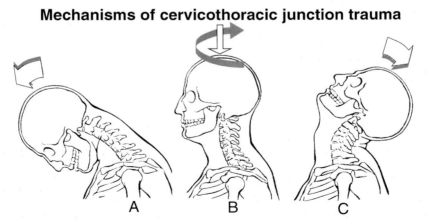

A   B   C

Fig. 3.8 The typical mechanisms of injury resulting in fracture–dislocations at the cervicothoracic junction is extreme flexion (A). B shows axial compression with or without rotation. Hyperextension (C) can result in posterior joint complex compression fractures.

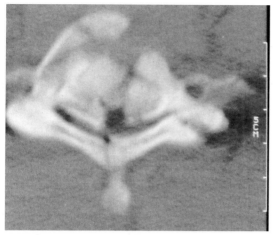

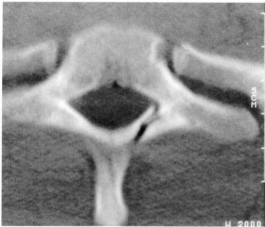

Fig. 3.9 Transverse plane computed tomographic scan of the cervicothoracic junction from an 18-year-old male involved in a rollover motor vehicle accident. Scan A demonstrates a comminuted burst fracture of C7 with almost complete ablation of the spinal canal and involvement of the articular processes. Scan B demonstrates a cleaved fracture of the body of T1 with associated fractures of the left lamina and central spinous process. The neurological lesion resulted in an incomplete quadriplegia below C6 and complete quadriplegia below T1. This case illustrates the violent nature of cervicothoracic junction injury.

dislocations at the cervicothoracic junction require careful scrutiny. The difficulty lies in the inability of routine lateral radiographs to identify lesions unless a 'swimmer's projection' technique is used (Fig. 3.10). The lateral X-ray is taken with the patient's arm elevated above the head with the other arm perpendicular to the body. Despite better visualization of the upper thoracic spine with this technique, tomography is considered essential to reflect the true status of the vertebral body and the posterior

elements. In the large patient, magnetic resonance imaging of the cervicothoracic junction provides a more detailed investigation and is considered the examination of choice if fracture or fracture–dislocation is suspected (Kerslake *et al.*, 1991). An added advantage is that magnetic resonance imaging is also capable of demonstrating oedema and haemorrhage within the spinal cord.

Complications following trauma to the cervicothoracic region are common, with An *et al.* (1994) reporting 28 out of 35 cases presenting with neurological deficits. In the 14 cases reported by Evans (1983), 11 were associated with a complete lesion of the spinal cord, and all remained complete. These findings may, in part, be reflective of the decrease in canal size in the thoracic spine.

Fracture of the vertebral body of the first thoracic vertebra is very rare and usually involves great force. This is thought to reflect the stabilizing effect of the first rib (Jones *et al.*, 1984). Fractures of the spinous processes of either C7 or T1, more commonly known as shoveller's fractures are thought to be stress fractures due to repetitive muscular action. First rib fractures can be either anterior or posterior, with the latter often involving the costotransverse articulation and the transverse processes of C7 and T1 (Jones *et al.*, 1984).

The question arises as to whether the morphological variations evident in the transitional regions of the spine influence the patterns of trauma and degenerative changes. In the thoracolumbar transitional region Singer *et al.* (1989) compared a series of 630 normal patient computed tomographic scans with scans of 44 patients with thoracolumbar injuries. They concluded that individuals with an abrupt transition had a greater predisposition to torsional injuries at this junction. A higher incidence of thoracolumbar junction mortice joints was demonstrated in the injury group. There has not been a similar investigation of the cervicothoracic junction reported.

Clinical anatomy

The cervicothoracic transition appears consistent with the other junctional regions of the spine. Marked changes in vertebral morphology occur at the transition as the cervical spine assumes the features of the thoracic region. Changes occur in the orientation of the zygapophysial joints through the transition and the incidence of facet tropism is such that care when interpreting passive manual testing of individual segments is necessary. Additionally, accessory gliding of these segments may test with variations in range and quality of movement irrespective of the presence of pathology. Grieve

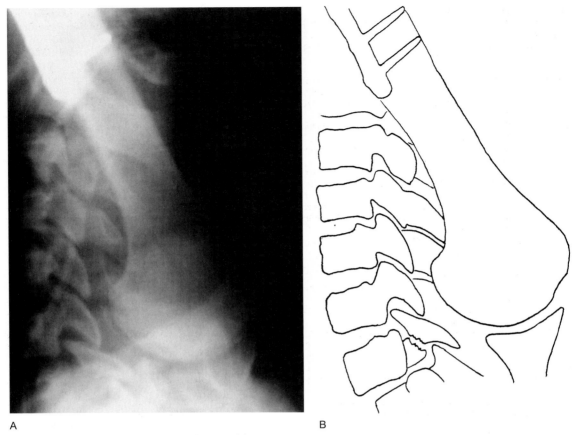

A   B

Fig. 3.10 Swimmer's view X-ray (A), with associated outline (B), to illustrate a bilateral dislocation and fracture of C7 on T1 in a 26-year-old male following a motor vehicle accident.

(1994) recommends caution, both in interpreting apparent abnormal motion, and in the nature of treatment using manual therapy at the thoraco-lumbar transition. The same advice is suggested for the cervicothoracic junction.

Despite the transitional variations in vertebral morphology, it would be spurious to associate the variations described here with increased likelihood of degenerative changes in either the zygapophysial joints or intervertebral disc. Given the relatively high incidence of degenerative disc changes and zygapophysial joint degeneration reported, the cervicothoracic junction should not be overlooked as a possible cause of patients' symptoms. Based on upper thoracic vertebral body morphology, and the postulated weight transmission, this region is potentially an area of localized spinal stress. The upper thoracic spine and the ribs assist with this increased loading. Deterioration in posture with an increasing thoracic kyphosis could be looked upon as further accentuating the stress in this transitional region.

References

Allen, B.L., Ferguson, R.L., Lehmann, R.R. *et al.* (1982) A mechanistic classification of closed, indirect fractures and dislocations of the lower cervical spine. *Spine* **7**: 1–27.

An, H.S., Gordin, R., Renner, K. (1991) Anatomic considerations for plate screw fixation of the cervical spine. *Spine* **16**: S548–551.

An, H.S., Vaccaro, A., Cotler, J.M., Lin, S. (1994) Spinal disorders at the cervicothoracic junction. *Spine* **19**: 2557–2564.

Bernhardt, M., Bridwell, K.H. (1984) Segmental analysis of the sagittal plane alignment of the normal thoracic and lumbar spines and thoracolumbar junction. *Spine* **14**: 717–721.

Bland, J.H. (1994) *Disorders of the Cervical Spine*, 2nd edn. Philadelphia: Saunders.

Boyle, J.J.W., Singer, K.P., Milne, N. (1996) Morphological survey of the cervicothoracic junctional region. *Spine* **21**: 544–548.

Boyle, J.J.W., Singer, K.P., Milne, N. (1997) Intervertebral disc degeneration in the cervicothoracic junctional region. *Manual Therapy* (in press).

Bull, J.W.D. (1948) Discussion on rupture of the intervertebral disc in the cervical region. *Proc. R. Soc. Med.* **41**: 513–516.

Curylo, L.J., Lindsey, R.W., Doherty, B.J. *et al.* (1996) Segmental variations of bone mineral density in the cervical spine. *Spine* **21**: 319–322.

Dalton, M.B. (1989) The effect of age on cervical posture in a normal female population. In: *Manipulative Therapists Association of Australia* (Jones, H.M., Jones, M.A., Milde, M.R., eds) **6**: 34–44, Adelaide, South Australia: MTAA.

Ecklin, U. (1960) *Die Altersveranderungen der Halswirbelsaule.* Berlin: Springer-Verlag.

Evans, D.K. (1983) Dislocations at the cervicothoracic junction. *J. Bone Joint Surg.* **65-B**: 124–127.

Farfan, H.F., Sullivan, J.D. (1967) The relation of facet orientation to intervertebral disc failure. *Can. J. Surg.* **10**: 179–185.

Fletcher, G., Haughton, V.M., Ho, K.C. *et al.* (1990) Age-related changes in the cervical facet joints: studies with cryomicrotomy, MR and CT. *A.J.R.* **154**: 817–820.

Fon, G.T., Pitt, M.J., Thies, A.C. (1980) Thoracic kyphosis: range in normal subjects. *A.J.R.* **134**: 979–983.

Francis, C.C. (1955a) Dimensions of the cervical vertebrae. *Anat. Rec.* **122**: 603–609.

Francis, C.C. (1955b) Variations in the articular facets of the cervical vertebrae. *Anat. Rec.* **122**: 589–602.

Francis, C.C. (1956) Certain changes in the aged male white cervical spine. *Anat. Rec.* **125**: 783–787.

Friedenberg, Z.B., Miller, W.T. (1963) Degenerative disc disease of the cervical spine. *J. Bone Joint Surg.* **45-A**: 1171–1178.

Gilad, I., Nissan, M. (1986) A study of vertebra and disc geometric relations of the human cervical and lumbar spine. *Spine* **11**: 154–157.

Giles, L.G.F. (1987) Lumbo-sacral zygapophyseal joint tropism and its effect on hyaline cartilage. *Clin. Biomechanics* **2**: 2–6.

Gladstone, R.J., Wakeley, C.P.G. (1932) Cervical ribs and rudimentary first thoracic ribs considered from the clinical and etiological standpoints. *J. Anat.* **66**: 334–370.

Griegel-Morris, P., Larson, K., Mueller-Klaus, K. *et al.* (1992) Incidence of common postural abnormalities in the cervical, shoulder, and thoracic regions and their association with pain in two age groups of healthy subjects. *Phys. Ther.* **72**: 425–430.

Grieve, G.P. (1994) Bony and soft tissue anomalies of the vertebral column. In: *Grieve's Modern Manual Therapy: The Vertebral Column*, 2nd edn (Boyling, J.D., Palastanga, N., eds). Churchill Livingstone, pp. 240–241.

Hägg, O., Wallner, A. (1990) Facet joint asymmetry and protrusion of the intervertebral disc. *Spine* **15**: 356–359.

Hall, M.C. (1965) *Luschka's Joint.* Springfield, IL: Thomas.

Jefferson, G. (1927) Discussion on spinal injuries. *Proc. R. Soc. Med.* **20**: 625–637.

Jones, M.D., Edwards, K.C., Ong, E. (1984) The cervicothoracic junction on chest radiograph. *Radiol. Clin. North Am.* **22**: 487–496.

Kazarian, L. (1981) Injuries to the human spinal column: biomechanics and injury classification. *Ex. Spts. Sci. Rev.* **9**: 297–352.

Kerslake, R.W., Jaspan, T., Worthington, B.S. (1991) Magnetic resonance imaging of spinal trauma. *Br. J. Radiol.* **64**: 386–402.

Liguoro, D., Vandermeersch, B., Guerin, J. (1994) Dimensions of cervical vertebral bodies according to age and sex. *Surg. Radiol. Anat.* **16**: 149–155.

Luschka, H. (1858) *Die Halbgelenke des menschlichen Korpers.* Berlin: Reimer.

Lysell, E. (1969) Motion in the cervical spine. An experimental study on autopsy specimens. *Acta Orthop. Scand. Suppl.* **123**: 1–61.

Malmivaara, A., Videman, T., Kuosma, E. *et al.* (1987) Facet joint orientation, facet and costovertebral joint osteoarthrosis, disc degeneration, vertebral body osteophytosis and Schmorl's nodes in the thoracolumbar junctional region of cadaveric spines. *Spine* **12**: 458–463.

Med, M. (1972) Articulations of the thoracic vertebrae and their variability. *Folia Morph.* **20**: 212–215.

Med, M. (1973) Articulations of the cervical vertebrae and their variability. *Folia Morph.* **21**: 324–327.

Mestdagh, H. (1976) Morphological aspects and biomechanical properties of the vertebroaxial joint (C2–C3). *Acta Morph. Neerl-Scand.* **14**: 19–30.

Milne, N. (1990) Zygapophysial joint orientation reflects the role of uncinate processes in the cervical spine. In: *Fourth Conference of the Australasian Society for Human Biology* (O'Higgins, P., ed.). Nedlands, Western Australia: Centre for Human Biology, UWA, pp. 171–185.

Milne, N. (1991) The role of zygapophyseal joint orientation and uncinate processes in controlling motion in the cervical spine. *J. Anat.* **178**: 189–201.

Milne, N. (1993a) *Comparative anatomy and function of the uncinate processes of cervical vertebrae in humans and other mammals.* PhD thesis, University of Western Australia.

Milne, N. (1993b) Composite motion in cervical disc segments. *Clin. Biomechanics* **8**: 193–202.

Nachemson, A. (1960) Lumbar intradiscal pressure. *Acta Orthop. Scand. Suppl.* **43**: 25–104.

Nathan, H. (1962) Osteophytes of the vertebral column. An anatomical study of their development according to age, race and sex with considerations as to their etiology and significance. *J. Bone Joint Surg.* **44-A**: 243–268.

Oegema, T.R., Bradford, D.S. (1991) The inter-relationship of facet joint osteoarthritis and degenerative disc disease. *Br. J. Rheumatol.* **30**: 16–20.

Overton, L.M., Grossman, J.W. (1952) Anatomical variation in the articulations between the second and third cervical vertebrae. *J. Bone Joint Surg.* **34-A**: 155–161.

Pal, G.P., Routal, R.V. (1986) A study of weight transmission through the cervical and upper thoracic regions of the vertebral column in man. *J. Anat.* **148**: 245–261.

Panjabi, M.M., Brand, R.A., White, A.A. (1976) Mechanical properties of the human thoracic spine. *J. Bone Joint Surg.* **58-A**: 642–652.

Panjabi, M.M., Duranceau, J., Goel, V. *et al.* (1991a) Cervical human vertebrae. Quantitative three-dimensional anatomy of the middle and lower regions. *Spine* **16**: 861–869.

Panjabi, M.M., Takata, K., Goel, V. *et al.* (1991b) Thoracic human vertebrae. Quantitative three-dimensional anatomy. *Spine* **16**: 888–901.

Penning, L. (1988) Differences in anatomy, motion, development and ageing of the upper and lower cervical disc segments. *Clin. Biomechanics* **3**: 37–47.

Penning, L., Wilmink, J.T. (1987) Rotation of the cervical spine. *Spine* **12**: 732–738.

Rogers, L.F., Thayer, C., Weinberg, P.E. *et al.* (1980) Acute injuries of the upper thoracic spine associated with paraplegia. *A.J.R.* **134**: 67–73.

Schmorl, G., Junghanns, H. (1971) *The Human Spine in Health and Disease*, 2nd edn (Besemann, E.F., trans.). Grune & Stratton.

Scoles, P.V., Linton, A.E., Latimer, B. *et al.* (1988) Vertebral body and posterior element morphology: the normal spine in middle life. *Spine* **13**: 1082–1086.

Shore, L.R. (1935) On osteo-arthritis in the dorsal intervertebral joints. A study in morbid anatomy. *Br. J. Surg.* **22**: 833–849.

Singer, K.P. (1996) Clinical anatomy of the thoracolumbar junction. In: *Clinical Anatomy and Management of Low Back Pain* (Giles, L.G.E., Singer, K.P., eds). Oxford: Butterworth-Heinemann (in press).

Singer, K.P., Willén, J., Breidahl, P.D. *et al.* (1989) Radiologic study of the influence of zygapophyseal joint orientation on spinal injuries at the thoracolumbar junction. *Surg. Radiol. Anat.* **11**: 233–239.

Singer, K.P., Giles, L.G.F., Day, R.E. (1990a) Influence of zygapophyseal joint orientation on hyaline cartilage at the thoracolumbar junction. *J.M.P.T.* **13**: 207–214.

Singer, K.P., Jones, T.J., Breidahl, P.D. (1990b) A comparison of radiographic and computer-assisted measurements of thoracic and thoracolumbar sagittal curvature. *Skel. Radiol.* **19**: 21–26.

Singer, K.P., Edmondston, S., Day, R.E., Breidahl, P.D., Price, R. (1995) Prediction of thoracic and lumbar vertebral body compressive strength: correlations with bone mineral density and vertebral region. *Bone* **17**: 167–174.

Stanescu, S., Ebraheim, N.A., Yeasting, R. *et al.* (1994) Morphometric evaluation of the cervico-thoracic junction. Practical considerations of posterior fixation of the spine. *Spine* **19**: 2082–2088.

Stokes, I.A.F. (1997) Biomechanics of the thoracic spine and rib cage. In: *The Clinical Anatomy and Management of Thoracic Spine Pain* (Singer, K.P., Giles, L.G.F., eds). Oxford: Butterworth-Heinemann (in press).

Taylor, J.R., Twomey, L.T. (1984) Sexual dimorphism in human vertebral body shape. *J. Anat.* **138**: 281–286.

Ten Have, H.A.M.J., Eulderink, F. (1980) Degenerative changes in the cervical spine and their relationship to its mobility. *J. Pathol.* **132**: 133–159.

Töndbury, G. (1959) La colonne cervicale: son développement et ses modifications durant la vie. *Acta Orthop. Belg.* **25**: 602–627.

Töndury, G. (1972) The behaviour of the cervical discs during life. In: *Cervical Pain* (Hirsch, C., Zotterman, Y., eds). Pergamon Press, pp. 59–66.

Veleanu, C. (1971) Vertebral structural pecularities with a role in the cervical spine mechanics. *Folia Morph.* **19**: 388–393.

Veleanu, C., Grün, U., Diaconescu, M. *et al.* (1972) Structural peculiarities of the thoracic spine: their functional significance. *Acta Anat.* **82**: 97–107.

White, A.A. (1969) Analysis of the mechanics of the thoracic spine in man. An experimental study of autopsy specimens. *Acta Orthop. Scand. Suppl.* **127**: 1–92.

White, A.A., Panjabi, M.M. (1990) Kinematics of the spine. In: *Clinical Biomechanics of the Spine*, 2nd edn. Philadelphia: Lippincott.

4

Normal kinematics of the cervical spine

L. Penning

This chapter deals with a radiological analysis of normal motion of the cervical spine followed by a functional anatomical correlation.

Functional radiographic studies

Kinematics is the study of motion without taking into account the influences of force and mass (as opposed to kinetics). Spinal kinematics have been profoundly studied by radiological methods. This chapter deals with the radiological analysis of normal motion of the cervical spine, followed by a comparative review which relates the anatomy with function.

Motion takes place in the separate motion segments of the craniovertebral junction, occiput to C2 (occipitoatlantal segment occiput–C1, atlantoaxial segment C1-2), and of the cervical spine proper C2–T1, including the cervicothoracic junction C7–T1.

Only movements in the three main planes are described: flexion–extension in the sagittal plane; lateral bending to the right and left in the frontal plane; and rotation to the right and left in the transverse (or axial) plane. The head may also move parallel to itself, which is called translation (White and Panjabi, 1978; Penning 1992a). Such translatory head motion is virtually limited to the sagittal plane.

The *range of flexion–extension motion* is determined by superimposition of radiographs of the cervical spine in both end-positions (Penning, 1968, 1978). Details are given in Figure 4.1. In superimposition, both the outlines of the vertebral bodies and the spinous processes should match. Only these midline structures may be used as landmarks, not, for

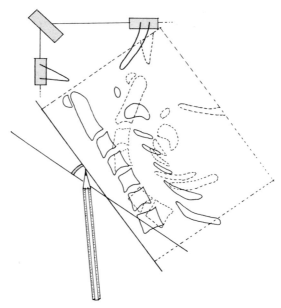

Fig. 4.1 Determination of ranges of motion between vertebrae. Flexion film is taped (shaded area) to the viewing box (occipital and vertebral outlines occiput to C7 in solid lines). Part of the outline of the film edges is shown. To determine flexion–extension range of motion of, e.g. C4-5, an extension view film (vertebral outlines and film edges shown in interrupted lines) is superimposed on a flexion film with the images of C5 matching. Then a line is drawn along one edge of the extension film on the underlying flexion film and viewing box. Next, images of C4 are made to match and a new line is drawn along the corresponding edge of the extension film. The angle between both lines is the range of flexion–extension motion at C4-5.

example, the articular processes. Both images should have the same radiological enlargement factor. Differences in lateral projection (due to concomitant rotation and/or lateral bending) interfere with reliable superimposition and enhance measurement error. If radiographs are too dark to allow reliable superimposition, the contours of vertebral bodies and spinous processes on one film are redrawn on a transparent paper, which is subsequently superimposed on the other film; this likewise enhances measurement error.

Ranges of flexion–extension motion are listed in Tables 4.1–4.3. Range of motion in children is larger than in adults (Markuske, 1971). In adults ranges decrease with increasing age, except at C6–7 (Vortman, 1992). Average range of motion is larger in passive motion (brought about by investigator) than in active motion (Dvorak *et al.*, 1988). According to

Vortman (1992), the average difference in each segment is 1.5°. Ranges show wide variations (Buetti-Bäuml, 1954; Dvorak *et al.*, 1988; Penning, 1968).

When only end-positions are taken into consideration, *sequence of contribution* of different regions of the cervical spine to total flexion–extension motion remains unknown. Such sequence can be studied by cineradiography, but small size and poor definition of individual frames interfere with detailed analysis. Using larger frames (100 × 100 mm) and lower speed (4 images/s), Van Mameren *et al.* (1990) were able to show that motion commences and ends in the lower part of the cervical spine (and never in the mid cervical part), and that sequences of contribution in normal subjects are rather constant.

During motion of the cervical spine as a whole, individual segments may temporarily move in opposite direction (so-called *paradox motion*, or inver-

Table 4.1 *Ranges of flexion–extension motion (in degrees) according to several authors*

	A	B	C	D	E	F
Occiput–C1					−10–30	3–31
C1–2			12 (5–20)	15 (8–22)	7–26	8–27
C2–3	5–18	5–16	10 (5–15)	12 (6–17)	9–16	10–16
C3–4	13–23	13–26	15 (7–23)	17 (10–24)	11–23	12–22
C4–5	16–28	15–29	19 (13–26)	21 (14–28)	15–26	14–25
C5–6	18–28	16–29	20 (13–28)	23 (16–31)	17–27	18–26
C6–7	13–25	6–25	19 (11–26)	21 (13–29)	9–23	7–23
C7–T1		4–12				

A = Buetti-Bäuml (1954): *n* = 30; 13–42 years, spread of ranges.
B = Penning (1960): *n* = 20; 15–30 years, spread of ranges.
C = Dvorak *et al.* (1988): *n* = 28; 22–47 years, active motion, average range (± 2 × s.d.).
D = Same group as C, passive motion, average range (± 2 × s.d.).
E = Van Mameren *et al.* (1990): *n* = 10; 19–22 years, spread of ranges, extension → flexion; negative values occiput–C1 indicate paradox motion.
F = Same group as E, flexion → extension.

Table 4.2 *Ranges of flexion–extension motion (average value ± 2 s.d., in degrees) according to Vortman (1992)*

	A	B	C	D	E	F	G
C2–3	7–15	8–17	6–19	6–16	6–15	4–14	5–15
C3–4	11–23	15–24	13–20	12–22	8–23	8–19	8–21
C4–5	15–25	15–29	12–27	14–26	8–25	12–20	12–21
C5–6	16–24	17–25	15–29	15–26	13–24	13–26	13–25
C6–7	12–23	15–23	13–22	13–22	12–20	10–24	11–22

A = 9 males 18–28 years, average age 22 years, active motion.
B = Same males as in A, passive motion.
C = 8 females 18–28 years, average age 22 years, active motion.
D = Groups A and C together.
E = 10 males 29–55 years, average age 41 years, active motion.
F = 10 females 29–55 years, average age 41 years, active motion.
G = Groups E and F together.

Passive motion increases the range of motion by an average 1.5° per segment. There is no difference between men and women, except for C2–3 (larger range in women). Smaller range of motion in elderly group, significant at C2–5, less significant at C5–6 and not significant at C6–7.

Table 4.3 *Average ranges of flexion-extension motion according to Markuske (1971)*

	A	B	C	D	E	F	G
C2-3	16.9	16.0	17.7	18.1	17.9	15.8	10.5
C3-4	21.0	21.7	22.3	22.5	22.5	21.7	16.6
C4-5	21.3	21.7	22.4	22.8	22.8	26.1	20.7
C5-6	21.6	22.6	22.8	24.6	24.6	26.4	22.2
C6-7	21.4	20.0	21.1	22.9	22.9	22.8	18.5

A = 20 boys 3-6 years; B = 20 girls 3-6 years; C = 20 boys 7-10 years; D = 20 girls 7-10 years; E = 20 boys 11-14 years; F = 20 girls 11-14 years; G = comparison with average values of Buetti-Bäuml (1954) (25 adults 20-38 years).

sion). Paradox motion was first described by Gutmann (1960) as an extension motion, occiput to C1, during the end-phase of flexion of the cervical spine. It occurs only in flexion of the whole cervical spine, not in flexion of the upper part alone (such as in nodding yes). Arlen (1977) noted paradox, occiput to

C1, motion in 90% of people under the age of 40, and in 40% of people over 40 years of age. With a dynamic method, Van Mameren *et al.* (1990) were able to show that paradox motion is a physiological phenomenon, not only occurring at occiput to C1, but occasionally also at C1-2, and in the lower cervical spine at C6-7 and occasionally at C5-6 (Van Mameren *et al.*, 1990).

Flexion-extension of separate segments can also be studied by comparing lateral radiographs of the cervical spine in maximal backward translation (chin-in position) and in maximal forward translation (chin-out position) of the head (Fig. 4.2). During this *chin-in/chin-out manoeuvre* the upper and lower cervical spine move in opposite directions (Table 4.4). In the chin-in position the upper part is flexed and the lower part extended, and vice versa. Reversal of direction of motion takes place anywhere between C2 and C5; range of motion in and around the region of reversal is reduced (Penning, 1992a). As flexion-extension occiput to C2 is maximal, without paradox motion occiput to C1, mobility of the craniovertebral junction is

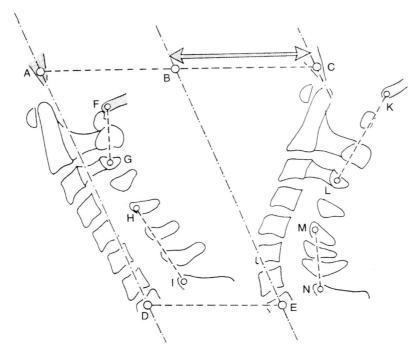

Fig. 4.2 Motion during chin-out/chin-in manoeuvres. Left: Lateral view of cervical spine occiput to T1 in chin-out position. Right: chin-in position. Line AC = translation distance of head (basiocciput). Because of co-motion of the upper thoracic spine (the centre of vertebral body T1 moves over distance DE), actual head translation with respect to the centre of the T1 body is over the distance BC (AB = DE). Corrected for radiological enlargement of 15%, this distance is 75 mm (upper normal limit). In chin-out position (left), the upper cervical spine occiput to C3 is in extension (small distance FG) and the lower cervical spine C5 to T1 is in flexion (large distance HI). In chin-in position (right), the reverse is true: large distance KL and small distance MN.

Table 4.4 *Cervical spine motion during head translation*

Occiput–C1	–29.0	–19 – –40
C1–2	–16.0	–6 – –30
C2–3	–4.8	–12 – +5
C3–4	–1.9	–10 – +10
C4–5	+5.6	0 – +15
C5–6	+13.1	+5 – +19
C6–7I	+13.2	+2 – +19

Mean ranges (in degrees) and spread of ranges of flexion (+) or extension (–) motion during chin-in → chin-out manoeuvres in 11 normal adults (5 women, 6 men, mean age 36 years, range 25–45 years; Patijn and Penning, unpublished data, 1994).

preferably studied by the chin-in/chin-out manoeuvre. Flexion–extension C5–T1 is not maximal, motion being more equally distributed over several segments, including the upper thoracic segments.

Practically performed, the chin-in/chin-out manoeuvre seems to allow a considerable degree of head translation, but for a large part this is due to co-motion of the upper thoracic spine (Fig. 4.2). With the centre of vertebral body T1 remaining in place, the range of head translation proves to be limited to an average of 45 mm with a spread of 2–75 mm (Penning, 1992a). This implies that already relatively small but sudden translatory movements of the head, as in backward acceleration in rear-end collisions, may theoretically result in damaging hyperflexion of the craniovertebral region (Penning, 1992b).

The pattern of motion between two vertebrae is represented by a *movement diagram*, demonstrating vertebral relationship in both end-positions of movement, range of motion and location of the instantaneous centre of motion. A flexion–extension movement diagram type I is shown in Figure 4.3 left, and type II in Figure 4.3 right.

The movement diagram serves as a starting point for further elaboration of vertebral kinematics (Penning, 1960, 1968). Motion is described as rotation about an axis perpendicular to the plane of motion; this axis is represented on the film or movement diagram as a point, and called the *instantaneous centre of motion*. The designation instantaneous indicates that the centre relates the end-positions of flexion and extension only, and does not suggest that motion in between is a circular motion about this centre. Centres tend to shift during motion along a certain path (centrode; Gertzbein *et al.*, 1985). Vortman (1992) has shown that centres of the cervical spine proper for motion from maximal extension to mid-position differ in place from those for motion from mid-position to maximal flexion. However, in radiographically normal spines, these differences in position prove to be negligibly small.

Figure 4.4 demonstrates how the instantaneous centre of motion can be constructed from the movement diagram. Another method to construct the instantaneous centre of motion from flexion–extension radiographs is elucidated in Figure 4.5. This method, used by different authors (Pennal *et al.*, 1972, Vortman, 1992), has less measurement error (Vortman, 1992).

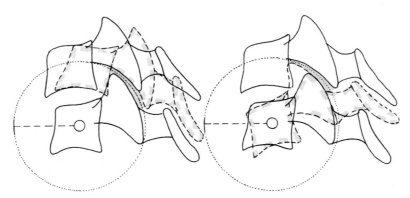

Fig. 4.3 Movement diagrams with instantaneous centre of motion. Left: Movement diagram C5–6 type I, with lower vertebra C6 in fixed position and upper vertebra C5 in end-positions of flexion (solid lines) and extension (broken lines). Dotted circle, with the instantaneous centre of flexion–extension motion (small circle in lower vertebral body) as centre point, passes through the intervertebral joint spaces (shaded). Right: Movement diagram C5–6 type II, with the upper vertebra C5 in a fixed position and the lower vertebra C6 in end-positions of flexion (solid lines) and extension (broken lines). The dotted circle, with the instantaneous centre of flexion–extension motion (small circle in lower vertebral body) as centre point, passes through the intervertebral joint spaces (shaded).

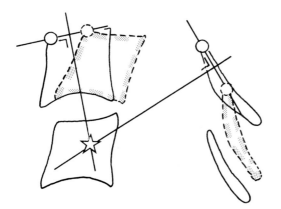

Fig. 4.4 Construction of instantaneous centre of motion (I). Left: Identical landmarks (small circles) of the upper vertebral body and arch in flexion (solid lines) and in extension (interrupted lines) are connected; perpendicular lines constructed from their midpoints converge on the instantaneous centre of motion (star). As inherent measurement error is considerable, the result should be checked by superimposing images of the lower vertebra, marking the constructed centre of motion on both films. Pierce a needle through the superimposed centres of motion, and rotate the upper film upon the lower film (Penning, 1978). If the centre of motion has been correctly determined, rotation out of the superimposed position of the lower vertebra will result in exact superimposition of the outlines of the upper vertebra.

The anatomist Fick (1904, 1911), described the *centres of cervical flexion-extension motion C2-7* as located in the caudal vertebral bodies, not in the intervertebral discs. In 1931, Dittmar concluded from functional radiological studies that the centres were located in the nuclei pulposi of the intervertebral discs. Exner (1954) confirmed this and added that the centres moved with the nuclei, backwards in flexion and forwards in extension. The author of this chapter proved radiologically that the instantaneous centres of flexion-extension motion are located in the caudal vertebral bodies (Penning, 1960), with a typical segmental difference: at C2-3 in the lower posterior half of the body of C3; and at C6-7 at the midpoint of the upper end-plate of the body of C7. The results in 20 cervical spines of young adults are shown in Figure 4.6 left. By optimization of technical errors, Amevo *et al.* (1991a,b,c) were able to locate the instantaneous centres more precisely (Fig. 4.6 right). Van Mameren *et al.* (1990) and Vortman (1992) achieved comparable results.

The *instantaneous axis of flexion-extension motion occiput-C1* traverses both anterior condyloid foramina (Spalteholz, 1953; Werne, 1959). The distance of this axis from the occipitoatlantal joints is about 15 mm. On lateral radiographs the centre of

motion is projected about the centre of a circle encompassing the outline of the occipital condyles (Fig. 4.7 bottom). The *instantaneous centre of flexion-extension motion C1-2* is projected in the dorsal half of the dens, or immediately dorsal to the dens (Van Mameren *et al.*, 1990; Fig. 4.8).

As shown by paradox occiput-C1 motion, flexion-extension in the occiput-C1 and C1-2 segments are not obligatory coupled motions. Consequently, the posterior arch of the atlas may be found somewhere between the occiput and spinous process of the axis, and not necessarily halfway between (Penning, 1978).

By systematically comparing lateral radiographs of the cervical spine in the neutral position and in

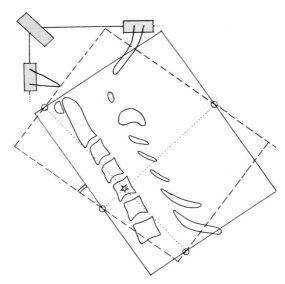

Fig. 4.5 Construction of instantaneous centres of motion (II). Flexion film (occipital and vertebral outlines shown) is taped onto the viewing box. Part of the upper and left film edges is shown. To determine instantaneous flexion-extension centre of motion of, for example, C4-5, the extension film (vertebral outlines not shown) is superimposed with outlines of C5 vertebra exactly matching, after which edges of the extension film are drawn on the underlying flexion film and the viewing box (solid lines). Next, outlines of C4 are made to match and the edges of the extension film again are drawn (interrupted lines). After the extension film has been removed, a line is drawn from the intersection (small circle) of both drawn upper edges of the extension film to the intersection of both drawn lower edges of the extension film. Another line is drawn from the intersection of the left drawn edges of the extension film to the intersection of the right drawn edges. Intersection of both lines (star) is the centre of flexion-extension motion at C4-5. The angle between the drawn edges of both extension films is the range of flexion-extension motion at C4-5.

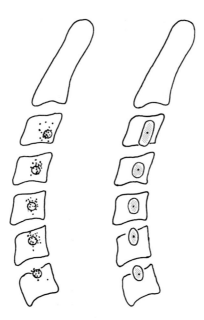

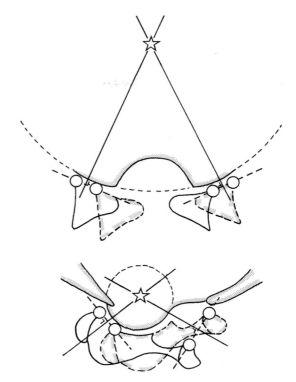

Fig. 4.6 Instantaneous centres of flexion–extension motion C2–7. Left: Instantaneous centres of flexion–extension motion C2–7 (dots), with estimated mean instantaneous centres (small circles), as determined by the author in 20 healthy subjects (Penning, 1960). Right: Instantaneous centres as determined by Amevo *et al.* (1991a,b,c) in 40 normal subjects (dots = mean centres; shaded areas = two s.d. distribution of centres; solid lines = superimposed range of technical errors).

flexion, occasionally *parallel motion (translation) of the axis with respect to the occiput* may be observed (Penning, 1995). As Figure 4.8 top shows, backward translation of the axis vertebra (with respect to the occiput) is accompanied by upward motion of the posterior atlantal arch (extension occiput–C1, flexion C1–2); forward translation (Fig. 4.8 bottom) moves the posterior atlantal arch downwards (flexion occiput–C1, extension C1–2). Parallel occiput to C2 motion is limited by unequal distribution of elastic tension over the posterior occipito-atlantal–axial ligaments.

As rotation takes place in the transverse (axial) plane, computed tomography (CT) is an appropriate modality to study it. *Ranges of rotation occiput to T1* may be determined by scanning the cervical spine in the supine position of the body with the head actively maximally rotated to the right or the left, and subsequently measuring on the obtained radiographs the difference in rotation of each of the vertebrae C1 up to T1 with respect to the occiput (Penning and Wilmink, 1987). From these measurements rotation of each of the segments can be calculated. The results in young adults are presented in Table 4.5.

Fig. 4.7 Instantaneous centres of occiput–C1 motion. Top: Anteroposterior projection (frontal plane) of basiocciput (presumed to be fixed) with outlines of occipital condyles, and of lateral masses of atlas in lateral bending to right (solid lines) and lateral bending to left (interrupted lines). Construction of the instantaneous centre of motion (star) is as in Figure 4.4. Instantaneous centre is projected in the mid sagittal plane high above the foramen magnum. A circle drawn from the centre of motion passes through the outlines of the occipital condyles. Bottom: Lateral projection (parasagittal plane) of the basiocciput (presumed to be fixed) with an outline of superimposed occipital condyles, and of atlas in flexion (solid lines) and extension (interrupted lines). Construction of the instantaneous centre of motion (star) is as in Figure 4.4. The instantaneous centre corresponds more or less with the axis through both anterior condyloid foramina (canales nervi hypoglossi). A circle drawn from the centre of motion passes through the outline of the occipital condyles (outline more curved than outline in frontal plane, typical of ovoid-shaped joint). Note that instantaneous centres of motion for flexion–extension and lateral bending are on the same side of the occipitoatlantal joint.

In this study, full rotation (i.e. both sides together) between occiput and upper thoracic vertebra T1 averages 144.4°. Occiput–C1 rotation is negligibly small. In accordance with the literature (White and Panjabi, 1978), 55% of total rotation of the cervical spine occurs at C1–2 (in our measurements 81°, or

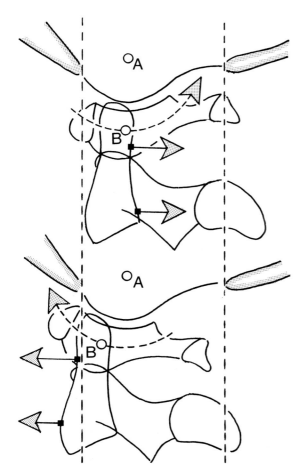

Table 4.5 *Ranges of rotation in 26 healthy adults 21-26 years (Penning and Wilmink, 1987)*

	A	B	C
Occiput–C1	1	−2–5	
C1–2	40.5	29–46	
C2–3	3.0	0–10	6.0
C3–4	6.5	3–10	9.8
C4–5	6.8	1–12	10.3
C5–6	6.9	2–12	8.0
C6–7	5.4	2–10	5.7
C7–T1	2.1	−2–7	4.7
Occiput–T1	72.2	61–84	
C2–T1	30.7	22–38	44.5

A = Mean ranges (in degrees) of rotation to left or right; B = same group as A, upper and lower limits rotation to left or right; C = Lysell (1969), *in vitro* study, mean values of rotation to left and right together.

head in fixed anteroposterior (AP) position, and the atlas and axis vertebra in both end-positions of rotation to the right and left. However, for better understanding of kinematics, motion of the head with respect to the atlas and axis vertebrae should be

Fig. 4.8 Parallel motion occiput to C2. Parallel motion occiput to C2 is occasionally observed when radiographs in the neutral position and flexion are systematically compared. Top: Occiput to C2 region of flexed cervical spine. Occiput–C1 segment is in extension (due to paradox motion); C1–2 is in normal flexion. Bottom: Occiput to C2 region of the cervical spine in the neutral position. Compared with the flexion radiograph (top), the axis vertebra has translated anteriorly with respect to the head (follow vertical lines drawn along anterior and posterior rims of the foramen magnum). This example shows forwards translation of the axis vertebra, to be accompanied by downwards motion of the posterior atlantal arch, and vice versa. A: instantaneous centre of flexion–extension motion; occiput to C1. B: instantaneous centre of flexion-extension motion; C1–2.

56%). Rotation C2–T1 (both sides together) averages 61.4°. Rotation here proves to be largest in the C3–7 region, and smallest at C2–3 and C7–T1. Figure 4.9 presents a drawing of the superimposed vertebral images as obtained during CT scanning of the cervical spine in head rotation to the right.

The *pattern of rotation occiput to C2* is best depicted as shown in Figure 4.10, with the rotated

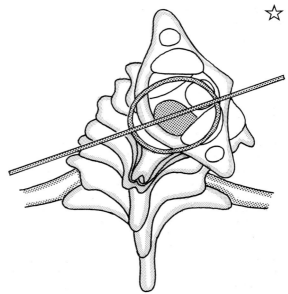

Fig. 4.9 Computed tomographic reconstruction of the rotated cervical spine. Top-view of vertebrae C1–T1 (with adjoining parts of the first rib). The head is rotated to the right side (star). The head is represented by the foramen magnum and a line corresponding with the mid sagittal plane of the head. With respect to the atlas, the head has shifted to the right but it is virtually not rotated. The total range of rotation occiput–T1 in this example, is 70°.

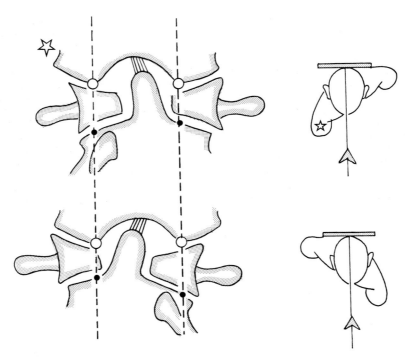

Fig. 4.10 Pattern of rotation occiput to C2 (I). Left: Drawings from anteroposterior (AP) radiographs of the head rotated on the cervical spine (with only the foramen magnum and the lateral condyles depicted). The right side is indicated by a star. Right: Views from above, showing film plane, direction of X-ray beam and the position of the head and shoulders. The right shoulder is indicated by a star. Note the strict (AP) projection of the head. Top left: Head rotation to the right. Head and atlas in AP projection with no occiput to C1 rotation. With respect to the head and atlas, the axis vertebra has rotated to left (shift of spinous process to the right). Occiput to C2 region is laterally bent to the left: the vertical line between the inner border of the occipital condyle (small circle) and the lateral mass of the axis vertebra (black dot) is shorter on the left side, with shift of the atlas to the left side with respect to the head. Bottom left: Head rotation to the left. With respect to the head and atlas, the axis vertebra has rotated to the right (shift of spinous process to the left). Occiput to C2 region is laterally bent to the right (the vertical line is shorter on the right side), with a shift of the atlas to the right side with respect to the head.

considered. Head rotation to the right (Fig. 4.10 top left) then proves to be attended by occiput to C2 rotation to the right (which is the same as C2 rotation to the left); by occiput to C2 lateral bending to the left; and by lateral sliding of the head upon the atlas to the right. Head rotation to the left (Fig. 4.10 bottom left) is attended by occiput to C2 rotation to the left; by occiput to C2 lateral bending to the right; and by lateral sliding of the head upon the atlas to the left.

Head rotation is thus attended by occiput to C2 rotation in the same direction (which has to be expected as the whole cervical spine is rotated in the same direction); and by occiput to C2 lateral bending in the opposite direction (which will be explained). The head always slides laterally upon the atlas away from the direction of lateral bending; this is related to

the triangular lateral masses of the atlas being wedged laterally during approximation of the corresponding occipital condyle and lateral mass of the axis vertebra. During rotation, the head thus slides in the direction of the rotation.

According to the CT study of rotational motion (Penning and Wilmink, 1987), average occiput to C2 rotation to the right or left of 40° produces an average lateral sliding of the occipital condyles upon the atlas of 4.5 mm (spread 3–6 mm), both sides together total 9 mm. Lateral shift with respect to the odontoid process is slightly less: both sides together total 7.8 mm. Consequently, average lateral shift of the odontoid process during rotation within the atlas is negligibly small, averaging 1.2 mm. Thus, in agreement with classical anatomical textbooks (Fick, 1904,

1911; Spalteholz, 1953), the centre of atlantoaxial rotation may be located about the centre of the odontoid process.

The *range of lateral bending occiput to C2* (both sides together) in the study of Werne (1959) averaged 5.5° (spread 1–14°), and in the study of Lewit *et al.* (1964) 8° (a spread of 4–13.5°).

The pattern of lateral bending occiput to C2 is best depicted in the way shown in Figure 4.11, with the laterally bent head in the fixed AP position, and the atlas and axis vertebrae in both end-positions of lateral bending to the right and left. However, for better understanding, the kinematics of motion of the head with respect to the atlas and axis vertebrae should also be considered. Lateral head bending to

the right (Fig. 4.11 top left) then proves to be attended by occiput to C2 rotation to the left (which is the same as axis vertebra rotation to the right); by occiput to C2 lateral bending to the right; and by lateral sliding of the head upon the atlas to the left. Lateral head bending to the left (Fig. 4.11 bottom left) is attended by occiput to C2 rotation to the right, occiput to C2 lateral bending to the left, and lateral sliding of the head upon the atlas to the right.

Thus lateral head bending is attended by lateral occiput to C2 bending in the same direction (which has to be expected as the whole cervical spine is laterally bent in the same direction), and by occiput to C2 rotation in the opposite direction (which will be explained). As has been explained in the previous

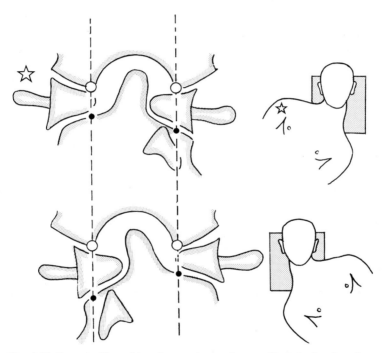

Fig. 4.11 Pattern of lateral bending motion occiput to C2. Left: drawings from radiographs of lateral bending of the head and cervical spine (only the foramen magnum and lateral condyles are depicted). The right side is indicated by a star. Right: Bird's-eye views showing film plane, shoulders and the laterally bent head and neck. The right shoulder is indicated by a star. Strict upright and anteroposterior position of the head with respect to film (non-rotated). Top left: Lateral head and neck bending to the right. The vertical line between the inner border of the occipital condyle (small circle) and the lateral mass of the axis vertebra (black dot) is shorter on the right side. With respect to the head, the atlas has shifted to the right. With respect to the head and atlas, the axis vertebra has rotated to the right (shift of spinous process to the left). This situation is comparable to that of head rotation to the left (Fig. 4.10 bottom). Bottom left: Lateral head and neck bending to the left. The vertical line is shorter on the left side. With respect to the head, the atlas has shifted to the left. With respect to the head and atlas, the axis vertebra has rotated to the left (shift of spinous process to the right). This situation is comparable to that of head rotation to the right (Fig. 4.10 top).

section, the head always slides laterally upon the atlas away from the direction of lateral bending.

It is tempting to attribute the *coupling of rotation and contralateral bending occiput to C2* (and vice versa) to the functional anatomy of the craniovertebral region itself (Reich and Dvorak, 1986). However, the explanation of the coupling has to be found in the biomechanical behaviour of the cervical spine proper C2–T1, which is described below.

Rotation and lateral bending C2–T1 are coupled motions. In 28 autopsy specimens C2–T3 of ages ranging between 11 and 67 years, Lysell (1969) found an average full rotation C2–T1 of 45° to be associated with 24° lateral bending to the same side. Full lateral bending C2–T1 of 49° proved to be coupled with 28° rotation to the same side (Table 4.6). If the thoracic spine with T1 is supposed to be fixed, the coupled rotation–lateral bending is gradually built up from C7 upwards, to reach a maximal value at C2. Lateral bending and rotation C2–T1 thus are obligatorily coupled, although in full lateral bending full rotation is not achieved; in full rotation, full lateral bending is not achieved.

The study of Lysell (1969) proves that C2 motion is the result of the behaviour of the cervical spine proper, C2–T1, as the craniovertebral segments occiput–C1 and C1–2 did not form part of the specimens. This is further substantiated by studies in the dog (Penning and Badoux, 1987). In this quadrupedal mammal, C2 does (virtually) not rotate during lateral bending of the craniovertebral junction, despite the fact that craniovertebral anatomy is comparable to that in humans. The explanation is the virtual inability of the canine cervical spine proper (C2–T1) to rotate: lateral bending C2–7 does not produce an appreciable amount of C2 rotation.

As opposed to C2 motion, head motion is relatively independent of motion of the cervical spine proper, due to the possibility of *compensatory counter-movements in the occipitoatlantoaxial segments*. In occiput to T1 rotation, the axis vertebra is laterally bent (with respect to T1) in the direction of rotation, but the head is kept in an erect position by contralateral bending in the occiput to C2 segment. As has been shown in Figure 4.10, rotation occiput to C2 is attended by lateral bending occiput to C2 in the opposite direction.

In occiput to T1 lateral bending, the axis vertebra is rotated in the direction of lateral bending, but the head is kept in the non-rotated position by counter-rotation in the C1–2 segment. As has been demonstrated in Figure 4.11, lateral bending occiput to C2 is attended by occiput to C2 rotation in the opposite direction. Thus, the seemingly coupled motions of contralateral bending occiput to C2 in rotation C1–2, and of counter-rotation C1–2 in lateral bending occiput to C2, are compensatory movements needed to keep the head in the imposed erect or non-rotated position (Figs 4.10 and 4.11 right).

Functional anatomy

Functional anatomy is the study of form and properties of the anatomical structures in the light of their kinematics. Having gained insight into the normal kinematics of the cervical spine, it is of interest to have a retrospective look at the form and orientation of bones and joints, at properties of discs and ligaments, and at the course and function of muscles.

The alar ligaments, connecting the (odontoid process of) the second vertebra with the (inner sides of the) occipital condyles, allow movements between the head and axis vertebra in all directions. Ranges and patterns of these movements are regulated by the interposed atlas, which articulates with the occipital condyles and the axis vertebra in the occipitoatlantal and atlantoaxial joints, respectively. Tightness of the alar ligaments ensures firm contact between the joint surfaces. Further stability is ensured by the tectorial membrane (Oda *et al.*, 1992).

The *occipitoatlantal joints, occiput to C1*, are relatively stable joints, guiding their own movements due to the markedly rounded and congruent anatomy of the ovoid joint surfaces. They allow flexion–extension and, to a far lesser degree, lateral bending, but rotation is hardly possible. If, in an anatomical specimen, the head is forcibly rotated with respect to the atlas (or vice versa), the occipital condyles are lifted out of the superior atlantal joint sockets. Such occipitoatlantal lifting (and hence rotation) is normally prevented by the tightness of the alar ligaments and the tectorial membrane. Experimental transection of these ligaments results in significant increase of occiput–C1 rotation (Dvorak *et al.*, 1987).

The *lateral atlantoaxial joints C1–2* have opposed convexity of their joint surfaces, the gaps between the anterior and posterior margins being

Table 4.6 *Coupled ranges of rotation/lateral bending, and lateral bending/rotation*

	A	B	C	D
C2–3	6.0	5.4	7.9	6.1
C3–4	9.8	6.8	9.8	6.8
C4–5	10.3	5.7	9.1	6.1
C5–6	8.0	4.5	9.0	4.7
C6–7	5.7	3.7	8.4	3.4
C7–T1	4.7	2.0	6.3	2.0

Values (in degrees) determined by Lysell (1969), in an *in vitro* study of 28 cervical spine specimens C2–T3 (11–67 years).

A = Mean values of rotation to left and right together; B = coupled lateral bending during rotation in A; C = mean values of lateral bending to left and right together; D = coupled rotation during lateral bending in C.

filled by large triangular meniscoid structures (Schonstrom *et al.*, 1993). Due to their opposed convexity, the joints lack inner stability, but this enables them to perform movements in all directions: flexion–extension, lateral bending and, above all, rotation.

During flexion–extension the joint surfaces make tilting movements and during lateral bending they slide laterally over small distances (average 2.4 mm, both sides together; Lewit *et al.*, 1964). Rotation is characterized by sliding movements over larger distances (20 mm or more), where the joint surfaces on each side are moving in opposite directions. Changing incongruities between the joint surfaces may be compensated for by the triangular meniscoid structures which, due to their contents (venous blood, fluid, fat) are easily remodelled and/or distended or compressed.

Stability of the *atlantoaxial relationship* is ensured by the nave formed by atlas and transverse ligament, keeping the odontoid process of the axis vertebra *in situ* during rotational movements. The freedom of movement of the odontoid process in lateral or anteroposterior directions is limited to 1–2 mm. In children, the freedom of anteroposterior motion of the odontoid process is larger (2–5 mm; Paul and Moir, 1949).

As may be derived from Figure 4.10, C2 rotation is attended by lateral shift of the odontoid process in the direction of C2 rotation. Figure 4.12 makes clear that this shift with respect to the occiput has a 'wheeling' character (Penning, 1978). This can be attributed to the more posteriorly placed insertion of the alar ligaments on the odontoid (Spalteholz, 1953), keeping the posterior portion of the odontoid *in situ*; the centre of motion is found here.

The possibility of parallel motion (translation) occiput to C2 (Fig. 4.8) provides, it seems, the craniovertebral junction with *elastic resistance* against sudden head acceleration. As shown in Fig. 4.13, sudden backward translation of the head with respect to C1 and C2 is absorbed by passive flexion occiput–C1, and does not immediately result in posterior occipitoatlantal dislocation. The same seems to be valid for sudden forwards translation of the head with respect to C1 and C2 (Fig. 4.14).

While in the spine proper, attaching muscles bridge several segments, part of the attaching *muscles in the craniovertebral junction* are restricted to one segment (occiput–C1 or C1–2), or to two segments (occiput–C2; Table 4.7). The function of these muscles can be understood from their course with respect to the centres of motion. A muscle cannot be effective if its course is radial (in the direction of the centre of motion): a wheel cannot be turned by pulling at the centre of its axle. A muscle will be maximally effective if its course is tangential with respect to the centre of motion.

Figure 4.15 shows the mentioned craniovertebral muscles projected in the three main planes, defining

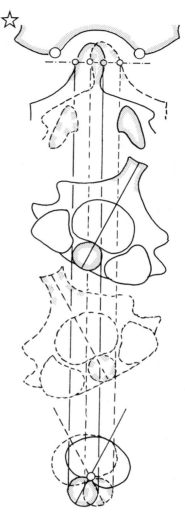

Fig. 4.12 Pattern of rotation occiput to C2 (II). Top: Superimposition of drawings of Figure 4.10 with outlines of foramen magnum with condyles, and axis vertebra in rotation to the right (solid lines) and rotation to the left (interrupted lines). The lateral borders of the dens are marked by small circles. The right side is indicated by a star. Central drawings: Axis vertebra shown in the transverse plane, with the position of the dens correlating with the position of the dens in the top drawing (vertical lines). Upper central drawing: axis vertebra rotation to the right (solid lines); lower central drawing: rotation to the left (interrupted lines). Bottom: superimposition of both central drawings with outlines of the dens and spinal canal only. The dens is seen to rotate (wheel) about a centre at its posterior wall (small circle).

their course with respect to the corresponding centres of motion. Table 4.7 shows that the predicted function of each of the muscles, as derived from its course with respect to the corresponding centre of

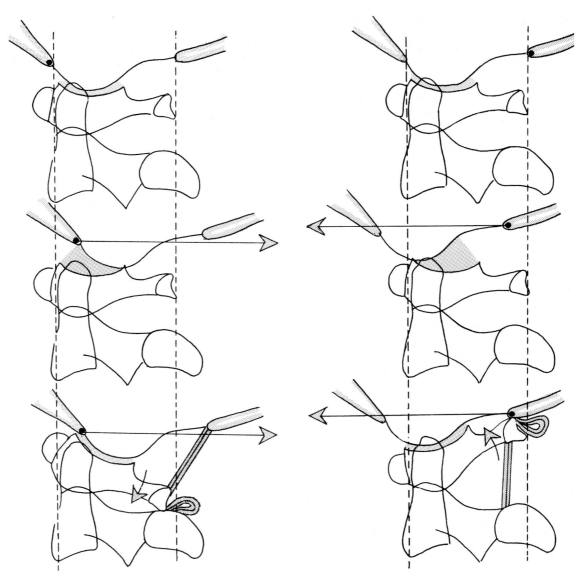

Fig. 4.13 Elastic absorption of sudden backward translation of the head. Top: Lateral view of the craniovertebral region in the neutral position. The black dot indicates the anterior rim of the foramen magnum (basion). The occipitoatlantal joint is shaded. Centre: In (sudden) backwards acceleration of the head (long arrow), inertia keeps the axis vertebra in place (compare along vertical lines); without motion of the atlas, posterior occipitoatlantal dislocation would occur (large shaded area). Bottom: Due to the downwards movement of the posterior atlantal arch (i.e. flexion of occiput to C1 and extension of C1–2; short arrow), sudden backwards acceleration of the head (over the same distance as in the central drawing) is elastically absorbed by stretching of the posterior occipitoatlantal ligamentous and muscular structures; there is no occipitoatlantal dislocation.

Fig. 4.14 Elastic absorption of sudden forwards translation of the head. Top: Lateral view of the craniovertebral region in the neutral position. The black dot indicates the posterior rim of foramen magnum (opisthion). The occipitoatlantal joint is shaded. Centre: In (sudden) forwards acceleration of the head (long arrow), inertia keeps the axis vertebra in place; without motion of the atlas, anterior occipitoatlantal dislocation would occur (large shaded area). Bottom: Due to upward movement of the posterior atlantal arch (i.e. extension occiput to C1 and flexion C1–2; short arrow), sudden backwards acceleration of the head (over the same distance as in the central drawing) is elastically absorbed by stretching of the posterior atlantoaxial ligamentous and muscular structures; there is no occipitoatlantal dislocation.

motion in Figure 4.15, is in good agreement with the data provided by anatomists (Spalteholz, 1953).

Due to the more or less parallel orientation of their joint surfaces, the *zygapophysial joints* C2–T1 lack inner stability. Stability is ensured by the intervertebral disc and flaval ligaments. The joints perform only sliding movements, not tilting movements. Like the atlantoaxial joints, they contain easily deformable meniscoid structures which are presumed to compensate for changing incongruences between the articular surfaces during motion (Penning and Töndury, 1963).

Figure 4.16 demonstrates that the *superior articular processes* C2–T1 from T1 upwards decrease in height with respect to the superior end-plates of the vertebral bodies, but the distances between these tops and the instantaneous centres of flexion–

extension motion remain about the same. We therefore suspected the difference in location of the centres of motion at C2–3 and C7–T1 (with gradual transitions in between) to be related to differences in height of the superior articular processes (Penning, 1960, 1968). Nowitzke *et al.* (1994) proved that this conjecture was correct, and also established that there was no relationship between the location of the centres and the slope of the superior articular facets (Table 4.8).

The difference in location of centres of motion is related to a different pattern of motion in the intervertebral disc: at C2–3 a more *sliding type*, at C7–T1 a more *tilting type* (Fig. 4.17; Penning, 1988). The tilting type of motion is typical of the *prototype disc*, resembling the classical (Greek) disc shape. Such prototype-like discs are found in the human

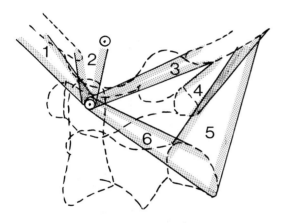

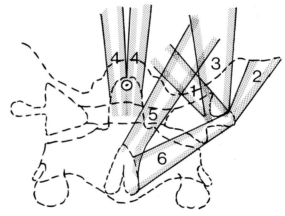

Fig. 4.15 Function of the craniovertebral muscles. Geometric representation of six muscles of the upper cervical region in the sagittal plane (top left), with instantaneous centres of flexion–extension motion of occiput to C1 and C1–2 (indicated by small circles); in the frontal plane (top right), with instantaneous centre of lateral bending motion at occiput to C2; and in the transverse plane (bottom right), with instantaneous centre of rotational motion at C1–2 (axis vertebra is shown in interrupted lines; atlas vertebra, only partly drawn, hatched). Names of the muscles are listed in Table 4.8. A muscle causes motion if its course in a corresponding plane is tangential with respect to the centre of motion: muscles 3 and 4 cause extension, muscles 2 and 3 lateral bending to the same side, and muscles 5 and 6 rotate to the same side (Table 4.8). A muscle is not effective if its course is radial with respect to the centre: muscle 6 is unable to flex or extend and muscle 4 to bend laterally. A more radial course with respect to the centre of rotation makes muscle 5 less effective in rotation than muscle 6. Bilateral action of muscles differs from unilateral action; for instance, bilateral contraction of muscle 6 will stabilize the C1–2 segment (with no flexion or extension, and no lateral bending or rotation); unilateral contraction will cause rotation of C1–2.

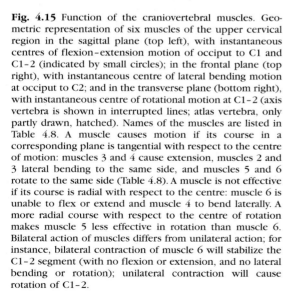

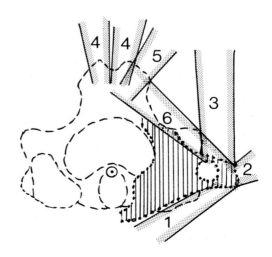

Table 4.7 *Function of muscles of the craniovertebral junction*

No.	Muscle name	Segment	F	E	Lr	Ll	Rr	Rl
1	Rectus capitis anterior	Occiput–C1	+	–	–	–	–	–
2	Rectus capitis lateralis	Occiput–C1	–	–	–	+	–	–
3	Obliquus capitis superior	Occiput–C1	–	+	–	+	–	–
4	Rectus capitis posterior minor	Occiput–C1	–	+	–	–	–	–
5	Rectus capitis posterior major	Occiput–C2	–	+	–	–	–	+
6	Obliquus capitis inferior	C1–2	–	–	–	–	–	+

This table lists muscles of the craniovertebral junction serving segments occiput–C1 (numbers 1–4), occiput to C2 (number 5) and C1–2 (number 6). + indicates that corresponding left-sided muscle causes flexion (F), extension (E), lateral bending to right (Lr) or left (Ll) and/or rotation (of head with respect to C2) to right (Rr) or left (Rl); – indicates no effect (data extracted from the anatomical textbook of Spalteholz, 1953).

lumbar spine, and the cervical and lumbar spine of quadrupedal mammals (Fig. 4.18 left; Penning, 1989). The slightly bulging anulus fibrosus of such a disc allows only tilting movements of the adjoining vertebral end-plates, attended by stretching of the anular fibres on one side and increased bulging of the anular fibres on the opposite side. In the sagittal plane the tilting movements correspond with flexion–extension, and in the frontal plane with lateral

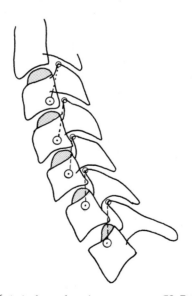

Fig. 4.16 Articular and uncinate processes C2–7. Drawing from a lateral radiograph of the cervical spine. Tops of the superior articular processes (smaller circles) rise higher above the corresponding cranial vertebral end-plates at C7 than at C3. Instantaneous centres of motion (larger circles) are nearer to the corresponding intervertebral disc at C6–7 than at C2–3. Distances between the tops of the articular processes and the instantaneous centres of motion at all levels are about equal. Uncinate processes (shaded) are smaller at C7 than at C3 (with intermediate sizes in between).

Table 4.8 *Height of articular processes and slope of intervertebral joints*

Vertebra	A	B
C3	6.2 (0–14)	36.4 (24–51)
C4	8.7 (4–15)	40.3 (28–53)
C5	10.2 (7–15)	41.7 (22–59)
C6	11.7 (7–18)	39.7 (26–64)
C7	13.6 (8–18)	31.4 (17–46)

Results of measurements of Nowitzke *et al.* (1994) of:

A = Mean height (and spread, in mm) of superior articular facets C3–7 with respect to cranial end-plates of vertebral bodies;
B = mean orientation (and spread, in degrees) of superior articular facets C3–7 with respect to posterior borders of the vertebral bodies.

bending. The cross-wise arrangement of the anular fibres makes parallel (sliding) movements and rotation virtually impossible (not more than 2 mm and 2°, respectively; Rolander, 1966).

The *cervical disc* has a quite different shape. The typical uncinate processes have given the cervical disc marked upwards concavity in the frontal plane (Fig. 4.18 right). This combination with slight upwards convexity in the sagittal plane grants the cervical disc a saddle shape. Saddle-shaped joints have two axes of motion, perpendicular to each other and located on opposite sides of the joint. The flexion–extension axis of the cervical disc is in the lower vertebral body, and the lateral bending–rotation axis is in the upper vertebral body. In contradiction, the two axes of ovoid joints (like the occiput–C1 joints) are located on the same (concave) side of the joint (Fig. 4.7).

The oblique orientation of the upper axis is in accordance with the coupling of rotation and lateral bending. If the orientation were parallel to the transverse plane, motion would be pure rotation; if the orientation were parallel to the frontal plane,

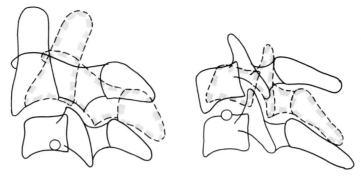

Fig. 4.17 Sliding and tilting types of motion. Left: Flexion–extension at C2–3 (range of motion 20°). Instantaneous centre of motion (indicated by small circle) is far from the intervertebral disc C2–3. Sliding of the C2 body upon the C3 body with marked step-off in end-positions of flexion (solid lines) and extension (interrupted lines). Right: Flexion–extension at C6–7 (range of motion 20°). Instantaneous centre of motion (indicated by small circle) is near the intervertebral disc of C6–7. Tilting of the C6 body upon the C7 body without step-off in end-positions of flexion (solid lines) and extension (interrupted lines).

motion would be pure lateral bending. Since the orientation is in between, motion is a combination of rotation and lateral bending in the same direction.

On anatomical grounds, the *rotation–lateral bending axis* is expected to lie in the mid sagittal plane, and to be oriented more or less perpendicular to the plane of the intervertebral joints (Penning and Wilmink, 1987; Penning, 1989). Precise localization and orientation of the axis were determined by Milne (1993). The steepness of the axis proves to be

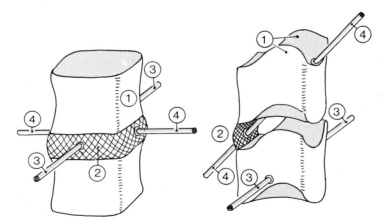

Fig. 4.18 Instantaneous axes of motion in prototype disc and cervical disc. Left: Prototype disc (resembling classic disc) between two vertebral bodies. 1 = Posterior aspect of vertebral body; 2 = anulus fibrosus with cross-wise arrangement of anular fibres, allowing tilting movements only; 3 = instantaneous axis for flexion–extension; 4 = instantaneous axis for lateral bending to right and left. The lumbar disc compares functionally with the prototype disc. Right: Saddle-shaped cervical disc and uncovertebral joints between two cervical vertebral bodies. 1 = Site of uncovertebral joints indicated by uncinate processes; 2 = anterior part of anulus fibrosus; 3 = instantaneous axis for flexion–extension; 4 = instantaneous axis for coupled lateral bending and rotation. Steepness of the latter axis varies, depending on the primary movement – steeper in rotation, less steep in lateral bending (Milne, 1993). Note that axes for flexion–extension, and lateral bending–rotation, are on opposite sides of the disc.

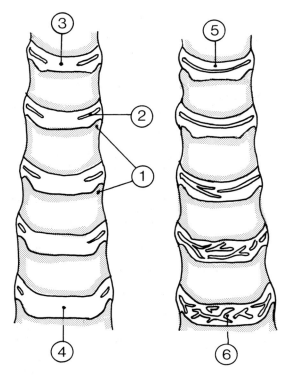

Fig. 4.19 Uncovertebral joints and disc ageing. Left: Frontal section of adult cervical spine with uncinate processes (1) and uncovertebral joint spaces (2). The C2–3 disc (3) has relatively large uncovertebral joints while the C6–7 disc has relatively small uncovertebral joints (4). Right: frontal section of elderly spine. C2–3 disc has been fissured by medial extension of uncovertebral joint spaces (5); C6–7 has been crumbled by irregular fissuring, starting at the centre (6).

uncovertebral joints is reflected by the size of the uncinate processes, at C3 covering the whole lateral aspect of the vertebral body, while at T1 only covering its posterior part (Fig. 4.19).

According to Töndury (1958) and Ecklin (1960), *natural ageing of the cervical disc* is related to the uncovertebral joints. At the C2–3 and C3–4 levels advancing age tends to extend the relatively large joint spaces medially and split the cartilaginous disc into cranial and caudal halves of about equal thickness (Fig. 4.19 right). As this leaves the cartilage intact, disc height remains preserved without development of spondylosis. At the lower levels, notably C5–6 and C6–7, the small or absent joint spaces do not serve as a starting point for regular splitting of the disc. Fissuring here tends to start at the centre of the disc, radiating into all directions (Fig. 4.19 right). When fissures become confluent, sequestra are formed, followed by disappearance of cartilage, decrease of disc height and

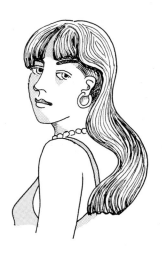

dependent on the primary movement: less steep in primary lateral bending, more steep in primary rotation. The variation in steepness is small at C2–3 and large at C7–T1 (Lysell, 1969; Milne, 1993).

An essential part of the saddle-shaped cervical discs are the *uncovertebral joints*, first described by von Luschka in 1858 (Hall, 1965). In childhood, these joints start as fissures in the posterolateral anular fibres of the cervical discs, between the developing uncinate processes and the corresponding excavations in the cranial vertebral bodies (Fig. 4.19), and evolve into diarthrotic joints in adult life (Töndury, 1958). They allow the typical cervical sliding and rotation movements, virtually impossible in proto-type-like discs. Uncovertebral joints are best developed at C2–3 and C3–4, and least, or not at all, at C5–6 and C6–7 (Töndury, 1958; Ecklin, 1960). This is in accordance with the extent of sliding movements between cervical vertebrae which are maximal at C2–3 and minimal at C6–T1. The size of the

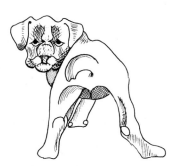

Fig. 4.20 Looking backwards in bipeds and quadrupeds. Top: Biped looking backwards by rotating the cervical spine. Bottom: Quadruped looking backwards by lateral bending of the cervical spine.

development of sclerosis and osteophytosis of the adjoining vertebral bodies. Seen in the light of kinematics, disc degeneration thus seems to be promoted by a tilting type of flexion–extension motion, and retarded by a sliding type.

Although the canine cervical spine proper, C2–T1, as opposed to the human cervical spine proper, is virtually unable to rotate (rotation C1–2 having about the same range as in humans; Penning and Badoux, 1987), its range of lateral bending C2–T1 largely exceeds that of humans: about 30° per segment (both sides together; Penning and Badoux, 1987), as opposed to 12° per segment in the human spine (Penning, 1968). The human cervical spine proper thus has acquired its ability of rotation, it seems, at the cost of lateral bending.

In a comparative anatomical study of dried cervical vertebrae, Hall (1965) established that *uncinate processes (and hence also uncovertebral joints) are absent in quadrupedal animals*, like the dog, but present in obligatory or facultative bipeds, like primates, rodents and marsupials. All these bipedal animals have to rotate their neck to look about them in the upright position, whereas quadrupeds do this by bending their necks laterally (Fig. 4.20).

According to Milne (1992), all species with uncinate processes have a hand capable of manipulation, prehension and bringing food to the mouth, the upper limb being supported by an ossified clavicle (species without uncinate processes lack a clavicle). He suggests that uncinate processes function to stabilize the neck against the turning effects of laterally directed muscles supporting the upper limbs (scalenus, levator scapulae, trapezius and sternomastoideus).

References

Amevo, B., Worth, D., Bogduk, N. (1991a) Instantaneous axes of rotation of the typical cervical motion segments. I. An empirical study of technical errors. *Clin. Biomechan.* **6:** 31–37.

Amevo, B., Worth, D., Bogduk, N. (1991b) Instantaneous axes of rotation of the typical cervical motion segments. II. Optimization of technical errors. *Clin. Biomechan.* **6:** 38–46.

Amevo, B, Worth, D., Bogduk, N. (1991c) Instantaneous axes of rotation of the typical cervical motion segments. III. A study in normal volunteers. *Clin. Biomechan.* **6:** 111–117.

Arlen, A. (1977) Die "paradoxe Kippbewegung des Atlas" in der Funktionsdiagnostik der Halswirbelsäule. *Man. Med.* **15:** 16–22.

Buetti-Bäuml, C. (1954) *Funktionelle Röntgendiagnostik der Halswirbelsäule.* Stuttgart: Thieme.

Dittmar, O. (1931) Röntgenstudien zur Mechanologie der Wirbelsäule. *Z. Orthop. Chir.* **55:** 321–351.

Dvorak, J., Panjabi, M.M., Gerber, M., Wichmann, W. (1987) CT-Functional diagnostics of the rotatory instability of the upper cervical spine. 1. An experimental study on cadavers. *Spine* **12:** 197–205.

Dvorak, J., Froehlich, D., Penning, L., Baumgartner, H., Panjabi, M.M. (1988) Functional radiographic diagnosis of the cervical spine. Flexion–extension. *Spine* **13:** 748–755.

Ecklin U. (1960) *Die Altersveränderungen der Halswirbelsäule.* Berlin: Springer.

Exner, G. (1954) *Die Halswirbelsäule. Pathologie und Klinik.* Stuttgart: Thieme.

Fick, R. (1904, 1911) *Handbuch der Anatomie und Mechanik der Gelenke.* Jena: Fischer.

Gertzbein, S.D., Seligman, J., Holtby, R. *et al.* (1985) Centrode patterns and segmental instability in degenerative disc disease. *Spine* **10:** 257–261.

Gutmann, G. (1960) Die Wirbelblockierung und ihr radiologischer Nachweis. *Die Wirbelsäule in Forschung und Praxis*, vol. 15. Stuttgart: Hippokrates, pp. 83–102.

Hall, M.C. (1965) *Luschka's Joint.* Springfield, IL: Charles C. Thomas.

Lewit, K., Krąusová, L., Kneidlová, D. (1964) Mechanismus und Bewegungsausmasz der Seitneigung in den Kopfgelenken. *Fortschr. Röntgenstr.* **101:** 194–201.

Lysell, E. (1969) Motion in the cervical spine. An experimental study on autopsy specimens. *Acta Orthop. Scand. (Suppl)* **123:** 5–61.

Markuske, H. (1971) Untersuchungen zur Statik und Dynamik der kindlichen Halswirbelsäule. Der Aussagewert seitlicher Röntgenaufnahmen. *Die Wirbelsäule in Forschung und Praxis*, vol. 50. Stuttgart: Hippokrates.

Milne, N. (1992) The effect of uncinate processes on motion in the neck. *Proc. Australas. Soc. Hum. Biol.* **5:** 345–357.

Milne, N. (1993) Composite motion in cervical disc segments. *Clin. Biomechan.* **8:** 193–202.

Nowitzke, A., Westaway, M., Bogduk, N. (1994) Cervical zygapophyseal joints. Geometrical parameters and relationship to cervical kinematics. *Clin. Biomechan.* **9:** 342–348.

Oda, T., Panjabi, M.M., Crisco, J.J., Bueff, H.U., Grob, D., Dvorak, J. (1992) Role of tectorial membrane in the stability of the upper cervical spine. *Clin. Biomechan.* **7:** 201–207.

Paul, L.W., Moir, W.M. (1949) Non pathologic variations in the relationship of the upper cervical vertebrae. *A.J.R.* **62:** 519–524.

Pennal, G.F., Conn, G.S., McDonald, G., Dale, G., Garside, H. (1972) Motion studies of the lumbar spine. *J. Bone J. Surg.* **54B:** 442–452.

Penning, L. (1960) *Functioneel röntgenonderzoek bij degeneratieve en traumatische aandoeningen der laagcervicale bewegingssegmenten.* Thesis, Groningen.

Penning, L. (1968) *Functional Pathology of the Cervical Spine.* Baltimore: Williams & Wilkins.

Penning, L. (1978) Normal movements of the cervical spine. *A.J.R.* **130:** 317–326.

Penning, L. (1988) Differences in anatomy, motion, development and aging of the upper and lower cervical discs and apophyseal joints. *Clin. Biomechan.* **3:** 37–47.

Penning, L. (1989) Functional anatomy of joints and discs. In: *The Cervical Spine*, 2nd edn. Philadelphia: Lippincott, pp. 33–56.

Penning, L. (1992a) Acceleration injury of the cervical spine by hypertranslation of the head. Part I. Effect of normal translation of the head on cervical spine motion. A radiological study. *Eur. Spine J.* **1:** 7–12.

Penning, L. (1992b) Acceleration injury of the cervical spine by hypertranslation of the head. Part II. Effect of hypertranslation of the head on cervical spine motion. discussion of literature data. *Eur. Spine J.* **1**: 13–19.

Penning, L. (1995) Craniovertebral kinematics in man and some quadrupedal mammals. An anatomico-radiological comparison. *Neuro-Orthopedics* **17/18**: 3–20.

Penning, L., Badoux, D.M. (1987) Radiological study of the movements of the cervical spine in the dog compared with those in man. *Anat. Hist. Embryol.* **16**: 1–20.

Penning, L., Töndury, G. (1963) Entstehung, Bau und Funktion der meniskoiden Strukturen in den Halswirbelgelenken. *Z. Orthop.* **8**: 1–14.

Penning, L., Wilmink, J.T. (1987) Rotation of the cervical spine. A CT study in normal subjects. *Spine* **12**: 732–738.

Reich, C., Dvorak, J. (1986) The functional evaluation of craniocervical segments in sidebending using x-rays. *Man. Med.* **2**: 108–113.

Rolander SD. (1966) Motion of the lumbar spine with special reference to the stabilizing effect of posterior fusion. An experimental study on autopsy specimens. *Acta Orthop. Scand. Suppl.* **90**, 1–144.

Schonstrom, N., Twomey, L., Taylor, J. (1993) The lateral atlanto-axial joints and their synovial folds. An *in vitro* study of soft tissue injuries and fractures. *J. Trauma* **35**: 886–892.

Spalteholz, W. (1953) *Handatlas und Lehrbuch der Anatomie des Menschen. I. Bewegungsapparat*, 15th edn, Spanner, R. (ed.) Amsterdam: Scheltema and Holkema.

Töndury, G. (1958) *Entwicklungsgeschichte und Fehlbildungen der Wirbelsäule*. Stuttgart: Hippokrates.

van Mameren, H., Drukker, J., Sanches, H., Beursgens, J. (1990) Cervical spine motion in the sagittal plane. I. Range of motion of actually performed movements; an X-ray cinematographic study. *Eur. J. Morphol.* **29**: 47–68.

van Mameren, H., Drukker, J., Sanches, H., Beursgens, J. (1992) Cervical spine motion in the sagittal plane. II. Position of segmental averaged instantaneous centers of rotation; a cineradiographic study. *Spine* **17**: 467–474.

Vortman, B.J. (1992) *Bewegingscentra van de lagere halswervelkolom* (Motion centres of the lower cervical spine, summary in English). Thesis, Groningen.

Werne, S. (1959) The possibilities of movement in the craniovertebral joints. *Acta Orthop. Scand.* **28**: 165–173.

White, A.A., Panjabi, M.M. (1978) *Clinical Biomechanics of the Spine*. Philadelphia: Lippincott.

5

Whiplash injuries

R. W. Teasell and A. P. Shapiro

Whiplash injuries are a controversial clinical entity and represent a perplexing problem for both patient and treating clinician. In 1990, the Société d'Assurance Automobile du Québec, a provincial government no-fault insurance carrier in Canada's second largest province, commissioned a group of clinicians, scientists and epidemiologists to review the scientific literature exhaustively and make public policy recommendations regarding the prevention and treatment of whiplash and its associated disorders. The stated reasons for commissioning this study reflected a grievous concern with both the magnitude of the problem and the paucity of strategies to address it effectively:

> The frequency of the clinical entity labelled as whiplash is high; the residual disability of victims appears significant in magnitude, and the costs of care and indemnity are high and rising. There is considerable inconsistency about diagnostic criteria, indications for therapeutic intervention, rehabilitation and the appropriate role of clinicians at all phases of the syndrome. Little is known about primary prevention of the condition, and virtually nothing is known about tertiary prevention of serious disability (Quebec Task Force, 1995).

Moreover, in their conclusion, the Quebec Task Force on Whiplash Associated Disorders noted that the scientific evidence regarding whiplash was 'sparse and generally of unacceptable quality' and they were forced to rely on consensus opinion for treatment recommendations.

Patients suffering whiplash injuries often present with symptoms that appear out of proportion to objective signs, numerous psychological and behavioural sequelae of chronic pain, and a poor response to conventional therapeutic interventions. Patients are often misclassified as hysterical or malingerers and many clinicians fail to regard whiplash as a legitimate injury. This is further complicated by pending litigation which engenders doubt regarding the veracity of patients' complaints or the degree of associated disability. Nevertheless, experimental and clinical evidence continues to provide compelling support for the concept that whiplash injuries have a physiological basis (Bogduk, 1986; Barnsley *et al.,* 1993a, 1995; Lord, 1996). At the same time there is a growing appreciation among medical practitioners that illness, as it presents to the clinician in the form of the sick or injured person, is a complex bio-psychosocial phenomenon that cannot be truly understood as simply a physiological entity (Engel, 1977; Cassell, 1991; Shapiro and Roth, 1993).

Definition and scope of the problem

The Quebec Task Force (1995) adopted the following definition of whiplash: 'Whiplash is an acceleration–deceleration mechanism of energy transfer to the neck. It may result from rear end or side-impact motor vehicle collisions, but can also occur during diving or other mishaps. The impact may result in bony or soft tissue injuries (whiplash injuries), which in turn may lead to a variety of clinical manifestations (Whiplash-Associated Disorders)'.

In the last few decades there has been a growing appreciation of the magnitude of whiplash injuries secondary to motor vehicle collisions. In 1971, the National Safety Council estimated that there were approximately 4 million rear-end collisions in the USA, resulting in as many as 1 million reported injuries per year (National Safety Council, 1971; Croft, 1988). In that same year the Insurance Institute for Highway Safety reported a 24% incidence of these injuries following rear-end collisions. Similarly, Macnab (1964, 1969, 1971, 1982) estimated that neck injuries occurred in one-fifth of all accidents involving rear-end collisions. Schutt and Dohan (1968) calculated the number of neck injuries sustained in automobile accidents to be 14.5 per 1000 industrial employees.

The cost of whiplash injuries is high. In British Columbia and Saskatchewan, two Canadian provinces with single-payer motor vehicle insurance programmes, 68% and 85% respectively of all claims paid out were for whiplash injuries (Sobeco *et al.,* 1989; Giroux, 1991; Quebec Task Force, 1995). The Quebec Task Force (1995) estimated that the annual incidence of compensated whiplash in the province of Quebec in 1987 was 70 per 100 000 inhabitants.

Biomechanics and pathophysiology of whiplash injuries

Typically the injured individual is the occupant of a stationary vehicle which is struck from behind (Commack, 1957; Macnab, 1964, 1969, 1971, 1973, 1982; Hohl, 1974; Frankel, 1976; LaRocca, 1978; Bogduk, 1986; Deans, 1986) although injury frequently occurs following side and head-on collisions (Deans, 1986). Injury results when neck musculature is unable to compensate for the rapidity of head and torso movement resulting from the acceleration forces generated at the time of impact (Hohl, 1989). When the physiological limits of cervical structures are exceeded, anatomical disruption of the soft tissues of the neck (including muscles, ligaments and joint capsules) results.

While the mechanism of injury is relatively well-understood and generally agreed upon, the actual *pathological lesions* accounting for chronically symptomatic whiplash injuries are by no means certain. Possible pathological lesions following whiplash injuries are listed in Table 5.1. Injuries occurring to the

Table 5.1 *Possible pathological lesions in whiplash injuries*

Muscle strain
Zygapophysial joint sprain or fracture
Anterior and/or posterior longitudinal ligament strain or tear
Intervertebral ligament sprain or tear
Intervertebral disc herniation
Retropharyngeal haematoma
Sympathetic trunk injury
Vertebral artery ischaemia
Concussion or mild traumatic brain injury
Thoracic outlet syndrome
Temporomandibular joint dysfunction

muscles of the neck, including stretching, tearing and haemorrhaging of the longus colli, longus capitis, scalenes and sternocleidomastoids, have long been thought to be the primary reason for pain (Lieberman, 1986). Recent work utilizing surface electromyography has demonstrated, within the limitations of this technology, that neck muscles following injury are abnormal in terms of their functioning (Donaldson, 1995). A critical element of the debate about persistent pain revolves around the normal anticipated time for musculoligamentous healing to occur. The Quebec Task Force (1995) notes:

> Apart from anatomic studies, much of the scientific understanding of soft tissue injury and healing is derived from animal models, and there is little information on the normal recuperation period. In the animal model of soft tissue healing, there is a brief period (less than 72 hours) of acute inflammation and reaction, followed by a period of repair and regeneration (approximately 72 hours to up to 6 weeks), and finally by a period of remodeling and rematuration that can last up to 1 year.

Supporting structures around facet joints may also be sprained or suffer cartilaginous damage or fracture (Lord *et al.,* 1993; Barnsley *et al.,* 1994). This was elegantly demonstrated in a carefully controlled trial with diagnostic local anaesthetic blocks. In this double-blind study, over half of consecutively referred whiplash patients experienced temporary relief from injections and the expected temporal difference in symptom relief was observed between injections of long-acting or short-acting local anaesthetics (Barnsley *et al.,* 1993b, 1995; Lord *et al.,* 1993). The anterior and posterior longitudinal spinal ligaments can theoretically undergo stretching and possible tearing (Macnab, 1964, 1969, 1971, 1973, 1982; Clemens and Burrow, 1972; Bogduk, 1986) although the recent introduction of magnetic resonance imaging (MRI) scanning has failed to reveal major injuries to these structures. Esophageal and laryngeal damage as well as injury to the cervical sympathetic chain have also been reported (Macnab, 1964, 1969, 1971, 1973, 1982), although evidence that these injuries are common or significant is lacking. Finally, injury to the brain (discussed later), temporomandibular joints and low back following whiplash has been reported but remains controversial. The pathophysiology of whiplash injuries is discussed in more detail elsewhere (Bogduk, 1986; Barnsley *et al.,* 1993a; Lord *et al.,* 1993).

The clinical picture of whiplash injuries

The clinical picture of whiplash is dominated by head, neck, and upper thoracic pain and is often associated with a variety of poorly explained symptoms such as dizziness, tinnitus and blurred vision. The symptom complex is remarkably consistent from patient to patient and frequently is complicated by psychological sequelae such as anger, anxiety, depression and concerns over litigation or compensation. In their cohort study, the Quebec Task Force (1995) found the highest incidence of whiplash claims among the 20–24-year age group. The potential array of physical and psychosocial complaints is listed in Table 5.2.

Females appear to experience whiplash injuries more often than men (Balla, 1980; Quebec Task Force, 1995). Women generally have slimmer, less muscular necks which, theoretically, are less able to resist damaging acceleration forces generated at the time of impact. Other possible reasons for the sex difference are that women may be more likely to seek medical attention; be sent to medical specialists for complaints of pain; respond to their injuries in a way that aggravates their condition; or be subjected to more external stressors making it more difficult for them to cope. At present, the sex difference with respect to those presenting with whiplash symptoms remains unexplained.

A delay in onset of symptoms of several hours following impact is characteristic of whiplash injuries (Dunsker, 1982; Deans *et al.,* 1987; Evans, 1992). Most patients feel little or no pain for the first few minutes following injury, after which symptoms gradually intensify over the next few days. In the first few hours findings on examination are generally minimal (Hohl, 1975). After several hours, limitation of neck motion, tightness, muscle spasm and/or swelling and tenderness of both anterior and posterior cervical structures become apparent (Hohl, 1975; Wickstrom and LaRocca, 1975). This delay is likely due to the time required for traumatic oedema and haemorrhage to occur in injured soft tissues (Jeffreys, 1980; Lieberman, 1986).

Table 5.2 *Potential presenting problems in whiplash*

Neck and shoulder pain
Headache
Arm pain/paraesthesiae/weakness
Dysphasia
Visual symptoms
Dizziness/vertigo
Tinnitus
Low back pain
Temporomandibular joint symptoms
Depression
Anxiety (including panic attacks)
Anger and frustration
Loss of job and income
Marital and family disruption
Drug dependence

Radiological findings

Radiological studies of the cervical spine taken at the time of the accident are generally unremarkable or reveal evidence of pre-existing degenerative changes. The most commonly reported abnormal X-ray finding is straightening of the normal cervical lordotic curve (Hohl, 1974). However, Hohl (1989) noted that straightening of the cervical spine was not necessarily indicative of a pathological condition (Borden *et al.,* 1960; Rachtman *et al.,* 1961; Hohl, 1974) and can be regarded as a normal variant (Hohl, 1989). Rarely, X-rays may reveal evidence of bony injury such as posterior joint crush fractures or minimal subluxation (Macnab, 1971). Radiological investigations are of limited value in diagnosis and prognosis and their main use is in ruling out surgically correctable anatomical injuries. Computed tomographic (CT) scanning and MRI should be reserved for cases where cervical disc protrusion or spinal cord injury is suspected. Radionucleotide bone scanning is warranted if there is significant clinical suspicion of an undiagnosed fracture (Hohl, 1989).

Clinical features of whiplash injuries

Local tenderness and referred pain

Local tenderness and pain referred to areas distal to the original injury are two hallmark features of the whiplash syndrome. The aetiology of these two clinical features remains enigmatic. Myofascial pain, although a poorly understood clinical entity, is felt by many (arguably most) clinicians to account for the majority of persistent neck, head and upper thoracic pain following whiplash injury (Fricton, 1993). The trigger point is regarded as the characteristic feature of myofascial pain (Travell and Simons, 1983). Myofascial trigger points are circumscribed, 2–5 mm in diameter, self-sustaining, hyperirritable foci of tenderness reported to be located within a taut band of skeletal muscle or its associated fascia. Compressing this trigger point is locally painful and may give rise to characteristic referred pain, tenderness and autonomic phenomena. The area of pain referral, which is often surprisingly consistent across patients, is termed the zone of reference.

Myofascial pain is thought to result from an acute muscle strain or overload which occurs at the time of impact. One hypothesis is that a small area of neuromuscular irritability develops and becomes self-sustaining, resulting in a trigger point (Travell and Simons, 1983). Aggravating factors are usually related to activities or postures which lead to contraction or tension of involved muscles while alleviating factors often contribute to relaxation of the involved muscles. *Myofascial trigger points* throughout the cervical and upper thoracic musculature often send referred pain and paraesthesiae down the ipsilateral arm when pressed on during palpation. Nerve conduction studies, F-wave and needle electromyographic studies are invariably normal.

Although the diagnosis of myofascial pain requires the presence of these palpable trigger points, it often proves difficult to establish reliably the presence or absence of trigger points on physical examination. This diagnostic unreliability, when combined with the psychological sequelae typically associated with chronic pain, has contributed to the confusion and controversy over myofascial pain syndrome. Empirical support for myofascial pain derives primarily from experimental studies involving mechanical irritation of deep tissues, i.e. muscles, deep fascia, etc.; such studies resulted in poorly localized aching or burning, often associated with muscle soreness and tenderness over bony prominences (Inman and Saunders, 1944; Feinstein *et al.,* 1954; Feinstein, 1977; Croft and Foreman, 1988). This referred pain, although often delayed in onset, was reproducible and often accompanied by autonomic phenomena. Mense (1994) has noted in animal experiments that persistent nociceptive input from muscle (in the form of an experimental myositis) results in an expansion of those rat dorsal horn neurons responding to electrostimulation of peripheral nerves. This is seen as indicative that the population of neurons which can be activated by nociceptive afferent input from a muscle increases in size over time. The spread of excitability or central sensitization to adjacent neuron populations in the dorsal horn may result in a subjective sensation of spreading or radiating pain and account for referral or spread of pain beyond the original injury.

Neck pain

Patients with whiplash injuries invariably complain of an achy discomfort in the posterior cervical region radiating out over the trapezius muscle and shoulders, down to the interscapular region, up to the occiput, and/or down the arms. This deep aching discomfort is often associated with burning and stiffness, with the latter typically being most apparent in the morning. Tenderness is often present over the posterior spinous prominence of the sixth cervical vertebra and the posterior paracervical musculature. Initially, there is marked restricted range of motion of the cervical spine which may be associated with muscle spasm.

Headaches

Headache is a common symptom following whiplash injury. Within 24 h of the accident, many patients complain of diffuse neck and head pain. The headache may be limited to the occipital area or may spread to the vertex, temporal frontal and retro-orbital areas (Speed, 1987). The pain may be a dull pressure or a squeezing sensation and include pounding and throbbing (migrainous) components (Balla and Moraitis, 1970; Speed, 1987). Muscle contraction and vascular headaches are often present simultaneously (post-traumatic mixed headache). Patients may experience concomitant nausea, vomiting and photophobia. The frequency of these various forms of headache in whiplash is not known. However, the incidence of unspecified headache in a retrospective analysis of 320 cases referred for medicolegal assessment was 55% (Wiley *et al.,* 1986). In our experience, vascular-like headaches are common following whiplash injuries and often occur in individuals with no previous history of migraines. They often respond, albeit incompletely, to pharmacological treatments directed at migrainous symptoms.

Visual disturbances

Whiplash patients may complain of intermittent blurring of vision (Horwich and Kasner, 1962; Macnab, 1971, 1982; LaRocca, 1978). Blurring of vision by itself is not believed to have diagnostic significance unless associated with damage to the cervical sympathetic trunk. Such damage, if severe, may lead to a Horner's syndrome (Macnab, 1971).

Dizziness

Complaints of dizziness or vertigo-like symptoms are common following whiplash injuries (Oosterveld *et al.,* 1991). Many patients complain of suddenly veering to one side or feeling dizzy if they turn the head or change posture quickly. Several theories have been postulated to explain these features, including vertebral artery insufficiency, inner ear damage, injury to the cervical sympathetic chain and an impaired neck-righting reflex (Toglia, 1976; Bogduk, 1986). The reflex or neuromuscular theory proposes that interference with normal signals coming from the upper cervical joints, muscles or nerves to the inner ear produces a feeling of ataxia (Macnab, 1971; DeJong *et al.,* 1977). Posture-related vertigo generally disappears once painless neck range of motion is restored. The entire concept of chronic vertigo arising from the cervical region has been questioned because of the relatively small cervical afferent input to the vestibular nuclei and the capacity of the system for making adjustments (Balch, 1984; Evans, 1992).

Tinnitus

Tinnitus or problems with auditory acuity are frequently reported in association with whiplash injuries (Chrisman and Gervais, 1962; Macnab, 1971;

Lieberman, 1986). Tinnitus may be due to vertebral artery insufficiency, injury to the cervical sympathetic chain or inner ear damage (Medical News, 1965; Bogduk, 1986). Tinnitus alone does not appear to have prognostic significance (Macnab, 1971) although anecdotally we have noted it to be common with more severe injuries. Additional auditory complaints include decreased hearing and loudness recruitment (Gibson, 1974; Lieberman, 1986). Electronystagmographic abnormalities have been reported in a number of whiplash victims in uncontrolled studies (Compere, 1968; Pang, 1971).

Arm pain and thoracic outlet syndrome

Arm pain and paraesthesiae are frequently reported following whiplash injury. Historically, these symptoms were attributed to cervical disc herniation and nerve root compression following whiplash trauma (Gay and Abbott, 1953). However, modern imaging techniques have shown that disc herniations occurring in association with whiplash injuries are distinctly uncommon. Even when present, their significance is uncertain given the significant number of asymptomatic individuals who exhibit disc herniations or foraminal stenosis on MRI (Boden *et al.,* 1990). Arm symptoms also have been attributed to thoracic outlet syndrome (TOS) secondary to intermittent or transient compression of the brachial plexus (Capistrant, 1977). However, objective evidence for TOS as a pathophysiological entity is lacking causing some authors to dispute its existence (Nelson, 1990; Wilbourn, 1990). Attributing symptoms to TOS may lead to surgery to decompress the brachial plexus, which is of dubious efficacy (Cherington *et al.,* 1986).

A frequent extracervical complaint of whiplash victims is numbness or a 'pins and needles' sensation down the arm, most commonly noted along the ulnar aspect of the forearm and hand. Macnab (1971) speculated that these symptoms may be the result of a form of TOS with spasm of the scalene muscles compressing the trunks of the brachial plexus. No data supporting this hypothesis have emerged. Trauma to the zygapophysial or facet joint which may have been fractured or had its capsule injured at the time of the accident has also been suggested as a cause (Bogduk, 1986). This hypothesis proposes that during the acute stage, oedema of this joint, or surrounding haemorrhage, may compromise the adjacent nerve roots posteriorly. In the chronic stage, nerve root fibrosis may ensue from pericapsular exudates. Objective evidence for this proposed pathophysiology is also lacking.

Low back pain

During motor vehicle accidents the lumbar and thoracolumbar spine may be suddenly forced into extension or flexed forwards as the torso moves in an arc over a fixed pelvis. In selected groups of whiplash patients the incidence of low back pain ranges from 25 to 60% (Braaf and Rosner, 1955; Hohl, 1974; Wiley *et al.,* 1986; Hildingsson and Toolanen, 1990). Factors which have been reported to increase the risk of low back pain include side-on collisions, a soft seat back and a lap belt with no shoulder strap (McKenzie and Williams, 1971; Croft and Foreman, 1988). Low back pain usually resolves before the neck symptoms but in some cases may persist indefinitely and in some patients may become the prominent complaint. A particularly confusing group of patients are those with onset of low back pain some time after the initial development of neck pain following motor vehicle accident.

Psychosocial problems

Psychosocial problems frequently develop as a reaction to chronic pain and disability. Depression, anxiety, anger, frustration, preoccupation with somatic complaints, marital stress, financial pressures and difficulty maintaining employment are common.

Pain attributed to a psychological aetiology

Unfortunately, the psychosocial sequelae of chronic pain are often misinterpreted as the cause of pain. This belief has enjoyed significant, albeit declining, popularity and has resulted in patients with chronic pain and disability secondary to whiplash injuries being labelled as hysterical, somatizers, hypochondriacs, psychogenic pain sufferers, and malingerers. Attribution of whiplash symptoms to a psychological aetiology persists for many reasons, including: a high selection bias with the poorest copers over-represented in tertiary specialty clinics; excessively strict adherence to the medical model of disease; a lack of appreciation for psychological sequelae; and frequent involvement with adversarial legal or insurance systems which is not only stressful but tends to encourage more extreme viewpoints among health care professionals. It is of note that the only study to follow prospectively a representative sample of whiplash patients from injury onset did not find that personality (neuroticism) or premorbid psychiatric history predicted non-resolution of symptoms (Radanov *et al.,* 1991). Although we regard whiplash as a physiologically based pain problem, it is inappropriate to disregard the potential impact of psychosocial factors or to forget that we diagnose and treat *people* with whiplash injuries. The constellation and interplay of physical symptoms, disability and emotional concomitants can only be truly understood if one understands the personality, lifestyle and social setting of the individual patient. This is illustrated by one particularly difficult and troubling group of patients, the excessively busy perfectionist with chronic whiplash pain.

The excessively busy perfectionist

The influence of a person's personality or life-coping skills in dealing with the pain and subsequent disability of a whiplash injury cannot be underestimated. In our practice the most common dysfunctional coping style is seen among whiplash patients who premorbidly were excessively busy perfectionists. Research on perfectionism and its significant role in psychological disorders, particularly depression, is relatively new (see Blatt, 1995, for a review). One type of perfectionism, referred to as self-oriented (Hewett and Flett, 1991) is particularly germane. Self-oriented perfectionists have exceedingly high, self-imposed and often unrealistic standards. Premorbidly, this is associated with some very adaptive traits and associated accomplishments. However, there is an underlying self-scrutiny and self-criticism with an attendant inability to accept personal flaws or failures. These individuals are particularly vulnerable to react to experiences of failure with significant levels of depression (Blatt and Zurloff, 1992) and stress (Gruen *et al.*, in press).

Self-oriented perfectionists have an intense need to maintain their excessively high standards which post-injury are no longer realistic given pain-imposed limitations. When the physical limitations imposed by their pain do not allow them to maintain their exceedingly high levels of productivity, they experience considerable distress and try even harder to push themselves despite their pain. Sustained high levels of activity in the face of pain combined with high levels of anxiety further increase their pain, thus requiring sustained periods of rest. However, these periods of rest are viewed as non-productive, leading to more anxiety and compelling the individual to make up for lost time with further overactivity. This continues until pain again becomes overwhelming, requiring the individual to rest. Rest is again viewed as non-productive and again generates anxiety and overactivity. The injured individual cycles between periods of overactivity followed by underactivity with escalating levels of anxiety as overall productivity/activity levels continue to drop. Depression ensues, as self-esteem in these individuals is dependent on their excessively high standards of productivity.

Although the role of emotional distress in exacerbating musculoskeletal pain is controversial, evidence suggests that stress-induced elevations in muscle tension over an extended period of time lead to increased pain in patients with facial, back and head pain. This tension may increase pain through reflex muscle spasm, ischaemia and/or the release of pain-eliciting neurotransmitters (Turk and Flor, 1984).

As well, since the perception of pain represents an interaction of sensory, affective and cognitive processes (Melzack and Wall, 1983), depression and/or anxiety may heighten the affective component of pain perception. Thus increased anxiety, depression, and continuous attempts to 'push through' the pain often result in significant emotional and physical deterioration. The perfectionist patient may become increasingly depressed and irritable as goals are blocked. Emotional distress may lead to interpersonal and occupational difficulties which further increase anxiety. Marital, financial and job security stressors may further compound the problem.

As a consequence of their high internal standards, perfectionists often see themselves as totally disabled. An inability to do their jobs perfectly is viewed as an inability to do their jobs at all. Emotionally, it is more acceptable to be physically disabled by pain than to do a less than perfect job with resultant feelings of inadequacy and self-denigration. A premorbidly successful and seemingly well-adjusted individual suddenly becomes an irritable, argumentative, anxious and depressed individual claiming total disability. A feeling of lack of control eventually leads to a sense of helplessness and defeat.

Third-party payers often inadvertently make the situation worse by withholding or delaying financial compensation, thus contributing to anxiety about meeting financial obligations and increasing feelings of inadequacy, helplessness and victimization. This decision to withhold benefits is often based on the belief that the patient is not disabled and the problem is really psychological or motivational. The perfectionist interprets any suggestion of psychological difficulty as tantamount to being viewed as emotionally inadequate and weak, resulting in a further assault on an already deteriorating self-esteem. Any suggestion that the problem is motivational is viewed with disbelief and outrage, especially in light of previous unsuccessful attempts to maintain premorbid levels of activity and productivity despite increasing pain. Moreover, perfectionists often expect others (including insurance representatives) to conform to the same unrealistically high standards that they expect from themselves. This further fuels their outrage and sense of victimization. The end result is that they vacillate between intense anger at the third-party payer, for withholding benefits and for questioning their adequacy and integrity, and intense anger at themselves for failing to overcome their physical and now mounting emotional difficulties. Self-directed anger is also experienced as very significant depression. In many cases, what appears to be an extreme preoccupation with the unfairness (albeit real) of the system and an inability to 'let go' of their anger is a self-protective mechanism (defence) against underlying intense feelings of inadequacy and worthlessness. This emotional turmoil, in turn, further exacerbates pain and disability.

Natural history and prognosis of whiplash injuries

It is difficult to be definitive regarding the natural history of whiplash as there is a paucity of longitudinal studies in anything but selected populations, e.g. individuals who attend specialists or who seek attention in a local emergency room. However, it appears that in many cases, the natural history of soft-tissue injuries following motor vehicle accidents is for recovery over a limited time period. It is only a minority of patients (fewer than 10%) who go on to develop chronic disabling pain (Nygren, 1984; Pearce, 1989) although, as discussed below, many more patients have persistent symptoms.

Defining recovery can be problematic. As part of the Quebec Task Force study (1995), a cohort of 4757 subjects who submitted claims in 1987 to the Quebec provincial (single-payer) insurance plan were reviewed. A significant number were excluded because of lack of police collision reports (1745) and because of a previous injury in another motor vehicle accident (204). This left 2810 patients. Cumulative recovery rates were 22.1% within 1 week, 53% within 4 weeks, 64% within 60 days, 87% by 6 months and 97% by 1 year. It was not clear whether patients had actually returned to work (or usual activities) or were simply deemed able to do so by the insuring agency. There was no indication whether patients suffered residual pain. It is of note that the percentage of motor vehicle claims paid out for whiplash under the Quebec no-fault system was only a fraction of that paid out by Canadian provinces with a tort system (Quebec Task Force, 1995). Accordingly, the high recovery rates in the Quebec Task Force cohort may simply reflect a higher threshold for allowing continued claims of disability.

Compare this to a study by Gargan and Bannister (1994) who studied 50 consecutive patients with soft-tissue neck injuries attending an emergency room within 5 days of the accident. At 3 months 15 patients were asymptomatic. Of these, 14 (93%) were still asymptomatic at 2 years. Thirty-five patients were symptomatic after 3 months; of these, 30 (86%) remained symptomatic after 2 years. After 1 year, 26 of the 50 (52%) reported they had recovered completely but only 19 (38%) at 2 years.

Radanov *et al.* (1994) studied 117 patients referred by primary care physicians with a diagnosis of whiplash. Patients were referred specifically for the study which limited selection bias. Initial assessment was conducted on an average of 7 days: 51 (44%), 36 (31%) and 28 (24%) of patients were symptomatic at 3, 6 and 12 months respectively. Hildingsson and Toolanen (1990) prospectively studied 93 consecutive cases referred acutely to an orthopaedic department because of a 'noncontact injury to the cervical spine resulting from car accidents'. At follow-up, an average 2 years after the accident, 42% recovered completely, 15% had minor discomfort, and 43% had discomfort sufficient to interfere with their capacity to work.

Bannister and Gargan (1993) reviewed both prospective and retrospective studies and concluded that symptoms present at 12 months post-collision were not likely to resolve further. In the only long-term study of note, Gargan and Bannister (1990) found that patients who were symptomatic at 2 years remained symptomatic 8–12 years later.

Mild traumatic brain injury associated with whiplash: the controversy

The presence of traumatic brain injury in association with whiplash has been postulated based on the observed similarities between the whiplash syndrome and post-concussion syndrome. Alves *et al.* (1986) reported that 6 months after injury the most common complaints following concussion in order of frequency were: headache, memory deficits, dizziness, tinnitus and hearing abnormalities, numbness, weakness, nausea and diplopia. Many of the complaints lasted for over 1 year with the majority of patients exhibiting at least one or two symptoms. In concussion there is evidence for a transitory impairment of information processing (Radanov and Dvorak, 1996). Like post-concussion syndrome patients, many whiplash victims report feeling dazed or in shock immediately post-trauma and whiplash amnesia has appeared in case reports in the neurological literature (Fisher, 1982).

In recent years, a number of researchers have argued that the cognitive difficulties reported by patients with whiplash are the result of a mild traumatic brain injury sustained as a consequence of the violent hyperflexion and hyperextension of the neck (Berstad *et al.*, 1975; Yarnell and Rossie, 1988; Olsnes, 1989; Kischka *et al.*, 1991; Radanov *et al.*, 1992). This has been postulated to occur on vehicular impact because the skull accelerates faster than the brain and subsequently impacts with the brain as it rotates backwards or accelerates forwards. Mild traumatic brain injury has been postulated to occur despite the fact that at the time of the accident patients with whiplash rarely experience loss of consciousness or post-traumatic amnesia, both considered by some authorities to be important diagnostic criteria for mild traumatic brain injury (Levin *et al.*, 1989; Gronwall, 1991; Kay *et al.*, 1992). Although some laboratory studies using non-human primates indicate brain damage can occur in simulated hyperextension–flexion or acceleration injuries without loss of consciousness (Ommaya *et al.,* 1968; Wickstrom *et al.,* 1970; Domer *et al.,* 1979; Liu *et al.,* 1984), the anatomy of non-human primates is markedly different from that of humans. This renders animal data suggestive but in need of confirmatory human research (Shapiro *et al.,* 1993).

A review of human research finds little or no evidence for enduring brain injury after whiplash (Shapiro *et al.,* 1993; Radanov and Dvorak, 1996). There is no conclusive evidence for neuropathological abnormalities after whiplash. A number of studies have reported electroencephalogram (EEG) abnormalities suggestive of brain injury in patients with whiplash; however, the reported incidence of these abnormalities ranges from 4 to 46% (Torres and Shapiro, 1961; Gibbs, 1971; Jacome, 1987). Although all of the EEG studies have methodological problems, the study reporting the highest incidence of EEG abnormalities (46%) is particularly flawed (Torres and Shapiro, 1961). Neuropsychological assessment is thought to be more sensitive for detecting mild brain injury, and a number of studies report poorer performance on neuropsychological measures of concentration and memory in groups of chronic whiplash patients 1 year or more after injury (Yarnell and Rossie, 1988; Olsnes, 1989; Kischka *et al.,* 1991; Radanov *et al.,* 1992). Patients in these studies are usually recruited from specialty clinics and typically represent a select sample with long-standing complaints of disabling pain, emotional distress and cognitive difficulties. These studies have failed to control for the documented effects of pain, medications, depression and anxiety/arousal on cognitive functioning (Shapiro *et al.,* 1993; Radanov and Dvorak, 1996).

The only prospective study to follow an un-selected sample of patients with whiplash found no evidence of cognitive deficit 6 months after injury (Radanov *et al.,* 1993). It is of note that the literature on mild traumatic brain injury suggests that difficulties in cognitive functioning as assessed by neuropsychological testing normalize by 3 months after injury (Gentilini *et al.,* 1985; Huggenholtz *et al.,* 1988; Gronwall, 1989; Ruff *et al.,* 1989). Given this literature on recovery of function in mild traumatic brain injury and research documenting the deleterious effect of pain and emotional distress on cognitive functioning (Stromgren, 1977; Weingartner and Siberman, 1982; Coyne and Gotlib, 1983; O'Hara *et al.,* 1986; Jamison *et al.,* 1988; Kewman *et al.,* 1991) one need not postulate a traumatic brain injury to account for *persisting* cognitive problems in samples of chronic whiplash patients (Shapiro *et al.,* 1993). The two prospective studies to assess neuropsychological functioning within a week of injury have failed to use adequate control groups (Ettlin *et al.,* 1992; Radanov *et al.,* 1993). Accordingly, a definite conclusion regarding *acute* cognitive deficits related to

mild traumatic brain injury awaits a prospective study that adequately controls for pain and emotional functioning.

Medical management of whiplash injuries

A wide variety of interventions are available to treat patients with whiplash injuries (Table 5.3). Unfortunately, there is a paucity of adequate clinical trials, and reports of efficacy remain largely anecdotal. *No treatment consistently cures the pain of whiplash injuries.* Treatment programmes should attempt to balance *pain control* with *increased function*, although in recent years there has been a trend towards focusing primarily on the latter. The concept that some injuries resulting in pain may be inaccessible to physical and pharmacological treatments is a difficult one for many patients (and some clinicians) to grasp and accept. Since there is a lack of good clinical trials the discussion that follows is based largely on our own anecdotal experience. Table 5.3 divides available treatments into those which first, are

Table 5.3 *Medical management of whiplash*

Treatments of obvious benefit
Education
Exercise-oriented physiotherapy
(stretching and aerobic exercises)

Treatments which decrease pain
Cervical collar
Physical modalities (e.g. local heat, ice, ultrasound, interferential current)
Analgesics, muscle relaxants, antidepressants, TENS
Manipulation
Cervical traction
Massage therapy
Relaxation therapy
Trigger point injections
Acupuncture

Treatments which improve coping skills
Psychological counselling
Vocational counselling

Treatments of dubious value
Occipital nerve blocks
Non-steroidal anti-inflammatory drugs
Intra-articular (facet joint) corticosteroid injections
Discectomy/surgical fusion
Magnetic necklace

Potential treatments that show some promise
Selective muscle retraining
Percutaneous facet joint denervation
Functional restoration programmes

TENS = Transcutaneous electrical nerve stimulation.

agreed to be of benefit; second, serve to decrease pain; third, improve coping skills; fourth, are of dubious value, and fifth, show potential promise.

Treatments generally agreed to be of benefit

Education

Education of the patient (and family) is a critical element of any treatment programme. Patients must clearly understand the goals of treatment – return of function, control of pain – and the likely prognosis. Education helps patients plan realistically for their future, provides them with a sense of control, and increases their confidence in the treating clinician. Patients must understand that 'hurt is not equal to harm'. Many patients excessively limit activities and movement of their neck in a logical attempt to avoid pain and by inference tissue damage. This may result in general deconditioning and constriction of neck muscles. McKinney *et al.* (1989) found that advice to mobilize, exercise, limit activity to pain tolerance and avoid dependence on collars and analgesics was as effective as a physiotherapy-directed programme. Information and advice regarding activities that aggravate pain (heavy lifting or maintaining prolonged postures) help prevent significant exacerbations of pain. For chronic whiplash patients, an emphasis on proper pacing of activities is helpful – often critical.

Exercise-oriented physiotherapy

Early mobilization of the neck which is gentle and graduated is thought to promote maximal healing of damaged soft tissues. Patients are then enrolled in a programme of stretching and aerobic exercise. Stretching of muscles and ligaments to their normal length has long been thought to maximize functioning. Strengthening exercises are controversial and often aggravate pain, particularly if introduced too early or too aggressively. Isometric strengthening exercises may be tolerated better. Theoretically, strong neck musculature is desirable to provide an active physiological splint which can potentially reduce pain. Formal exercise programmes should be time-limited with a shift over time to a home exercise programme. Exercise-oriented treatments were divided by the Quebec Task Force (1995) into mobilization and exercise. Regarding *mobilization* they noted: 'The cumulative evidence suggests that mobilization techniques can be used as an adjunct to strategies that promote activation. In combination with activating interventions, they appear to be beneficial in the short term but the long term benefit has not been established'. Regarding *exercise* they noted: 'The cumulative evidence suggests that active exercise as part of a multimodal intervention may be

beneficial in the short and long term. This suggestion should be confirmed in future studies'.

Two studies are of note. McKinney *et al.* (1989) reported that patients receiving 2 weeks of physiotherapy which combined McKenzie and Maitland mobilization techniques demonstrated greater improvement/recovery 1 week after treatment than patients prescribed rest and soft collars. However, there was no difference between the two groups at 2-year follow-up. Moreover, a third group simply given advice on early activation and a home programme of exercises did better than either group. Mealy *et al.* (1986) reported that patients receiving Maitland mobilization techniques had more short-term relief of pain and range of motion than patients prescribed rest and a soft cervical collar.

Treatments which serve primarily to decrease pain

These treatments, which are listed in Table 5.3, are the most commonly used treatments in the management of whiplash injuries. They provide subsets of patients with consistent relief of pain. Unfortunately, it is impossible to predict in advance whether a particular treatment will relieve pain for a given patient. As well, the benefits of these treatments are invariably short-lived. Patients often regard these treatments as their only consistent source of pain relief and many believe these treatments improve their quality of life, albeit for a short time. In contrast, third-party payers often view them as expensive, passive, and without proven long-term utility. Accordingly, they are reluctant to fund them. This raises the question as to how long one should fund measures that temporarily reduce pain with no evidence of prolonged efficacy. It is of note that some of these treatments are more readily funded (e.g. medications) than others. Passive treatments such as physical modalities, massage, manipulation and even medications, if not performed within the framework of an active rehabilitation programme may potentially result in greater dependence on the part of patients and discourage them from taking more active responsibility for their own rehabilitation.

Cervical collar

Initial use of a cervical collar still enjoys popularity, although its use appears to be declining. Research has failed to demonstrate its efficacy. A controlled, double-blind study demonstrated that patients mobilized early without a collar experienced a greater reduction of pain and improved cervical range of motion (Mealy *et al.*, 1986) relative to rest and use of a collar. This result was confirmed by McKinney (1989). However, another prospective study failed to demonstrate differences between early active treatment with traction and physiotherapy compared with rest in a collar and unsupervised mobilization (Pennie and Agambar, 1991). A soft cervical collar does not truly immobilize the neck (Colachis *et al.,* 1973; Fisher *et al.,* 1977; Johnson *et al.,* 1977). If a cervical collar is prescribed, continuous use for more than 2 weeks should be discouraged (Teasell and Shapiro, 1993). According to Lieberman (1986), *prolonged collar use* leads to a variety of complications including disuse atrophy of the neck muscles, soft-tissue contractures, shortening of muscles, thickening of subcapsular tissues, increased dependence and enhancement of feelings of disability. Although chronic collar use runs the risk of iatrogenic complications, anecdotally we have observed that whiplash patients frequently find that cervical collars help control pain when used judiciously for limited periods of time.

Physical modalities

Ice packs may be helpful in the early acute phase of whiplash (3-10 days after the accident) to limit muscle swelling. After the acute phase, local hot packs, ultrasound and interferential current or transcutaneous electrical nerve stimulation (TENS) may serve to reduce pain temporarily. Recent research on TENS in low back pain showed it to be no better than placebo; nevertheless it may assist specific subsets of patients (Deyo *et al.,* 1990). In patients who benefit initially from TENS, the positive effect generally decreases over time.

Moist heat tends to be more effective than dry heat. Many patients find it useful to apply ice for 3–5 min before stretching the involved regional muscles. There is some limited evidence that pulse electromagnetic treatment may be useful in the early stages of whiplash (Foley-Nolan *et al.,* 1992). The use of physical modalities serves primarily as an adjunct to therapeutic exercise and should not take the place of an active exercise programme (Teasell and Shapiro, 1993).

Medications

Drugs have a limited role in the management of whiplash injuries, despite their widespread use. They have significant potential for misuse and adverse side-effects. Medications are frequently overused in chronic whiplash injuries because the treating physician is uncertain how else to ease the pain and emotional distress of the suffering patient. *Analgesic medications* have their greatest application in the acute stage. Non-steroidal anti-inflammatory drugs (NSAIDs) are more likely of benefit due to their analgesic properties than their anti-inflammatory properties. Long-term usage carries with it a substantial risk of stomach ulceration. Muscle relaxants appear to work primarily through their anxiolytic effect and have not been adequately studied (Quebec Task Force, 1995). Narcotic analgesics must be carefully monitored and their use limited because of the risk of tolerance and addiction; the issue of narcotic use in chronic pain is not fully resolved (Brena and Sanders, 1991). Long-term narcotic use has traditionally been discouraged (Lieberman, 1986) and in our opinion patients are better served by avoiding them. Moulin *et al.* (1996), in a randomized controlled trial, found that although morphine reduced pain in chronic pain sufferers, many of whom had suffered whiplash injuries, there was no corresponding improvement in function. Anecdotally we suspect many patients take strong narcotic medications more for their mood-enhancing properties.

Tricyclic antidepressants (TCAs), either administered in small doses before bedtime or in full antidepressant doses, are often helpful in chronic pain patients, especially those with a non-restorative sleep pattern (Butler, 1984; Ward, 1986). TCAs have been shown to have an analgesic effect in animal studies (Spiegel *et al.,* 1983). TCAs' mechanism of action is not clear but may be related to their ability to block the reuptake of serotonin, thereby enhancing endogenous pathways of pain control, improving non-restorative sleep patterns and/or treating co-occurring depression. The major side-effects of TCAs are dry mouth, morning drowsiness and weight gain. Despite the fact that TCAs are regarded as the best medication for chronic pain, most patients experience significant side-effects which they find intolerable.

Manipulation

There is no definitive research on the efficacy of cervical manipulation in whiplash patients (Quebec Task Force, 1995). Anecdotal experience and one published study (Cassidy *et al.,* 1992) suggest it offers short-term relief of symptoms in chronic whiplash patients. Physicians are concerned most about the high-velocity/low-amplitude thrust manoeuvre and the rare but serious complication of vertebral artery dissection (Teasell and Marchuk, 1994).

Cervical traction

Although this treatment has been advocated for cervical whiplash injuries (Macnab, 1971; Jackson, 1978), there is no evidence it is of benefit in whiplash injuries. The only controlled trial failed to demonstrate any effect (Zylbergold and Piper, 1985). In our experience, mechanical cervical traction often aggravates symptoms. In the initial stage, traction is contraindicated because the distractive forces may increase pain and further damage healing tissue (Weinberger, 1976).

Massage

Massage therapy is a time-honoured treatment for musculoskeletal problems, in particular myofascial pain and muscle tension. There is no evidence that it produces long-lasting benefits and controlled trials are lacking. Massage can play a role in keeping the patient functional by providing temporary relief of pain. Anecdotally, benefits have been observed in some whiplash patients who are in situations in which muscle tension and pain gradually build up (i.e. an office worker or a student studying for an exam) because it promotes muscle relaxation and a decrease in pain. Massage therapy must be gentle because aggressive or deep friction massage is often poorly tolerated, resulting in increased pain.

Trigger point injections

Tender points within cervical and upper thoracic muscles can produce an abrupt onset of pain from the point of palpation with distal referral of pain in a characteristic pattern (Travell and Simons, 1983). Injection of local anaesthetics and corticosteroids is a popular, albeit unproven, treatment. It is not clear that anaesthetics are essential to the therapeutic effect since injections of sterile water, normal saline or dry needling into trigger points may also produce a therapeutic response. A recent study found that subcutaneous injections of sterile water were more effective than injections of normal saline in patients with chronic neck and shoulder pain from whiplash injury (Byrn *et al.,* 1991, 1993).

Treatments which improve coping skills

The Quebec Task Force (1995) found no quality research regarding psychosocial interventions in the treatment of whiplash injuries. Although this is surprising given the importance of psychosocial issues, it may reflect excessive reliance on the acute medical model on the part of both treating clinicians and whiplash patients. These treatments are usually employed to help patients cope better or move on with their lives in the face of chronic pain. They don't necessarily reduce pain *per se* although, in some cases, they can significantly decrease emotional distress and improve the patient's overall level of functioning. There may be greater acceptance on the part of third-party payers for these treatments because they offer some opportunity for long-term benefit. The need for these treatments varies widely among patients and does not necessarily correlate with the severity of injury.

Treatments of dubious value

Occipital nerve blocks have not been shown in any controlled study to be effective in treating whiplash injuries. *Cervical facet joint corticosteroid blocks* have recently been subjected to a randomized controlled double-blind study which failed to demonstrate effectiveness in whiplash patients with pain of greater than 3 months' duration. In this study, the level of facet joint pathology was identified using cervical facet joint diagnostic blocks (Barnsley *et al.,* 1994). Hamer *et al.* (1992) used *discectomy/fusion* in 0.5% of cases and found significant relief of pain in only 10% of those operated on. This lack of efficacy is consistent with our experience. The Quebec Task Force (1995) found no acceptable studies on surgical interventions in whiplash injuries. *Cervical epidural injections* have been reported to be beneficial in uncontrolled trials. Theoretically they should not be helpful because the damaged tissues are presumably outside the epidural space. The *magnetic necklace* is mentioned by the Quebec Task Force (1995) because of its widespread use among lay people. A controlled trial using active and sham treatment in chronic neck pain patients failed to demonstrate any benefit (Hong *et al.,* 1982).

Unproven treatments that show some promise

Selective muscle retraining

Some recent work with selective muscle retraining suggests that this form of treatment may offer benefits (Donaldson, 1995). Selective muscle retraining uses surface electromyogram to identify muscles which are not functioning properly, either because they are underactive when they should contract or overactive when they should relax. This technique not only provides objective evidence of muscle dysfunction but also has been reported to treat many patients successfully. The muscles that appear underactive are selectively exercised to achieve more symmetrical or appropriate muscle functioning.

Percutaneous facet joint denervation

These procedures have been reported to offer benefit to a subset of patients in uncontrolled studies. Hildebrandt and Argyrakis (1986) reported on 35 patients presenting with headache, neck, shoulder and arm pain who underwent zygapophysial joint or dorsal rami diagnostic blocks. The involved joints were then partially denervated using radiofrequency electrocoagulation. Thirteen of 35 patients reported significant relief, 10 some improvement, and 12 no benefit. Verkest and Stolker (1991) performed facet joint denervation procedures on 53 patients with cervical facet joint pain. They reported that over 80% received long-lasting improvement in this uncontrolled study.

Lord *et al.* (1996), using radiofrequency neuroanatomy of the dorsal cervical rami achieved virtually complete relief of chronic whiplash pain in patients with a medium pain duration of 34 months. In this randomized double-blind clinical trial, 7 of 12 patients receiving the active treatment obtained pain relief in excess of 6 months. Only 1 of 12 patients in the sham surgical placebal control was pain free. This treatment requires further evaluation but is very promising.

Functional restoration programmes

Functional restoration programmes (FRPs) have become very popular because of the limitations of current treatment programmes and the frequently observed discordance between pain, impairment and disability (Gatchel, 1994). Gatchel has noted that the hypothetical constructs of impairment, pain and disability defy objective outcome measurement and reliable assessment. In contrast, function can be observed and objectively measured, which allows rehabilitation treatment programmes to avoid reliance on subjective (and supposedly less reliable) self-reports of pain and disability (Gatchel, 1994). FRPs combine aggressive exercise regimens, discourage pain behaviours and attempt to address psychosocial issues. FRPs have arisen as a natural evolution of behavioural theories of pain (Fordyce, 1976, Fordyce *et al.*, 1985). Most FRPs provide a multidisciplinary approach designed to improve factors contributing to disability apart from the pain itself. FRPs have been described as a tertiary, medically directed, inter-disciplinary amalgam of a sports medicine approach to restoring physical capacity and a cognitive crisis intervention technique for disability management (Gatchel *et al.*, 1992). Unfortunately, there is a paucity of properly controlled evidence that FRPs actually work for chronic low back pain (Teasell and Harth, in press) and there are no published studies specific to whiplash. FRPs offer a promising approach but must be considered unproven until adequate controlled trials with whiplash patient support the uncontrolled low back pain studies currently available.

The medical dilemma: maximizing function vs relieving pain

For clinicians the goal of relieving pain (and suffering) often clashes with the goal of maximizing function. For example, maximizing function inevitably results in increased pain. The concept that increasing a patient's level of function reduces his or her overall level of suffering and, in some cases pain, has resulted in a proliferation of FRPs. While some patients may do well in functional restoration, for others increasing physical activities inevitably results in a significant increase in pain. Even those who benefit are left with significant limitations.

Treatment geared only towards pain control at the expense of maximizing function is inappropriate. Currently the focus of rehabilitation management has been and should remain increasing function. Some clinicians have argued that improved function should be the only goal (Clifford, 1993), if not the driving factor (Gatchel, 1994). While the term benign chronic pain is used to encourage patients to remain active despite the pain, one must be careful not to forget the often destructive effects of pain on a patient's life. Most clinicians take a middle road, encouraging increased function while providing restrictions to prevent significant exacerbations of pain. The validity of these restrictions has not been well-established for whiplash patients as a whole and is difficult to establish for any given individual. King *et al.* (1994) questioned the need for any restrictions in chronic pain. Balancing pain control and increased function (or decreased disability) has always been a major area of controversy in the management of these patients and will probably remain so for some time.

Future directions

Medicine is being paradoxically driven in two opposite directions which will direct the future of treatment of whiplash patients. The first trend is a natural progression of the science of medicine with its reliance on technology and the need to prove the efficacy of treatment utilizing randomized controlled clinical trials. This scientific emphasis not only removes the external biases of the treatment–patient interaction but is in keeping with the fiscal concerns of hard-pressed insuring or funding agencies. The second trend is patient-focused care, the so-called art of medicine which focuses on the person and not simply the injury. Such an approach deals with the physical, psychological, social and spiritual aspects, and sees the person as greater than the sum of his or her parts. This approach is also better equipped to deal with the many complicating factors including the patient's coping abilities and belief systems, family influences, work and employer-related issues, and the importance of litigation and compensation (Shapiro and Roth, 1993). As we begin to appreciate more the role of these factors and particularly the individual's coping strategies, such an approach is taking on a greater role. The challenge of the 21st century will be to integrate the science and art of medicine to treat whiplash patients successfully.

Summary

Patients with chronic whiplash injuries are difficult to treat. It is important to recognize that the natural history of acute whiplash is such that many patients will improve or recover relatively quickly. Supportive education and a progressive programme of exercises, involving stretching of the involved region as well as an aerobic exercise programme, are regarded as the mainstays of medical management. Other physical treatments (physical modalities, manipulation, TENS) and pharmacological treatments provide short-term pain reduction at best and should not be used in isolation. Injections and surgical interventions are rarely useful in uncomplicated whiplash. Psychosocial interventions, including vocational counselling, are becoming more popular as we recognize the importance of treating the person with a whiplash injury and not just the injury itself. However, psychosocial interventions remain unproven. New techniques such as selective muscle retraining or functional restoration programmes offer potentially new but unproven treatment approaches for subsets of patients. At present, the Quebec Task Force (1995), despite its self-acknowledged limitations and partisan funding, offers the best scientific guidelines for treating these patients. The challenge of treatment is to integrate the art and science of medicine efficiently and effectively to increase function and reduce pain and suffering.

References

Alves, W.M., Colohan, A.R.T., O'Leary, T.J., Rimel, R.W., Jane, J.A. (1986) Understanding post-traumatic symptoms after minor head injury. *J. Head Trauma Rehabil.* **1**: 1–12.

Balch, R.W. (1984) *Dizziness, Hearing Loss and Tinnitus, the Essentials of Neurology.* Philadelphia, PA: F.A. Davis, p. 152, discussed in Evans (1992).

Balla, J.I. (1980) The late whiplash syndrome. *Aust. N.Z. J. Surg.* **50**: 610–614.

Balla, J.I., Moraitis, S. (1970) Knights in armour. A follow-up study of injuries after legal settlement. *Med. J. Aust.* **2**: 355–361.

Bannister, G., Gargan, M. (1993) Prognosis of whiplash injuries: a review of the literature. In: *Spine: State of the Art Reviews. Cervical Flexion-Extension/Whiplash Injuries,* vol. 7, (Teasell, R.W., Shapiro, A.P. eds). Philadelphia: Hanley & Belfus, pp. 557–570.

Barnsley, L., Lord, S., Bogduk, N. (1993a) The pathophysiology of whiplash. In: *Spine: State of the Art Reviews Cervical Flexion - Extension/Whiplash Injuries,* vol. 7, (Teasell, R.W., Shapiro, A.P. eds). Philadelphia: Hanley & Belfus, pp. 329–353.

Barnsley, L., Lord, S., Bogduk, N. (1993b) Comparative anaesthetic blocks in the diagnosis of cervical zygapophysial joint pain. *Pain* **55**: 99–106.

Barnsley, L., Lord, S.M., Wallis, B.J., Bogduk, N. (1994) Lack of effect of intra-articular corticosteroids for chronic cervical zygapophysial joint pain. *N. Engl. J. Med.* **330**: 1047–1050.

Barnsley, L., Lord, S.M., Wallis, B.J., Bogduk, N. (1995) The prevalence of chronic cervical zygapophysial joint pain after whiplash. *Spine* **20**: 20–25.

Berstad, J.R., Baerum, B., Lochen, E.A., Mogstad, T.E., Sjaasta, O. (1975) Whiplash: chronic organic brain syndrome without hydrocephalus *ex vacuo. Acta Neurol. Scand.* **51**: 268–284.

Blatt, S. (1995) The destructiveness of perfectionism. *Am. Psychol.* **50**: 1003–1020.

Blatt, S.J., Zurloff, D.C. (1992) Interpersonal relatedness and self-definition: two prototypes for depression. *Clin. Psychol. Rev.* **12**: 527–562.

Boden, S.D., McCowin, P.R., Davis, D.O., Dina, T.S., Mark, A.S., Wiesel, S. (1990) Abnormal magnetic resonance scans of the cervical spine in asymptomatic subjects. *J. Bone Joint Surg. (Am.)* **72**: 1178–1184.

Bogduk, N. (1986) The anatomy and pathophysiology of whiplash. *Clin. Biomech.* **1**: 92–101.

Borden, A.G.B., Rechtman, A.M., Gershom-Cohen, J. (1960) The normal cervical lordosis. *Radiology* **74**: 806.

Braaf, M.M., Rosner, S. (1955) Symptomatology and treatment of injuries of the neck. *N.Y. J. Med.* **55**: 237.

Brena, S.F., Sanders, S.H. (1991) Opioids in nonmalignant pain: questions in search of answers. *Clin. J. Pain* **7**: 342–345.

Butler, S. (1984) Present status of tricyclic antidepressants in chronic pain therapy. In: *Advances in Pain Research and Therapy,* vol. 7 (Benedette C. *et al.* eds). New York: Raven Press, pp. 173–197.

Byrn, C., Borenstein, P., Linder, L.E. (1991) Treatment of neck and shoulder pain in whiplash syndrome patients with intracutaneous sterile water injections. *Acta Anesthesiol. Scand.* **35**: 52–53.

Byrn, C., Olsson, I., Falkheden, L. *et al.* (1993) Subcutaneous sterile water injection for chronic neck and shoulder pain following whiplash injuries. *Lancet* **341**: 449–452.

Capistrant, T.D. (1977) Thoracic outlet syndrome in whiplash injury. *Ann. Surg.* **185**: 175–178.

Cassell, E.J. (1991) *The Nature of Suffering and the Goals of Medicine.* New York: Oxford University Press.

Cassidy, J.D., Lopes, A.A., Yong-Hing, K. (1992) The immediate effect of manipulation versus mobilization on pain and range of motion in the cervical spine: a randomized controlled trial. *J. Manipul. Physiol Ther.* **15**: 570–575.

Cherington, M., Happer, I., Marchanic, B., Parry, L. (1986) Surgery for thoracic outlet syndrome may be hazardous to your health. *Muscle Nerve* **9**: 632–634.

Chrisman, O.D., Gervais, R.F. (1962) Otologic manifestations of the cervical syndrome. *Clin. Orthop.* **24**: 34–39.

Clemens, H.J., Burrow, K. (1972) Experimental investigation on injury mechanisms of cervical spine at frontal and rear-front vehicle impacts. Proceedings of the Sixteenth Stapp Car Crash Conference, pp. 76–104.

Clifford, J.C. (1993) Successful management of chronic pain syndrome. *Can. Fam. Phys.* **39**: 549–559.

Colachis, S.C., Strohm, B.R., Ganter, E.L. (1973) Cervical spine motion in normal women: radiographic study of effect of cervical collar. *Arch. Phys. Med. Rehabil.* **54**: 161–169.

Commack, K.V. (1957) Whiplash injuries to the neck. *Am. J. Surg.* **93**: 663–666.

Compere, W.E. (1968) Electronystagmographic finding in patients with 'whiplash' injuries. *Laryngoscope* **78**: 1226-1232.

Coyne, J.C., Gotlib, I.H. (1983) The role of cognition in depression: a critical appraisal. *Psychol. Bull.* **39**: 593-597.

Croft, A.C. (1988) Biomechanics. In: *Whiplash Injuries. The Cervical Acceleration Deceleration Syndrome* (Foreman, S.M., Croft, A.C., eds). Baltimore: Williams & Wilkins, p. 1072.

Croft, A.C., Foreman, S.M. (1988) Cited by Croft, A.C. Soft tissue injury: long-term and short-term effects. In: *Whiplash Injuries. The Cervical Acceleration Deceleration Syndrome,* (Foreman, S.M., Croft, A.C., eds). Baltimore: Williams & Wilkins, p. 293.

Deans, G.T. (1986) Incidence and duration of neck pain among patients injured in car accidents. *Br. Med. J.* **292**: 94-95.

Deans, G.T., McGailliard, J.N., Kerr, M., Rutherford, W.H. (1987) Neck pain - a major cause of disability following car accidents. *Injury* **18**: 10-12.

DeJong, P.T.V.M., DeJong, J.M.B.V., Cohen, B., Jongkees, L.B.W. (1977) Ataxia and nystagmus induced by injection of local anaesthetics in the neck. *Ann. Neurol.* **1**: 240-246.

Deyo, R.A., Walsh, N.E., Martin, D.C., Schoenfeld, L.S., Ramamurthy, S. (1990) A controlled trial of transcutaneous electrical nerve stimulation (TENS) and exercise for chronic low back pain. *N. Engl. J. Med.* **322**: 1627-1634.

Domer, F.R., Lin, Y.K., Chandran, K.B., Krieger, K.W. (1979) Effect of hyperextension-hyperflexion (whiplash) on the function of the blood-brain barrier of rhesus monkeys. *Exp. Neurol.* **63**: 304-310.

Donaldson, S. (1995) Testing for the existence of muscular injury in MVA victims using surface electromyography. *Med. Scope Monthly* Sept 1-13.

Dunsker, S.B. (1982) Hyperextension and hyperflexion injuries of the cervical spine. In: *Neurological Surgery,* 2nd edn (Youmans, J.R., ed.). Philadelphia, PA: WB Saunders, pp. 2332-2343.

Engel, G. (1977) The need for a new medical model: a challenge for biomedicine. *Science* **196**: 129-136.

Ettlin, T.M., Kischka, U., Reichman, S. *et al.* (1992) Cerebral symptoms after whiplash injury of the neck: a prospective clinical and neuropsychological study of whiplash injury. *Neurol. Neurosurg. Psychiatry* **55**: 943-948.

Evans, R.W. (1992) Some observations on whiplash injuries. In: *The Neurology of Trauma,* (Evans, R.W. ed.). Neurologic Clinics 10(4). Philadelphia: WB Saunders, pp. 975-995.

Feinstein, B. (1977) Referred pain from paravertebral structures. In: *Approaches to the Validation of Manipulation Therapy* (Buerger, A.A., Tobis, J.S., eds). Springfield, IL: Charles C Thomas, pp. 139-174.

Feinstein, B., Langton, J.N.K., Jameson, R.M., Schiller, F. (1954) Experiments of pain referred from deep somatic tissues. *J. Bone Joint Surg. (Am.)* **36**: 981-997.

Fisher, S.V., Bowar, J.F., Awad, E.A., Gullickson, G. (1977) Cervical orthoses effect on cervical spine motion: roentgenographic and gonometric method of study. *Arch. Phys. Med. Rehabil.* **58**: 109-115.

Fisher, C.M. (1982) Whiplash amnesia. *Neurology (NY)* **32**: 667-668.

Foley-Nolan, D., Moore, K., Codd, M., Barry, C., O'Connor, P., Coughlan, R.J. (1992) Low energy high frequency pulsed electromagnetic therapy for acute whiplash injuries. A double blind randomized controlled study. *Scand. J. Rehabil. Med.* **24**: 51-59.

Fordyce, W.E. (1976) *Behavioral Methods for Chronic Pain and Illness.* St Louis, MO: C.V. Mosby.

Fordyce, W.E., Roberts, A.H., Sternbach, R.A. (1985) The behavioural management of chronic pain: a response to critics. *Pain* **22**: 113-125.

Frankel, V.H. (1976) Pathomechanics of whiplash injuries to the neck. In: *Current Controversies in Neurosurgery* (Morley, T.P., ed.). Philadelphia: WB Saunders, pp. 39-50.

Fricton, J.R. (1993) Myofascial pain and whiplash. In: *Spine: State of the Art Reviews. Cervical Flexion-Extension/Whiplash Injuries,* vol. 7 (Teasell, R.W., Shapiro, A.P. eds). Philadelphia: Hanley & Belfus, pp. 403-422.

Gargan, M.F., Bannister, G.C. (1990) Long term prognosis of soft tissue injuries of the neck. *J. Bone Joint Surg.* **72B**: 901-903.

Gargan, M.F., Bannister, G.C. (1994) The rate of recovery following whiplash injury. *Eur. Spin. J.* **3**: 162-164.

Gatchel, R.J., Mayer, T.G., Hazard, R.G., Rainville, J., Mooney, V. (1992) Editorial: Functional restoration. Pitfalls in evaluating efficacy. *Spine* **17**: 988-995.

Gatchel, R.J. (1994) Occupational low back pain disability. Why function needs to 'drive' the rehabilitation process. *Am. Pain Soc. J.* **3**: 107-110.

Gay, J.R., Abbott, K.H. (1953) Common whiplash injuries of the neck. *J.A.M.A.* **152**: 1698-1704.

Gentilini, M., Nichelli, P., Schoenhuber, R. *et al.* (1985) Neuropsychological evaluation of minor head injury. *J. Neurol. Psychiatry* **48**: 137-140.

Gibbs, F.A. (1971) Objective evidence of brain disorder in cases of whiplash injury. *Clin. Electroencephalogr.* **2**: 107-110.

Gibson, J.W. (1974) Cervical syndromes: use of comfortable cervical collar as an adjunct in their management. *South. Med. J.* **67**: 205-208.

Giroux, M. (1991) Les blessures 'a la colonne cervicale; importance du problème. *Medicin Quebec* Sept 22-26.

Gronwall, D. (1989) Cumulative and persisting effects of concussion on attention and cognition. In: *Mild Head Injury* (Levin, H.S., Eisenberg, H.M., Benton, A.L., eds). New York: Oxford University Press.

Gronwall, D. (1991) Minor head injury. *Neuropsychology* **5**: 253-266.

Gruen, R.J., Silva, R., Ehrlich, J., Schweitzer, J.W., Friedhoff, A.J. (1997) Vulnerability to stress: self-criticism and stress-induced changes in biochemistry. *J Personal* **65**: 33-49.

Hamer, A.J., Prasad, R., Gargan, M.F. *et al.* (1992) Whiplash injury and cervical disc surgery. Presented at the British Cervical Spine Society Meeting. Bowness-on-Windermere, Nov 7, 1992 (cited by Bannister and Gargan, 1993).

Hewett, P.L., Flett, G.L. (1991) Perfectionism in the self and social contexts: conceptualization, assessment, and association with psychopathology. *J. Personal. Soc. Psych.* **60**: 456-470.

Hildebrandt, J., Argyrakis, A. (1986) Percutaneous nerve block of the cervical facets - a relatively new method in the treatment of chronic headache and neck pain. *Man. Med.* **2**: 48-52.

Hildingsson, C., Toolanen, G. (1990) Outcome after soft tissue injury of the cervical spine. *Acta Orthop. Scand.* **61**: 357-359.

Hohl, M. (1974) Soft tissue injuries of the neck in automobile accidents: factors influencing prognosis. *J. Bone Joint Surg.* **56A**: 1675–1682.

Hohl, M. (1975) Soft tissue injuries of the neck. *Clin. Orthop.* **109**: 42–49.

Hohl, M. (1989) Soft tissue neck injuries. In: *The Cervical Spine*, 2nd edn, The Cervical Spine Research Society Editorial Committee (eds). Philadelphia, PA: J.B. Lippincott, pp. 436–441.

Hong, C.Z., Lin, J.C., Bender, L.F., Schaeffer, J.N., Meltzer, R.J., Causin, P. (1982) Magnetic necklace: its therapeutic effectiveness on neck and shoulder pain. *Arch. Phys. Med. Rehabil.* **63**: 462–466.

Horwich, H., Kasner, D. (1962) The effect of whiplash injuries on occular functions. *South. Med. J.* **55**: 69–71.

Huggenholtz, H., Stuss, D.T., Stethem, L.L., Richard, M.T. (1988) How long does it take to recover from a mild concussion? *J. Neurosurg.* **22**: 853–858.

Inman, V.H., Saunders, J.B.deC.M. (1944) Referred pain from skeletal structures. *J. Nerv. Ment. Dis.* **99**: 660–667.

Jackson, R. (1978) *The Cervical Syndrome*, 4th edn. Springfield, IL: Charles C. Thomas.

Jacome, D.E. (1987) EEG in whiplash: a reappraisal. *Clin. Electroencephogr.* **18**: 41–45.

Jamison, R.N., Brocco, T.S., Parris, W.C. (1988) The influence of problems with concentration and memory on emotional distress and daily activities in chronic pain patients. *Int. J. Psychiatry Med.* **18**: 183–191.

Jeffreys, E. (1980) *Disorders of the Cervical Spine*. London: Butterworths.

Johnson, R.M., Hart, D.L., Simmons, E.F., Ramsby, G.R., Southwick, W.O. (1977) Cervical orthoses – a study comparing their effectiveness in restricting cervical motion in normal subjects. *J. Bone Joint Surg. (Am.)* **59**: 332–339.

Kay, T., Newman, B., Cavallo, M. *et al.* (1992) Towards a neuropsychological model of functional disability after mild traumatic brain injury. *Neuropsychology* **6**: 371–384.

Kewman, D.G., Vaishampayan, N., Zald, D., Han, B. (1991) Cognitive impairment in musculoskeletal pain patients. *Int. J. Psychiatry Med.* **21**: 253–262.

King, J.C., Kelleher, W.J., Stedwill, J.E., Talcott, G. (1994) Physical limitations are not required for chronic pain rehabilitation success. *Am. J. Phys. Med. Rehabil.* **73**: 331–337.

Kischka, U., Ettlin, T.H., Heim, S., Schmid, G. (1991) Cerebral symptoms following whiplash injury. *Eur. Neurol.* **31**: 136–140.

LaRocca, H. (1978) Acceleration injuries of the neck. *Clin. Neurosurg.* **25**: 205–217.

Levin, H.S., Eisenberg, H.M., Benton, A.L. (1989) (eds) *Mild Head Injury*. New York: Oxford University Press.

Lieberman, J.S. (1986) Cervical soft tissue injuries and cervical disc disease. In: *Principles of Physical Medicine and Rehabilitation in the Musculoskeletal Diseases* (Leek, J.C. *et al.*, eds) New York: Grune & Stratton, pp. 263–286.

Liu, K., Chandran, K.B., Heath, R.G. *et al.* (1984) Subcortical EEG changes in rhesus monkeys following experimental hyperextension–hyperflexion (whiplash). *Spine* **9**: 329–338.

Lord, S., Barnsley, L., Bogduk, N. (1993) Cervical zygapophyseal joint pain in whiplash. In: *Spine: State of the Art Reviews*, vol. 7 (Teasell, R.W., Shapiro, A.P., eds). Philadelphia: Hanley & Belfus, pp. 355–372.

Lord, S.M., Barnsley, L., Wallis, B.J. *et al.* (1996) Percutaneous radiofrequency neurotomy for chronic cervical zygapophyseal joint pain. *N. Engl. J. Med.* **335**: 1721–1726.

Macnab, I. (1964) Acceleration injuries of the cervical spine. *J. Bone Joint Surg. (Am.)* **46**: 1797–1799.

Macnab, I. (1969) Acceleration extension injuries of the cervical spine. In: *AAOS Symposium of the Spine*. St Louis: CV Mosby, pp. 10–17.

Macnab, I. (1971) The 'whiplash syndrome'. *Orthop. Clin. North Am.* **2**: 389–403.

Macnab, I. (1973) The whiplash syndrome. *Clin. Neurosurg.* **20**: 232–241.

Macnab, I. (1982) Acceleration extension injuries of the cervical spine. In: *The Spine*, 2nd edn (Rothman, R.H., Simeone F.A., eds). Philadelphia, PA: WB Saunders, pp. 647–660.

McKenzie, J.A., Williams, J.F. (1971) The dynamic behavior of the head and cervical spine during 'whiplash'. *J. Biomech.* **4**: 474–490.

McKinney, L.A. (1989) Early mobilization and outcome in acute sprains of the neck. *Br. Med. J.* **299**: 1006–1008.

McKinney, L.A., Dornon, J.O., Ryan, M. (1989) The role of physiotherapy in the management of acute neck sprains following road-traffic events. *Arch. Emerg. Med.* **6**: 27–33.

Mealy, K., Brennan, H., Fenelon, G.C.C. (1986) Early mobilization of acute whiplash injuries. *Br. Med. J.* **292**: 656–657.

Medical News (1965) Animals riding in carts show effects of 'whiplash' injury. *J.A.M.A.* **194**: 40–41.

Melzack, R., Wall, P.D. (1983) *The Challenge of Pain*. New York: Basic Books.

Mense, S. (1994) Referral of muscle pain. *Am. Pain Soc. J.* **3**: 10–12.

Merskey, H. (1993) Psychological consequences of whiplash. In: *Spine: State of the Art Reviews*, vol. 7 (Teasell, R.W., Shapiro, A.P., eds). Philadelphia: Hanley & Belfus, pp. 471–480.

Moulin, D.E., Iezzi, A., Amireh, R., Sharpe, W.K.J., Boyd, D., Merskey, H. (1996) Randomized trial of oral morphine for chronic non-cancer pain. *Lancet* **347**: 143–147.

National Safety Council (1971) *Accident Facts*. Chicago: National Safety Council, p. 47.

Nelson, D.A. (1990) Thoracic outlet syndrome and dysfunction of the temporomandibular joint: proved pathology or pseudosyndromes? *Perspect. Biol. Med.* **33**: 567–576.

Nygren, A. (1984) Injuries to car occupants: some aspects of the interior safety of cars. *Acta Otolaryngol. (Stockh.)* **395** (Suppl): 1–164.

O'Hara, M.W., Hinrichs, J.V., Kohout, F.J. *et al.* (1986) Memory complaint and memory performance in the depressed elderly. *Psychol. Aging* **1**: 208–214.

Olsnes, B.T. (1989) Neurobehavioral findings in whiplash patients with long-standing symptoms. *Acta Neurol. Scand.* **80**: 584–587.

Ommaya, A.K., Fass, F., Yarnell, P. (1968) Whiplash injury and brain injury: an experimental study. *J.A.M.A.* **204**: 285–289.

Oosterveld, W.J., Kortschot, H.W., Kingma, G.G. *et al.* (1991) Electronystagmographic findings following cervical whiplash injuries. *Acta Otolaryngol. (Stockh.)* **111**: 201–205.

Pang, L.Q. (1971) The otological aspects of whiplash injuries. *Laryngoscope* **81**: 1381–1387.

Pearce, J.M.S. (1989) Whiplash injury: a reappraisal. *J. Neurol. Neurosurg. Psychiatry* **52:** 1329-1331.

Pennie, B., Agambar, L. (1991) Patterns of injury and recovery in whiplash. *Injury* **22:** 57-99.

Quebec Task Force on Whiplash-Associated Disorders (1995) *Spine* **20:** 1S-73S.

Rachtman, A.M., Borden, A.G.B., Gershon-Cohen, J. (1961) The lordotic curve of the cervical spine. *Clin. Orthop.* **20:** 208.

Radanov, B.P., Dvorak, J. (1996) Impaired cognitive functioning after whiplash injury of the cervical spine. *Spine* **21:** 393-397.

Radanov, B.P., diStefano, G., Schnidrig, A., Ballinari, P. (1991) Role of psychosocial stress in recovery from common whiplash. *Lancet* **338:** 712-715.

Radanov, B.P., Dvorak, J., Valach, L. (1992) Cognitive deficits in patients after soft tissue injury of the cervical spine. *Spine* **17:** 127-131.

Radanov, B.P., DiStefano, G.D., Schnidrig, A. *et al.* (1993) Cognitive functioning after common whiplash. *Arch. Neurol.* **50:** 87-91.

Radanov, B.P., Sturzenegger, M., DeStefano, G., Schnidrig, A. (1994) Relationship between early somatic, radiological, cognitive and psychosocial findings and outcome during a one-year follow-up in 117 patients suffering from common whiplash. *Br. J. Rheumatol.* **33:** 442-448.

Ruff, R.M., Levin, H.S., Mattis, S. *et al.* (1989) Recovery of memory after head injury. A three centre study. In: *Mild Head Injury* (Levin, H.S., Eisenberg, H.M., Benton, A.L. eds). New York: Oxford University Press, pp. 176-188.

Schutt, C.H., Dohan, F.C.S. (1968) Neck injuries to women in auto accidents. A metropolitan plague. *J.A.M.A.* **206:** 2689-2692.

Shapiro, A.P., Roth, R.S. (1993) The effect of litigation on recovery from whiplash. In: (Teasell, R.W., Shapiro, A.P. eds). *Spine: State of the Art Reviews. Cervical Flexion-Extension/Whiplash Injuries,* vol. 7 Philadelphia: Hanley & Belfus, pp. 531-556.

Shapiro, A.P., Teasell, R.W., Steenhuis, R. (1993) Mild traumatic brain injury following whiplash. In: Teasell, R.W., Shapiro, A.P. (eds) *Spine: State of the Art Reviews. Cervical Flexion-Extension/Whiplash Injuries,* vol. 7. Philadelphia: Hanely & Belfus, pp. 455-470.

Sobeco, Ernst and Young (1989) Saskatchewan Government Insurance automobile injury study. Report to the Saskatchewan Government Insurance Office, March.

Speed, W.G. (1987) Psychiatric aspects of post-traumatic headaches. In: *Psychiatric Aspects of Headache* (Adler, C.S. *et al.* eds). Baltimore: Williams & Wilkins, pp. 210-216.

Spiegel, K., Kalb, R., Pasternak, G.W. (1983) Analgesic activity of tricyclic antidepressants. *Ann. Neurol.* **13:** 462-465.

Stromgren, L.S. (1977) The influence of depression on memory. *Acta Psychiatr. Scand.* **56:** 109-128.

Teasell, R.W., Harth, M. (1996) Functional restoration in returning patients with chronic low back pain to work: revolution or fad? *Spine* **21:** 844-847.

Teasell, R.W., Marchuk, Y. (1994) Vertebro-basilar artery stroke as a complication of cervical manipulation. *Crit. Rev. Phys. Rehabil. Med.* **6:** 121-129.

Teasell, R.W., Shapiro, A.P. (1993) Flexion-extension injuries and chronic pain. In: *Pain Research and Clinical Management: Progress on Fibromyalgia and Myofascial Pain,* vol. 6 (Merskey, H., Vaeroy, H., eds). Amsterdam: Elsevier, pp. 253-266.

Toglia, J.V. (1976) Acute flexion-extension injury of the neck. Electronystagmographic study of 309 patients. *Neurology* **26:** 808-814.

Torres, F., Shapiro, S.K. (1961) Electroencephalograms in whiplash injury. *Arch. Neurol.* **5:** 28-35.

Travell, J., Simons, D.G. (1983) *Myofascial Pain and Dysfunction: The Trigger Point Manual.* Baltimore: Williams & Wilkins.

Turk, D.C., Flor, H. (1984) Etiological theories and treatments for chronic pain. II. Psychosocial factors and interventions. *Pain* **19:** 209-233.

Verkest, A.C.M., Stolker, R.J. (1991) The treatment of cervical pain syndromes with radiofrequency procedures. *Pain Clin.* **4:** 103-112.

Ward, N.G. (1986) Tricyclic antidepressants for chronic low back pain. *Spine* **11:** 661-665.

Weinberger, L.M. (1976) Trauma or treatment? The role of intermittent traction in the treatment of cervical soft tissue injuries. *J. Trauma* **15:** 377-382.

Weingartner, H., Siberman, E. (1982) Models of cognitive impairment: cognitive changes in depression. *Psychol. Pharm. Bull.* **18:** 27-42.

Wickstrom, J.K., LaRocca, H. (1975) Management of patients with cervical spine and head injuries from acceleration forces. *Curr. Pract. Orthop. Surg.* **6:** 83.

Wickstrom, J.K., Martinez, J.L., Rodriguez, R. Jr *et al.* (1970) Hyperextension and hyperflexion injuries to the head and neck of primates. In: *Neckache and Backache.* (Gurdijian, E.S., Thomas, L.M., eds) Springfield, IL: Charles C Thomas, pp. 108-117.

Wilbourn, A.J. (1990) The thoracic outlet syndrome is overdiagnosed. *Arch. Neurol.* **47:** 328-330.

Wiley, A.M., Lloyd, J., Evans, J.G., Stewart, B.M., Sanchez, J. (1986) Musculoskeletal sequelae of whiplash injuries. *Advocates Q.* **7:** 65-73.

Yarnell, P.R., Rossie, G.V. (1988) Minor whiplash head injury with major debilitation. *Brain Inj.* **2:** 255-258.

Zylbergold, R.S., Piper, M.C. (1985) Cervical spine disorders. A comparison of three types of traction. *Spine* **10:** 867-871.

Diagnosis and Management

6

Diagnostic imaging of mechanical and degenerative syndromes of the cervical spine

L. J. Rowe

Introduction

Degenerative conditions of the cervical spine are the most common clinically significant pathological entities encountered in the cervical spine. They are readily depicted by various imaging modalities, including conventional radiography, computed tomography (CT) and magnetic resonance imaging (MRI). Each imaging method exhibits its own advantages and disadvantages dependent on the condition being imaged (Modic *et al.*, 1989). In this chapter imaging features of various degenerative syndromes of the cervical spine are examined.

Degenerative disc disease

Degenerative disc disease (DDD) is characterized by dehydration, fissuring, anular disruption and osteophytosis. The preferred term is degenerative disc disease, although alternative nomenclature is used, including spondylosis, discogenic spondylosis and spondylosis deformans. The term spondylosis deformans can be applied to advanced disc degeneration associated with radiographic findings of multilevel severe loss of disc height and large anterior osteophytes which pathologically buttress disc herniations producing deformed vertebral bodies (Resnick, 1985).

Degenerative disc disease is extremely common, occurring in up to 5% of women and 13% of men during the third decade, more than 90% of adults over the age of 50 years and almost 100% by 70 years (Irvine *et al.*, 1965, Schmorl and Junghanns, 1971). The most common levels are the C5-6, C6-7 and C4-5 interspaces respectively (Gore *et al.*, 1986).

This distribution most likely reflects the degree of biomechanical stresses and susceptibility to injury which is also mirrored in intersegmental differences in bone mineral density with C5 considered by Curylo *et al.* (1996) to be the most dense, followed by C6, C4 and C7.

The lack of clinicoradiological correlation in DDD has been well-documented (Heller *et al.*, 1983). MRI studies of the cervical spine in asymptomatic individuals have shown degenerative changes in almost 20% of these spines (Teresi *et al.*, 1987; Boden *et al.*, 1990a). Radiographically diagnosed DDD in the presence of neck pain is not a reliable outcome predictor for conservative or surgical intervention (Dillin *et al.*, 1986; Gore *et al.*, 1987; Ruggieri, 1995). In whiplash patients, degenerative changes present at the time of injury diminish the prognosis (Torg *et al.*, 1986; Maimaris *et al.*, 1988). Current literature supports the notion that whiplash injuries do predispose to premature disc disease (Davis *et al.*, 1991; Watkinson *et al.*, 1991; Rowe and Yochum, 1996a). Restricted post-traumatic cervical motion has been correlated with a high incidence of degenerative changes in the following 5 years (Hohl, 1974).

Imaging features

Conventional radiography

Degenerative disc changes are graphically depicted, such as a loss in disc height, osteophytes and displacement. In addition, they assist to exclude fractures, dislocations, neoplastic and other pathological processes.

Loss in vertical height is assessed by comparison with adjacent discs. Normally the disc height is less at C6-7 and C7-T1 as the transition is made to the thoracic spine. There is a lag time between dehydration as shown on MRI and loss of disc height. Bony outgrowths from vertebral bodies occur initially at the insertion of the anterior longitudinal ligament and the latent time between disc injury and the first appearance of radiographically detectable osteophyte formation may be demonstrated as early as 3 months following injury. Intersegmental subluxation as a sequel to DDD is common and most frequently is retrolisthesis (retrodisplacement, retropositioning, posterior translation). Any anterior displacement is typically related to deforming facet arthropathy.

Loss of lordosis occurs commonly from the segment above the DDD level due to segmental extension as the uncovertebral joints approximate (Eideken and Pitt, 1971; MacNab, 1975). Neck pain is more prevalent and most severe when the lordosis has

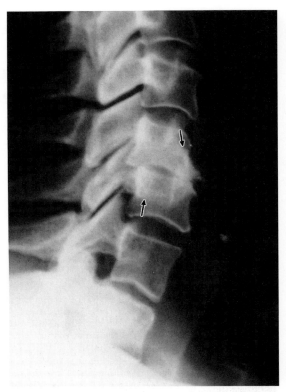

Fig. 6.2 Degenerative disc disease, end-plate sclerosis. A prominent increase in density of the end-plates and vertebral bodies adjacent to the narrowed intervertebral disc space is demonstrated (arrows). There is associated retrolisthesis of the superior segment and anterior osteophytes.

Comment: This appearance is uncommon and can mimic an osteoblastic bony process such as metastatic carcinoma. The distinctive convex superior border is typical of a degenerative process.

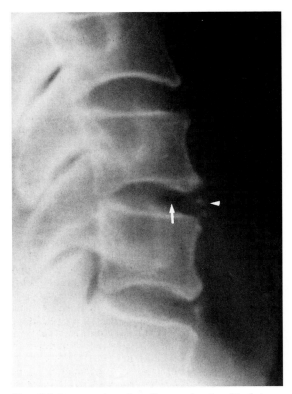

Fig. 6.1 Degenerative disc disease. At the C5–6 intervertebral disc level a loss of height is evident. Note the radiolucent linear density within the substance of the disc representing the accumulation of nitrogen gas within degenerative clefts (vacuum phenomenon; arrow). Anteriorly the calcifications lie within the anular fibres (intercallary bones; arrowhead).

Comment: These are common hallmarks of degenerative disc disease and can occur either in concert with each other or separately. The vacuum phenomenon is best demonstrated on extension views.

been lost (Batzdorf and Batzdorf, 1988). Vacuum phenomena are occasionally observed, usually on extension views, as a horizontal translucent cleft within the anterior aspect of the disc (Fig. 6.1). Until recently, such vacuum phenomena have been erroneously implicated as a soft-tissue sign for post-traumatic disc tear, which has now been shown to represent degenerative fissures (Reymond *et al.*, 1972; Bohrer and Chen, 1988). End-plate sclerosis is uncommon but periodically can be quite marked, mimicking an osteoblastic bony process such as metastatic carcinoma. Such sclerosis can display features reminiscent of hemispherical spondylosclerosis in the lumbar spine with a distinctive convex superior border which may or may not involve contiguous vertebrae across a single degenerative disc (Rowe, 1988; Rowe and Yochum, 1996b; Fig. 6.2). End-plate irregularity and poor definition may produce an appearance identical to that of infection. Occasionally, spontaneous ankylosis can be observed (Fig. 6.3).

Canal size can be estimated on the lateral view from the point of the posterior mid vertebral body to the adjacent spinolaminar line and normally is around 17 mm in anteroposterior diameter. A measurement of less than 13 mm suggests stenosis with cord impingement and less than 10 mm impingement will invariably be present (Edwards and LaRocca, 1985). Generally, spinal canal diameters of 17 mm or greater will need an osteophyte of at least 3.3 mm to impinge upon the cord, while those canals less than 17 mm will only need 2.1 mm spurs to create the same compression effect (Edwards and LaRocca, 1985). Patients with canal sizes of 10–13 mm are premyelopathic since the average spinal cord size from C1 to C7 averages 10 mm (Robinson *et al.*, 1977). Although these dimensions estimate canal size on plain films, CT or MRI provides more accurate assessment of the cord itself and its surrounding spaces (Rahim and Stambough, 1992).

Computed tomography

Axial images through degenerative cervical discs are especially useful for the depiction of osteophytes and the resultant canal stenosis. In contrast to the lumbar spine, inherent anatomical limitations in the cervical spine impair the detection of disc herniations, ligamentous hypertrophy, neural elements and extradural lesions. These include the paucity of epidural fat, low tissue differential densities and smaller-sized foramina. Utilising CT combined with myelography (CT myelography; CTM) and thin slices of 1.5–3 mm thickness, these shortcomings can be compensated for producing diagnostic accuracies approaching that of MRI (Larsson *et al.*, 1989; Wilson *et al.*, 1991). Myelography on its own has virtually no role in the evaluation of cervical spine DDD given its invasive nature and lack of sensitivity. Intravenous contrast-enhanced CT (IVCT) can be used to evaluate spinal canal size and its contents when MRI is not available (Baleriaux *et al.*, 1983; Russell, 1990). Degraded image quality due to the effects of the shoulder girdle can impair evaluation of the lower cervical discs.

CT features of DDD include osteophytes, sclerosis, end-plate irregularities, vacuum phenomena, calcification and disc bulging. Osteophytes are readily apparent on bone window images as rough and irregular bony excrescences from the vertebral body margins. Anterior osteophytes may be seen to displace or impress on the adjacent retropharyngeal wall. Posterior osteophytes extend into the central canal and may be seen contacting and deforming the adjacent cord. Sagittal reconstructions will assist in visualizing this effect. Posterolateral osteophytes originate from the uncovertebral and zygapophysial joints to compromise the lateral foramina (see Fig. 1.12).

Sclerosis occupies the subend-plate bone and may be interspersed with focal radiolucencies. These radiolucencies represent either focal end-plate depressions (Schmorl's nodes) or raised calcified end-plate foci. Intraosseous gas beneath the end-plate is rarely seen (vertebral pneumatocyst) and should not be confused with linear, wafer-like vacuum phenomena within a collapsed vertebral body due to corticosteroid induced osteonecrosis (Malghem *et al.*, 1993; Grunshaw and Carey, 1994; Laufer *et al.*, 1996). More frequently, vacuum phenomena can be seen in the periphery of the disc as expressions of anular tears and centrally within nuclear clefts. Extension into the spinal canal, with or without disc herniation, can occasionally be observed (Elster and Jensen, 1984). Calcification within the anulus is usually focal and near the circumference of the disc while nuclear calcifications are placed more internally. Bulging discs, unlike the lumbar spine, are uncommon and are recognized by a broad-based soft-tissue convexity

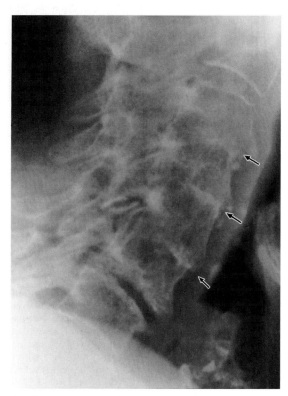

Fig. 6.3 Degenerative disc disease, spontaneous ankylosis. Observe the absence of intervertebral disc spaces at multiple levels in this octogenarian patient (arrows).

Comment: Fusion at degenerative discs is uncommon and most commonly occurs in the elderly. Differential considerations include rheumatoid arthritis, ankylosing spondylitis, post-trauma and post-infection.

extending less than 2 mm beyond the adjacent posterior vertebral bodies.

Magnetic resonance imaging

This is the imaging modality of choice for definitive examination of DDD in the cervical spine. In comparison with CT in lateral and central canal pathology, MRI sensitivity is at least 90%, in comparison to 75–80% for CT (Brown *et al.,* 1988; Wilson *et al.,* 1991; Rao and Williams, 1994).

The myriad of protocols that have been developed for cervical spine MRI reflect attempts to overcome the inherent anatomical complexities that make its imaging difficult. As a minimum, axial and sagittal views must be obtained. Pulse sequences should include T1 and those producing a T2 effect. In general, T1 and T2 axial and sagittal views are acquired. To reduce long acquisition times, and pulsation artefacts, to produce T2 images, it is usual to use gradient echo or fast spin echo pulses. As with CT, the reduced disc volume requires thin slice acquisition (3–4 mm).

The T1 images are most useful for delineating vertebral body marrow and spinal cord outlines. The posterior vertebral body cortex and protruding osteophytes can be masked by the pulsation of cerebrospinal fluid (CSF); therefore it is best appreciated on T2 images. These images produce an unmistakable myelogram effect which enhances the posterior vertebral surfaces, the extradural space, herniated discs and cord myelopathy. In herniated discs, T2 images show the extruded material as a relatively high signal allowing separation from low signal osteophytes. Where there is difficulty differentiating osteophytes from disc herniation, especially in the lateral canal, the intravenous injection of gadolinium, as with IVCT, enhances the adjacent epidural venous plexus and disc margin which can increase the signal of disc material (Ross *et al.,* 1992). Myelopathy requires CSF-gated T2 images to show the high signal of oedema, tumour or multiple sclerosis plaques and low signal of gliosis (Rao and Williams, 1994).

MRI hallmarks of DDD are readily identified. The intervertebral disc shows reduced signal, reflecting dehydration best seen on T2-weighted images. Loss of signal can be demonstrated within weeks following injury such as whiplash (Davis *et al.,* 1991). The presence of vacuum phenomenon will show a signal void, as will calcium on T1 and T2 (Berns *et al.,* 1991). Bulging of the posterior disc margin can be observed. Protruding osteophytes are low in signal on T1 and T2, while soft disc herniations will become higher in signal on T2, which allows their differentiation. Posterior cord impingement from thickened ligamentum flavum is best seen on mid sagittal images (Fig. 6.4). Paraspinal muscle atrophy is often observed in DDD with increased fatty replacement and diminished bulk, although no clinical correlative

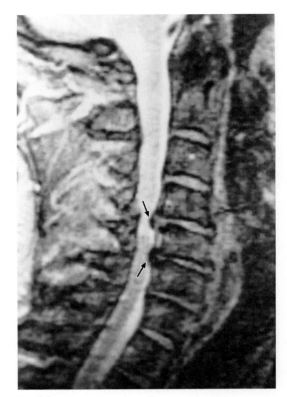

Fig. 6.4 Degenerative disc disease, magnetic resonance imaging. Protruding posterior osteophytes are visible as low signal extensions beyond the vertebral body margins (arrows). The effect on the adjacent spinal cord can be readily appreciated.

Comment: Differentiation of osteophytes from herniation can be achieved by noting on T2 images that disc herniations will exhibit higher signal. Posterior cord impingement from thickened ligamentum flavum can also be demonstrated, especially on mid sagittal images.

studies have been made to define its significance (Rao and Williams, 1994).

Vertebral bone marrow changes adjacent to the end-plates are extremely common findings in tandem with DDD. As in the lumbar spine, three patterns can be recognized reflecting altered vascularity, marrow conversion and bone density. Type 1 end-plate changes show decreased intensity on T1-weighted images and increased signal intensity on T2-weighted images (white–black). Type 2 end-plate changes show increased intensity on T1-weighted images and increased or isointense signal intensity on T2-weighted images (white–white). Type 3 end-plate changes show decreased intensity on T1-weighted images and decreased signal intensity on T2-weighted images (black–black; Modic *et al.,* 1988a,b).

Low signal of the end-plates on T1 correlates with inflammatory marrow (Toyone *et al.,* 1994). Conversely, high signal on T1 denotes the presence of fatty marrow (Lang *et al.*, 1990; Toyone *et al.*, 1994). Type 1 changes tend to progress to type 2 over time (hypervascular to fatty), whereas type 2 remain stable (fatty; Modic *et al.*, 1988a,b).

Cervical disc herniation

Cervical disc herniation occurs across a broad spread of age ranges from 20 to 60 years, being most common in individuals in their 30s (Kelsey *et al.*, 1984). Herniation after the age of 30 is unlikely to occur since the gelatinous nucleus pulposus has been replaced by fibrocartilage (Oda *et al.*, 1988; Bland and Boushey, 1990; Kokubun *et al.*, 1996; Mercer and Jull, 1996). The male-to-female ratio is approximately 1.4 to 1 (Kondo *et al.*, 1981; Kelsey *et al.*, 1984). Cervical disc herniations are less common than lumbar disc herniations and linked risk factors include smoking, diving and lifting heavy objects (Kelsey *et al.*, 1984). The most common levels of involvement are the C6–7 (60%) and C5–6 (30%) intervertebral discs respectively (Kondo *et al.*, 1981; Kelsey *et al.*, 1984).

Clinical manifestations are dependent on the size and location of the herniation and on other factors. Size cannot be a criterion for aggressive therapy since some herniations will diminish over time with conservative care (Maigne and Deligne, 1994). The incidence for asymptomatic herniations, even in a population which has never experienced neck pain, may be as high as or greater than 10% under the age of 40, and 5% over age 40, with an overall average incidence of 8% (Modic *et al.*, 1989; Boden *et al.*, 1990a; Lehto *et al.*, 1994). This compares with up to 28% of asymptomatic lumbar spines exhibiting herniations (Boden *et al.*, 1990b). In over 30% of autopsies a cervical disc herniation may be evident (Kokubun *et al.*, 1996).

Cervical disc herniations are often referred to according to their consistency, being soft when the gelatinous nucleus pulposus extrudes, and are unassociated with posterior bony osteophytes. So-called hard herniations are fibrocartilaginous anular bulges which occur in tandem with posterior osteophytes. Central and larger herniations can produce the same effects as a cord tumour, with mixed upper and lower motor neuron features involving multiple dermatomes and even the lower limbs. Lateral herniations are less common due to the relative anatomical barrier of the uncovertebral joints and tend to select a single nerve root producing features consistent with lower motor neuron involvement. Anterior herniations can uncommonly cause dysphagia (Lambert *et al.*, 1981; Bernado *et al.*, 1988). Multilevel herniations can occur in up to 12% of necks above the age of 30 years (Kokubun, 1996). Almost 50% of the posterior herniations are intraligamentous, lying between the deep and superficial layers of the ligament, 30% are transligamentous, and 20% epidural (Kokubun *et al.*, 1996). Re-herniation at the level of previous operation for a disc herniation is uncommon compared to lumbar spine discectomies (Ross, 1991).

Imaging features

Conventional radiography

This has a limited role in the detection of a herniation. It does detect loss of disc height, bony canal stenosis and other bony pathology, but does not directly image neural compression (Modic *et al.*, 1989).

Myelography

With the advent and increasing availability of MRI, myelography should be avoided wherever possible. The features are that of a smooth extradural filling defect in the ventral surface of the contrast column at the level of the disc, and there can be obliteration of the exiting axillary sleeve (Russell, 1995; Fig. 6.5A).

Computed tomography

CT is more sensitive and without the morbidity of myelography in detecting cervical disc herniation (Yu *et al.*, 1983). Thin-slice examinations (1.5–2 mm) are used to pass through the narrower disc spaces and avoid artifactual volume imaging of the adjacent endplates. Spiral CT is ideal for imaging disc herniations (Russell, 1995).

The inherent paucity of epidural fat reduces tissue plane differentiation of the intraspinal contents, and greatly reduces the sensitivity of non-contrast CT examinations; this is overcome by the introduction of contrast media. Conditions including cord tumours and disc herniations may not be seen on non-contrast CT due to this regional anatomical peculiarity (Penning *et al.*, 1986). This can be alleviated by combining CT with intrathecal (CTM). or intravenous contrast (IVCT). The administration of intravenous contrast enhances the herniation by opacifying overlying epidural veins (Russell *et al.*, 1984; Russell, 1995). Combining discography with CT (CT-discography; CTD) can delineate symptomatic internal disc derangements which, when removed by discectomy, produces relief of symptoms in up to 70% of cases (Whitecloud and Seago, 1987; Schellas *et al.*, 1996).

The CT features of a cervical disc herniation include a broad-based soft-tissue density contiguous with the posterior disc margin and distortion of the ventral surface of the thecal sac (Russell, 1995).

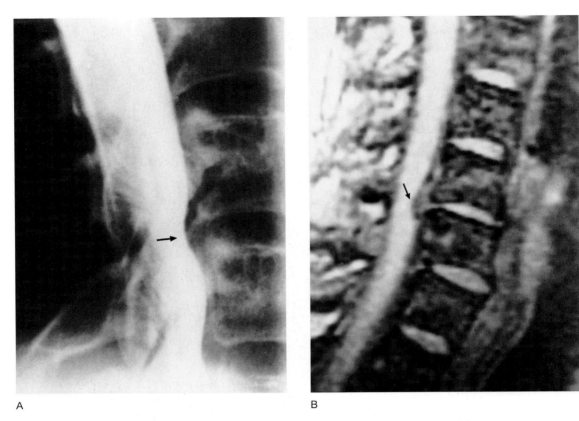

A   B

Fig. 6.5 Cervical disc herniation. (A) Myelogram. A smooth extradural filling defect in the ventral surface of the contrast column at the level of the disc can be seen (arrow). (B) Magnetic resonance imaging (MRI). At the C6–7 intervertebral disc note the posterior herniation, which is impinging directly on to the adjacent spinal cord (arrow).

Comment: Although the myelogram demonstrates compression of the spinal cord it does not distinguish between disc bulge, osteophyte or herniation. Such a study should be performed in conjunction with computed tomography, or not at all if MRI is available. On MRI the posterior discal extension is clearly visible. MRI generally cannot distinguish between asymptomatic and symptomatic disc herniations and may not detect significant anular tears.

CTM is particularly useful for demonstrating impingement upon the exiting nerve root with a failure for the axillary sleeve to fill with contrast. Both bone and soft-tissue windows must be utilized, otherwise calcification and osteophytes will be overlooked.

Magnetic resonance imaging

MRI is the most sensitive imaging modality in depicting cervical disc herniation and neural compression. It is the best method for evaluating the patient with radiculopathy or myelopathy (Modic *et al.*, 1989).

MRI generally cannot distinguish between asymptomatic and symptomatic disc herniations. At least 10% of an asymptomatic population under 45 years will have a disc herniation, and over 15% less than 64 years will have spinal cord impingement (Modic *et al.*, 1989; Boden, 1990a). Significant anular tears can escape detection with MRI and may only be demonstrated with discography (Schellas *et al.*, 1996). The MRI features of a cervical disc herniation include extension of nuclear material beyond the posterior margin of the vertebral body seen on T1 which, on sagittal images, has been referred to as the 'squeezed toothpaste' sign (Simon and Lukin, 1988; Fig. 6.5B). On T2-weighted images disc material is slightly higher in signal intensity, which allows differentiation from a protruding osteophyte (Fig. 6.6). Radiculopathy is best evaluated by oblique projections to demonstrate the intervertebral foramen and its contents and their relationship to any disc material or bony element (Modic *et al.*, 1987).

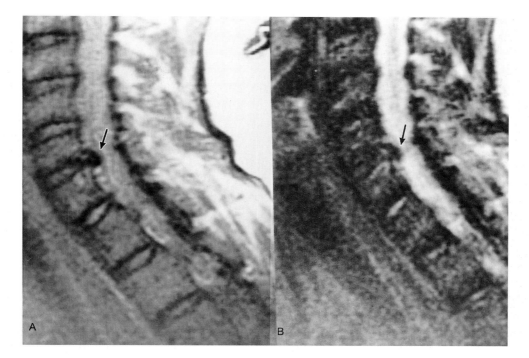

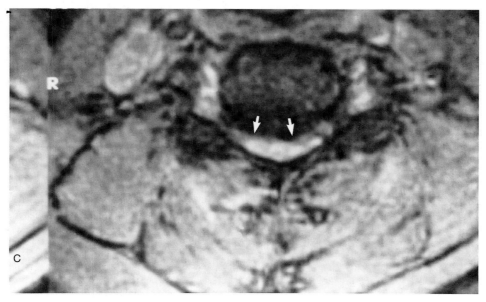

Fig. 6.6 Pseudodisc herniation, posterior osteophytes. (A) Magnetic resonance imaging (MRI) T1-weighted sagittal image. At the C5–6 posterior disc margin a low signal protuberance can be clearly seen (arrow). (B) MRI T2-weighted sagittal image. The protruding density does not change in its signal characteristics remaining low (arrow). The characteristic myelogram effect obtained with this sequence is readily appreciated as the cerebrospinal fluid becomes accentuated and clearly depicts the impingement. (C) MRI T1-weighted axial image. The effect on the adjacent spinal cord from the posterior osteophytes is graphically displayed (arrows).

Comment: Posterior osteophytes can simulate a disc herniation on T1-weighted images. On T2-weighted images disc material is slightly higher in signal intensity, which allows differentiation from a protruding osteophyte which remains low in signal. The presence of these osteophytes is occasionally referred to as a hard disc herniation.

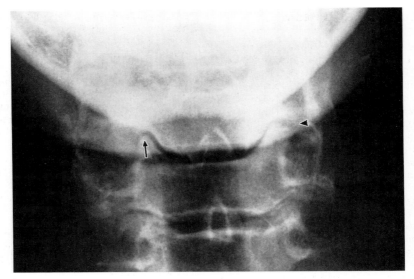

A

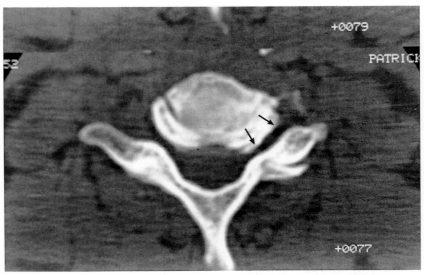

B

Fig. 6.7 Uncovertebral joint degeneration. (A) Plain film. There are early degenerative changes in the uncovertebral joint on the left side with the tip of the uncinate process being more pointed (arrow). Progression of degenerative changes is evidenced by the rounding of the tip to a bulbous form with the uncinate spur slanting laterally (arrowhead). (B) Axial computed tomographic scan. Proliferative changes at the uncovertebral joint extend into the adjacent intervertebral foramen creating stenosis (arrows).

Comment: The degree of uncovertebral joint arthrosis parallels the loss of disc height. Osteophytes from the uncovertebral joint can potentially impinge upon the adjacent exiting nerve root and can deflect the course of the vertebral artery (compare with Figures 1.4 and 1.12).

Uncovertebral joint disease

The uncovertebral joints are a unique anatomical feature of the cervical spine, consisting of an elevated lip originating from the posterolateral border of the inferior vertebral body (the uncus), which invaginates into a reciprocal depression on the superior vertebra (uncinate fossa). It was von Luschka (1850) who first called attention to these joints, to which his name has become inexorably linked; he referred to them as *eschencrure* (tailor-made).

The debate as to whether they represent a synovial joint or are extensions of the intervertebral discs has little relevance to their clinical significance and imaging findings. Early histopathological changes of the joints between the ages of 9 and 14 years are well-documented; they consist of a short horizontal cleft that appears bilaterally at the lateral margins of the disc, adjacent to the uncinate processes as a functional adaptation to axial rotation (Haughton, 1995; see Chapter 2 and Fig. 3.6). Eventually, this horizontal cleft coalesces across the midline to form a continuous horizontal fissure. Degenerative changes in these joints will always coexist with a level of degenerative disc disease.

Imaging features

Conventional radiography

Degenerative changes within the uncovertebral joints invariably coexist with DDD as the loss in disc height produces impaction of the uncinate process into the opposing fossa. The initial change is a sharpening of the uncinate process followed by a rounding of the tip to a bulbous form (Rowe and Yochum, 1996b). When the disc height is less than 50%, the uncinate spur slants laterally and begins to impinge into the adjacent foramen (Fig. 6.7A). Uncovertebral osteophytes do not impinge on nerve roots until they obliterate at least 50% of the foraminal volume (Dunsker, 1981; Rahim and Stambough, 1992; Fig. 6.7B). When osteophytes from the zygapophysial joint facet and the uncovertebral joint coexist, they create an hourglass configuration to the foramen. Uncovertebral osteophytes can deflect the course of the vertebral artery (Oga *et al.*, 1996; see Fig. 1.12). The combination of decreased disc height and uncovertebral joint arthrosis on the lateral view can combine to produce a linear pseudofracture appearance adjacent to the inferior end-plate, most commonly at C5 (Daffner *et al.*, 1986; Rowe, 1990; Fig. 6.8).

Additional imaging

The proximity of the uncovertebral joint to the exiting nerve root accounts for the frequency of nerve root compression as it degenerates, most commonly involving the C5-6 and C6-7 foramina. CT with thin axial images is the best method for accurately demonstrating mineralized uncovertebral osteophytes (Russell, 1995; Fig. 6.7B). MRI has the

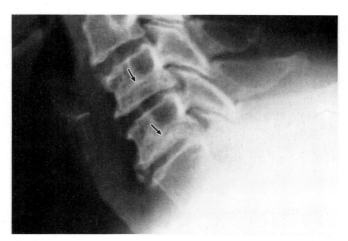

Fig. 6.8 Pseudofracture, uncovertebral joint arthrosis. The combination of decreased disc height and uncovertebral joint arthrosis on the lateral view combines to produce a linear trilaminar density which can simulate the presence of a fracture (arrows).

Comment: This pseudofracture appearance adjacent to the inferior end-plate is most commonly seen at the C5 vertebral body and is invariably associated with a loss in disc height.

added advantage of showing non-invasively the relationship to the exiting nerve root.

Zygapophysial joint degenerative disease

Clinical syndromes associated with the zygapophysial joints are well-documented and include radiculopathy, myelopathy, headaches and referred pain (Bogduk and Marsland, 1986; Heller, 1992). Imaging, in general, is highly sensitive and specific in identifying the presence of zygapophysial joint facet arthrosis.

Imaging features

Conventional radiography

Degenerative zygapophysial joints produce distinctive features which may include diminished joint space, blurred facet surfaces, osteophytes, sclerosis, subluxation and subchondral cysts (Rahim and Stambough, 1992; Russell, 1995; Rowe and Yochum, 1996b; Fig. 6.9). Osteophytes on frontal views can be seen to extend laterally, and on oblique views foraminal encroachment can be assessed. On the lateral study, osteophytes may be seen projecting from the superior or inferior tips of the articular pillars. Anterolisthesis of 2–9 mm from zygapophysial joint facet arthrosis (degenerative spondylolisthesis)

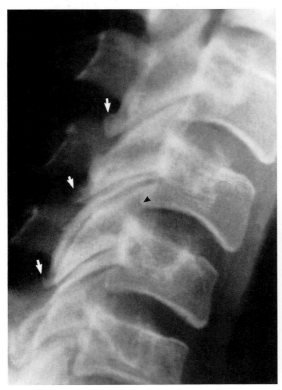

A

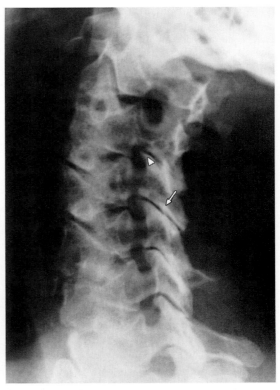

B

Fig. 6.9 Zygapophysial joint degenerative disease. (A) Lateral view. Osteophytes can be identified extending from the posterior zygapophysial joint margins (arrows). The zygapophysial joint spaces are also diminished and there is a small degree of anterolisthesis of C4 on C5 (arrowhead). (B) Oblique view. All zygapophysial joints show degenerative features with loss of joint space, osteophytes and subchondral sclerosis (arrow). Osteophytes may be displayed on this projection protruding into the dorsal aspect of the foramen (arrowhead).

Comment: Degenerative changes in the zygapophysial joints on conventional radiographs are most clearly depicted on oblique views. The characteristic features are diminished joint space, blurred joint surfaces, osteophytes, sclerosis, subluxation and, rarely, subchondral cysts.

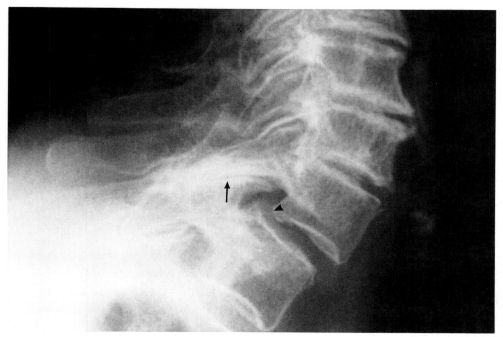

Fig. 6.10 Degenerative spondylolisthesis. The zygapophysial joints exhibit a combination of diminished joint space and remodelling of the facet surface to a more horizontal plane (arrow). Note the resultant anterolisthesis (arrowhead).

Comment: Degenerative anterolisthesis is most common in the lower cervical spine, especially at C7–T1. Usually there is 2–9 mm of displacement, which should not be confused with a traumatic subluxation or dislocation.

is due to a combination of diminished joint space and remodelling of the facet surface to a more horizontal plane; it is most common in the lower cervical spine, especially C7–T1 (Lee *et al.,* 1986; Rowe and Yochum, 1996b; Fig. 6.10).

Additional imaging

CT bone windows are ideal for demonstrating degenerative changes, especially surface irregularities, osteophytes and subchondral cysts. Compression of adjacent neural elements can be identified with accuracy rates as high as 96% when CT is combined with myelography (Bell and Ross, 1992). Myelography on its own can detect between 67 and 92% of nerve root compressions (Bell and Ross, 1992). Technetium-99m phosphate bone scans will show discrete focal uptake at the site of zygapophysial joint facet arthrosis but do not correlate clinically with a painful joint.

The normal MRI appearance of an intermediate signal of the zygapophysial joint space on T1-weighting which is hyperintense on T2-weighting, and clear definition of a hypointense zygapophysial joint facet cortical surface, are lost in the presence of arthrosis. The MRI appearance is that of a hypointense, blurred mass representing loss of joint cartilage, osteophytes and sclerosis. Hypertrophy of the joint capsule can also be seen. Although synovial folds (see Fig. 1.10) and menisci can be seen in normal cervical zygapophysial joint, altered appearances or positions have not been described to delineate their clinical significance (Yu *et al.,* 1987). MRI does not show osteophytes particularly well but neural compromise is well depicted with an accuracy of up to almost 90% (Bell and Ross, 1992; Ruggieri, 1995).

Evagination of hypertrophic synovium can form a synovial cyst, most commonly at C6–7, which has the potential to act as a space-occupying mass producing nerve root, or even cord, pressure (Patel and Sanders, 1988). On CT, a synovial cyst is seen as a rounded soft-tissue mass contiguous with a degenerative zygapophysial joint; the cyst may extend posterolaterally into the foramen. With CT and intravenous contrast the cyst's peripheral rim will enhance, and occasionally it is calcified (Nijensohn *et al.,* 1990). On MRI, the rim is well-defined and hypointense relative to the central zone which, on T2-weighting, remains low, often due to calcification or blood products (Nijensohn *et al.*, 1990). The rim will enhance with gadolinium administration (Snow and Scott, 1994) and the central core can be of high signal on T1-weighting due to contained protein or haemorrhage within the fluid.

Atlantoaxial degenerative joint disease

Degenerative joint disease at the atlantoaxial joint is a relatively uncommon, but clinically important, entity. Primary degenerative joint disease of the upper cervical complex is an underdiagnosed condition that carries significant patient morbidity though it may not be readily amenable to treatment (Halla and Hardin, 1987; Star *et al.*, 1992). At least 4% of individuals with spinal osteoarthritis will have atlantoaxial osteoarthritis (Halla and Hardin, 1987). Degeneration of the C1–2 joint may also be secondary to, and the only sign for, pre-existing pathology such as os odontoideum, agenesis of the odontoid or ununited fracture (Rowe and Yochum, 1996a). Unlike inflammatory arthropathies such as rheumatoid and psoriatic arthritis, the transverse ligament remains intact with no intersegmental instability (Rowe and Yochum, 1996b).

The atlantoaxial articulations are composed of two joint complexes, the paired lateral mass joints and the singular central atlanto-odontoid articulation. Each complex exhibits distinct clinical and imaging features. Imaging is pivotal in defining the diagnosis and is best determined on conventional lateral and open-mouth frontal projections and on CT.

Lateral mass degenerative joint disease

The lateral mass articulations are the zygapophysial joints of the atlas and axis. Clinically, degenerative changes afflict elderly patients who present with at least a 2-year history of severe occipitocervical pain which is frequently diagnosed as occipital neuralgia (Star *et al.*, 1992). The hallmarks of the disorder are loss of more than 50% rotation on the ipsilateral side of degeneration and localized unilateral occipitocervical tenderness. There may be additional complaints of postauricular headaches and joint crepitus. Conservative treatments are usually effective, though refractory cases may require surgical fusion (Harata *et al.*, 1981; Star *et al.*, 1992). Intra-articular injections may, at times, relieve symptoms (Busch and Wilson, 1989; Dreyfus *et al.*, 1994).

Imaging features
Conventional radiography

On the frontal open-mouth view the most frequently observed abnormalities are unilateral loss of joint space, subchondral sclerosis and osteophytes at the lateral joint margin (Fig. 6.11). Lateral subluxation of C1 on C2 towards the side of arthrosis can occasionally be observed. These features can sometimes be appreciated on the lateral film projected over the odontoid silhouette. Also, widening of the adjacent retropharyngeal space is occasionally observed due to an anteriorly projecting osteophyte or due to fibrocartilaginous debris (Star *et al.*, 1992). The atlantodental interspace should remain normal at less than 3 mm. In severe cases, some degrees of pseudo-basilar invagination may occur secondary to loss of joint space and compression remodelling of the lateral masses.

Additional imaging

CT with bone windows demonstrates osteophytes which may project anteriorly and deform the adjacent pharyngeal wall. Underlying atlantoaxial rotary subluxation can also be discerned. MRI can be used to exclude coexisting intraspinal pathology such as tumour, infection, spinal stenosis or disc disease. Uncommonly, degenerative changes of the atlantoaxial joint can be associated with cord compression, especially if occurring in conjunction with a congenitally narrowed canal, an abnormal odontoid process or degenerative changes in the adjacent cervical segments (Benitah *et al.*, 1994). MRI is particularly useful for isolating synovial cysts. Identifying atlantoaxial intra-articular meniscoids has been largely unrewarding (Yu *et al.*, 1987; Mercer and Bogduk, 1993). Technetium-99m phosphate bone scans will show discrete focal uptake at the site of atlantoaxial arthrosis (Star *et al.*, 1992).

Central atlanto-odontoid degenerative joint disease

The central atlanto-odontoid articulation is formed by the anterior surface of the odontoid process and the posterior surface of the opposing arch of the atlas. It remains unclear as to the clinical significance of its possible pain-producing capacity associated with degenerative changes within this joint, although synovial fluid communication with the lateral joints has been demonstrated (Mellstrom *et al.*, 1980). Degeneration appears to be more common at the central joint than at the lateral joints, with an incidence as high as 35% in the 40–50-year age group, increasing to almost 90% in the over-60-year age

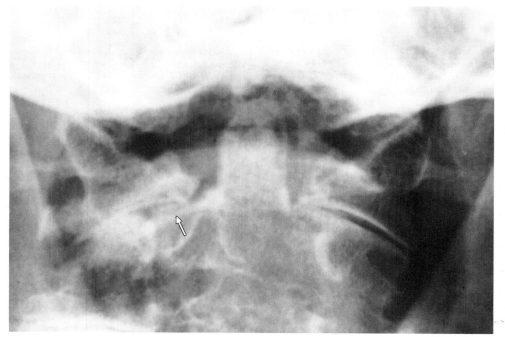

Fig. 6.11 Lateral mass degenerative joint disease. Observe the unilateral loss of joint space, subchondral sclerosis and osteophytosis at the lateral joint margin (arrow).

Comment: Degenerative joint disease of the atlantoaxial joint is a relatively uncommon but clinically important entity which is an underdiagnosed condition and carries significant patient morbidity. At least 4% of patients with spinal osteoarthritis will have atlantoaxial osteoarthritis.

group (Shore, 1935; von Torkulus and Gehle, 1972; Harata *et al.*, 1981).

Imaging features

Conventional imaging

On a lateral view study, narrowing of the atlanto-dental joint space to less than 1 mm, osteophytes at the superior and inferior margins of the atlas anterior arch, and some sclerosis of the opposing surfaces, are the main signs. Occasionally, an osteophyte can be identified extending from the tip of the dens. The anterior arch of the atlas may become ivory-like due to sclerosis. On flexion there will be no change in the atlantodental interspace.

Additional imaging

Lateral tomography and CT can show the degenerative features to advantage (Genez *et al.*, 1990). Axial and reconstructed CT bone window images accurately display the loss of joint space, osteophytes, sub-chondral cysts, small ossicles and calcification of the transverse ligament (Genez *et al.*, 1990). Osteophytes

most commonly project from the tip of the dens (80%), superior aspect of the atlas anterior arch (70%), atlas median facet (60%) and the inferior aspect of the atlas anterior arch (20%). Cystic radiolucencies are most common within the odontoid process (30%), with loose ossicles (35%) and calcification in the transverse ligament (10%; Genez *et al.*, 1990).

Degenerative disorders associated with congenital anomalies

Block vertebrae

Congenital block vertebra is a defect in spinal embryogenesis characterized by a failure in the vertebral segmentation process producing fusion of two or more contiguous vertebral segments (see Fig. 1.3B). Any segment of the spine can be involved, most commonly in the cervical spine, followed by the lumbar and thoracic spines respectively (Evans, 1932; Ramsey and Bliznak, 1971). The most common sites for cervical block vertebrae are at the C2–3 then C5–6 segments respectively (see Chapter 1).

A spectrum of clinical syndromes can emanate from degenerative changes involving at least six possible anatomical structures, e.g. posterior joint degenerative changes, intervertebral joint degenerative changes, spinal canal stenosis, intervertebral canal stenosis, various soft-tissue injuries (such as ligamentous and muscular) and altered vertebrobasilar blood flow (Scher, 1979; see Chapter 1). Most notably it is the immediately adjacent segments which are placed under greater biomechanical stress and become the focus for the majority of clinical manifestations. The site of canal stenosis is characteristically immediately below or above the fusion coexisting with degenerative osteophytic encroachment. In C2–3 block vertebrae, transverse ligament degeneration can produce atlantoaxial instability and cord compression (Barucha and Dastur, 1964; Holmes and Hall, 1978).

Imaging features

The fused vertebral bodies are small in their sagittal dimensions with the anterior surface notably concave near the site of the vestigial intervertebral disc (wasp waist or hourglass deformity) and this is the most reliable sign of congenital fusion (Brown *et al.*, 1964; Dolan, 1977; O'Connor *et al.*, 1991; Nguyen and Tyrrel, 1993). Immediately adjacent to the fusion site the first mobile vertebral body is often flattened and widened, depending on age. The intervertebral disc within the fusion is frequently calcified (Dussault and Kaye, 1977; Fig. 1.3B). At the immediately adjacent mobile intervertebral disc premature degenerative phenomena can be observed (Fig. 6.12). Judicious use of CT and MRI should assess for disc herniation and spinal stenosis when neurological findings are present.

Klippel–Feil syndrome

Klippel–Feil syndrome consists of a clinical triad of a short webbed neck (pterygium colli), low posterior hairline and reduced cervical motion. The underlying pathological defect is the presence of congenital fusions of multiple vertebrae; this has been considered to be linked to a wide variety of systemic abnormalities including deafness, and heart and genitourinary defects (Gray *et al.*, 1964; Hensinger, 1991). Complicating mechanical and degenerative cervical spine changes are common, including zygapophysial joint dysfunction and arthrosis, disc degeneration, disc herniation and spinal stenosis (Scher, 1979; Born *et al.*, 1988; Leyson, 1988).

Imaging features

The imaging hallmark is the presence of multiple segmentation defects with a short neck. Distinct

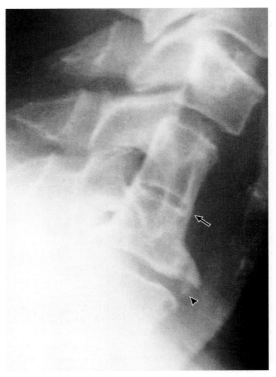

Fig. 6.12 Degenerative disc disease complicating block vertebrae. Congenital synostosis is evident, characterized by hypoplastic vertebral bodies and a vestigial intervertebral disc (arrow). At the disc space immediately below, observe the advanced degenerative disc disease with an anterior osteophyte and loss of disc height (arrowhead).

Comment: Complicating degenerative syndromes are common in the presence of block vertebrae and usually occur in immediately adjacent segments due to increased biomechanical loads. A spectrum of clinical syndromes can emanate from degenerative changes involving at least six possible anatomical structures, e.g. posterior joint degenerative changes, intervertebral joint degenerative changes, spinal canal stenosis, intervertebral canal stenosis, various soft-tissue injuries (such as ligamentous and muscular) and altered vertebrobasilar blood flow.

neurological compression syndromes secondary to degenerative disc and zygapophysial joint disease can produce radiculopathy and, in severe cases, myelopathy, which is best imaged with MRI (Ritterbusch *et al.*, 1991). A rare complication includes sudden catastrophic quadriplegia due to minor trauma causing dislocation at unfused levels (Elster, 1984; Born *et al.*, 1988; O'Connor *et al.*, 1991). Klippel–Feil syndrome patients most at risk for compressive degenerative lesions are those with extensive multilevel fusion, an abnormal cervico-occipital junction, occipitalization with a block vertebra at C2–3, and a single open interspace in an otherwise fused cervical spine (Nagib *et al.,* 1984). MRI may show an associated Chiari malformation where there is cerebellar herniation through the foramen magnum.

Occipitalization

Occipitalization is a congenital synostosis of varying degrees between the atlas and occiput (O'Connor *et al.,* 1991). Partial occipitalization (hemi-occipitalization). is more common, especially of the anterior arch. A wide range of clinical presentations exist, although the majority are asymptomatic and are identified incidentally on radiographic examination (Harcourt and Mitchell, 1990).

Imaging features

Conventional imaging shows the anomaly well. On the frontal view there is overlap of the occipital structures with the upper cervical complex (McRae and Barnum, 1953). Various structures will be fused to the skull, including articulations and transverse processes. The atlantoaxial joint planes are frequently asymmetrical and odontoid anomalies are common (McRae, 1953; Wackenheim, 1974; Hensinger, 1991).

The lateral view demonstrates varying degrees of atlas fusion, invagination and adjacent vertebral anomalies. In flexion, the posterior arch does not separate from the occiput. Up to 50% of occipitalizations will demonstrate atlantoaxial instability (McRae, 1953; Hinck *et al.,* 1961; Hensinger, 1991). Up to 70% of occipitalizations show a complete block vertebra at C2–3 (McRae, 1953; Hensinger, 1991).

CT and MRI clarify anatomical details and establish sites of neurological impingement (Geehr *et al.,* 1977; Malhotra and Leeds, 1984; Lufkin *et al.,* 1988). Vertebral artery angiography in selected patients with appropriate vertebrobasilar territory manifestations may show agenesis, hypoplasia or abnormal endpoints of at least one vessel in up to 25% of occipitalization anomalies (Janeway *et al.,* 1966; Bernini *et al.,* 1969).

Odontoid anomalies

The two most important variations of the odontoid process are a failure to form (agenesis) and non-union (os odontoideum).

Agenesis of the odontoid process

The lack of an odontoid process produces a striking appearance on conventional studies which is unmistakable. On the frontal film no odontoid is visible; a truncated, smooth-surfaced stump projecting above the atlantoaxial joints is most common and is designated as a hypoplastic odontoid process. Lateral

displacement of the atlas provides radiographic evidence of instability due to incompetent alar ligaments. The lateral projection allows assessment of the odontoid height, with less than 12 mm consistent with hypoplasia (McManners, 1983).

Varying degrees of enlargement and sclerosis of anterior and posterior tubercles of the atlas, as a compensation to atlantoaxial instability, is often seen (Holt *et al.,* 1989). The anterior tubercle rear surface is often rounded. Flexion–extension studies will elucidate the degree of instability present but do not necessarily correlate with the clinical presentation. Atlantoaxial instability often coexists with lateral mass degenerative changes.

Os odontoideum

Os odontoideum is most likely due to post-traumatic non-union of a fractured dens, usually during childhood (Fielding *et al.,* 1980) and frontal radiographs will usually demonstrate a hypoplastic and an adjacent separated ossicle (Hensinger, 1986, 1991). Some lateral displacement is occasionally seen; this can be accentuated on lateral bending. On flexion–extension the ossicle can be seen to move through an arc as it slides over the odontoid stump. Very rarely, fusion of the ossicle to the atlas ring may occur but this is only defined by CT examination (Hensinger, 1986). The atlas anterior arch is often enlarged and sclerotic and is a useful sign to exclude an acute fracture (Holt *et al.,* 1989; Hensinger, 1991). The posterior surface of the anterior arch may be round or even angular adjacent to the separating cleft.

Degenerative changes can occur at the non-union site with osteophytes and sclerosis. Most commonly there is thickening of the anteriorly sited ligaments which combine with the advancing posterior arch to create compromise of the central canal (Stratford, 1957), which can best be evaluated with MR imaging. CT and MRI are best performed in flexion to assess the degree of cord compression (Roach *et al.,* 1984).

Diffuse idiopathic skeletal hyperostosis

Diffuse idiopathic skeletal hyperostosis (DISH) is the second most common degenerative spinal disorder affecting as many as 12% of people beyond middle age (Resnick *et al.,* 1978a). DISH is a generalized spinal and extraspinal articular disorder which is characterized by ligamentous calcification and ossification, predominantly the anterior longitudinal ligament. DISH has been described by various names, including spondylosis hyperostotica, spondylitis ossificans ligamentosa, senile ankylosing hyperostosis and Forrestier's disease, as well as others (Rowe and Yochum, 1996b).

DISH is characterized clinically by its broad spectrum of presentations from asymptomatic to complaints of spinal stiffness and low-grade musculoskeletal pain. Up to 20% of individuals may experience dysphagia due to anterior proliferative bone growths from the cervical spine, or oesophageal obstruction due to anterior bone growths from the thoracic spine compressing the adjacent oesophagus (Resnick *et al.*, 1978a; Underberg-Davis and Levine, 1991). Removal of the offending bony plaques can be followed by regrowth within years (Suzuki *et al.*, 1991). There is an association with adult onset of diabetes mellitus in up to 13–32% (Julkunen *et al.*, 1966, 1971).

Imaging features

Conventional imaging

The radiographic hallmarks of DISH consist of exuberant hyperostosis from the anterior vertebral body margins which usually bridge the intervening disc spaces (Fig. 6.13). Definitive criteria for the diagnosis of DISH include four or more contiguous vertebrae involved with anterior hyperostosis, relative preservation of intervertebral disc height and an absence of zygapophysial joint ankylosis (Resnick *et al.*, 1975). The bony hyperostosis is most frequent and most exuberant in the lower segments (C4–7), usually beginning from the anteroinferior vertebral body margin and extending downwards, tapering at its distal extent. The thickness of this anterior hyperostosis may be over 1 cm and it is thicker at mobile levels and thinner at immobile levels (Suzuki *et al.*, 1991). Frequently the deep fibres of the anterior longitudinal ligament are the last to ossify; this produces a distinctive radiolucent zone of separation from the vertebral body (Resnick *et al.*, 1978a).

Horizontal radiolucent linear clefts due to anterior discal extrusions should not be confused with fractures or pseudarthroses. Ossification within the posterior longitudinal ligament (OPLL) can occasionally be observed (Goldwin, 1979). Despite the radiographic evidence of segmental ankylosis, paradoxically, the vertebral motion may be remarkably unaffected, most likely relative to the articular sparing of the zygapophysial joints.

Complicating fractures can occur through the ankylosing new bone, most commonly at C5–7 with severe neurological sequelae, including quadriplegia (Yagan and Karlins, 1986). In cases of fused lower segments, atlantoaxial instability rarely occurs (Chiba *et al.*, 1992). Additionally, fractures of adjacent uninvolved segments, such as odontoid fractures, may be seen with no effect on those involved with DISH (Fardon, 1978).

Additional imaging

CT and MRI are useful in defining coexisting spinal stenosis due to ossification of the posterior longitud-

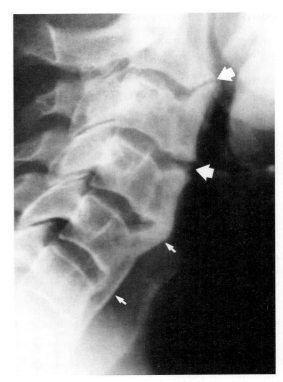

Fig. 6.13 Diffuse idiopathic skeletal hyperostosis (DISH). The radiographic hallmark of DISH is the exuberant hyperostosis from the anterior vertebral body margins bridging the intervening disc spaces (arrows). Horizontal radiolucent linear clefts due to anterior discal extrusions should not be confused with fractures or pseudarthroses (arrowheads).

Comment: Definitive criteria for the diagnosis of DISH include four or more contiguous vertebrae involved with anterior hyperostosis, relative preservation of intervertebral disc height and an absence of zygapophysial joint ankylosis. Despite the radiographic evidence of segmental ankylosis, paradoxically, the vertebral motion may be remarkably unaffected.

inal ligament (Ono *et al.*, 1977), hypertrophic posterior osteophytes (Alengat *et al.*, 1982) or ligamentum flavum hypertrophy (Kopman *et al.*, 1982).

Ligamentous ossifications

Ossifications within ligaments of the cervical spine are commonly observed radiographic findings, often with no clinical implications. These include ponticles of the atlas, stylohyoid ligament, nuchal bones, discal calcifications and ossification of the posterior longitudinal ligament.

Ponticles of the atlas

Calcification within the borders of the posterior oblique occipital membrane surrounding the vertebral arteries as they course adjacent to the lateral masses of the atlas have been referred to as ponticles, of which there are two, lateral and posterior (Buna *et al.*, 1984). The lateral ponticle is seen on frontal upper cervical radiographs as a curvilinear calcification extending from the upper lateral mass of the atlas toward the transverse process.

A posterior ponticle (pons posticus, retroarticular process) occurs in up to 15% of the population and is demonstrated on lateral radiographs. It may exist as an incomplete hook-like process (Kimmerle's anomaly), or as a complete bridge forming a distinct circular opening (arcual foramen; Kohler and Zimmer, 1968). The clinical significance of this finding remains in conjecture, though its common occurrence supports the contention that it plays no role. However, it has been suggested that it represents a risk factor for manipulation-induced vertebral artery dissection (Gatterman, 1981; Buna *et al.*, 1984), post-traumatic subarachnoid haemorrhage (Gross, 1990) and Barre–Lieou syndrome.

Nuchal ligament

Focal ossification within the ligamentum nuchae (nuchal bone) is a common age-related finding, the incidence increasing with age, and it is of doubtful clinical significance. The most common location is within the interspinous spaces from C4 to C7 (Kohler and Zimmer, 1968). Ossification is usually ovoid with the long axis orientated vertically and it exhibits a distinct cortical shell. Differentiation from an un-united secondary ossification centre and fracture of the spinous process (clay shoveller's fracture) should be made (Rowe, 1987).

Anulus fibrosus

Calcification within the outer anular fibres of the cervical disc is a very common finding noted in up to 70% of autopsies (Schmorl and Junghanns, 1971). Pathologically, hydroxyapatite crystals are deposited within degenerative anular fibres and they are often associated with a loss of disc height and have been called intercallary bones (Fig. 6.1). Radiographically these are most commonly seen at the C5 or C6 level at the anterior discal surface as a 1–2 mm thick linear density, usually not attached to the adjacent vertebral body margins.

Nucleus pulposus

Calcification within a cervical nucleus pulposus is uncommon, in contrast to the thoracic and lumbar spines. It is encountered in DDD, herniated disc, block vertebrae, in an idiopathic form and occasionally as part of a biochemical metabolic defect (Rowe and Yochum, 1996b).

Degenerative disc calcification within the nucleus is best seen on CT as a central conglomerate opacity or as fragmented dispersed densities. On CT, herniated discs may be seen to contain calcium and this dates the lesion as being of at least 6 months. The vestigial disc space between a congenital block vertebra is commonly observed to have calcified but this is considered to be of no significance. Idiopathic forms of disc calcification are most significant in children where, between the ages of 6 and 12 years, a painful neck, sometimes with torticollis and fever, can occur, with radiographs demonstrating dense nucleus pulposus calcification (Rowe and Yochum, 1996b; Fig. 6.14). Rarely, metabolic disorders such as gout, pseudogout, ochronosis and even hyperparathyroidism can underlie the calcification.

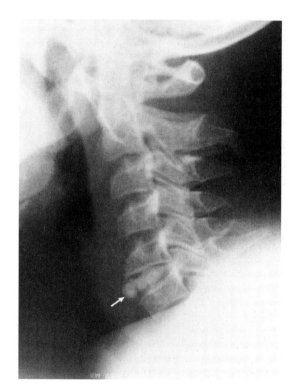

Fig. 6.14 Idiopathic nucleus pulposus calcification in children. Dense calcification can be seen within the C5–6 disc space (arrow).

Comment: Idiopathic calcification is a perplexing childhood condition typically presenting between the ages of 6 and 12 years with a painful neck, sometimes with torticollis and fever. As symptoms abate, so will the calcification, the only sequelae being slightly flattened adjacent vertebral bodies.

Stylohyoid ligament

The stylohyoid ligament traverses the soft tissues of the lateral aspect of the neck, between the styloid process and the hyoid bone, acting as a suspensory ligament. Ossification to varying degrees is common, especially with advancing age, and is occasionally seen to coexist with DISH. Symptoms associated with stylohyoid ligament ossification are very uncommon (Bolton, 1987). Pain in the pharynx, painful deglutition and referred otalgia, often initiated after tonsillectomy, and associated with elongation of the styloid process more than 2.5 cm due to ossification of the stylohyoid ligament, have been referred to as Eagle's syndrome (Eagle, 1949).

Conventional lateral radiographs show a band of ossification of variable length running obliquely from the skull base immediately anterior to the auditory meatus towards the hyoid bone. Union with the hyoid bone is typically at the lesser cornu (Fig. 6.15). Frontal views depict the ossification similarly as an oblique linear density originating just medial to the mastoid process and sloping medially. The bony mass often has a distinct shell of cortical bone, though some specimens are internally featureless. Most are thick, with diameters up to 1 cm and are of variable length. Complete ossification along its entire length is usually interrupted with linear lucencies and bulbous ends simulating pseudoarticulations (Mueller *et al.*, 1983; Bolton, 1987).

Posterior longitudinal ligament

Ossified posterior longitudinal ligament (OPLL) is an uncommon degenerative disorder of the spine characterized by thick bone formation within the

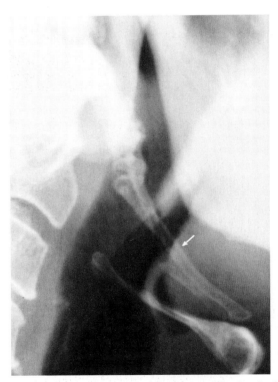

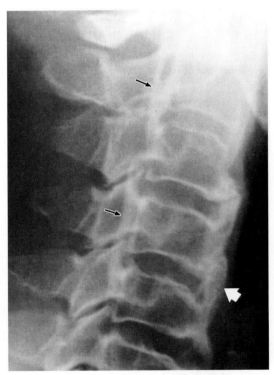

Fig. 6.15 Stylohyoid ligament ossification. The band of ossification within the ligament extends obliquely towards the hyoid bone (arrow). Along its length linear lucencies and adjacent bulbous ends mark pseudoarticulations (arrow).

Comment: Such calcification, of variable length, is commonly observed within the ligament and is usually of no clinical significance. Pain in the pharynx, painful deglutiltion and referred otalgia, often initiated after tonsillectomy, and associated with elongation of the styloid process more than 2.5 cm due to ossification of the stylohyoid ligament, have been referred to as Eagle's syndrome (Eagle, 1949).

Fig. 6.16 Ossified posterior longitudinal ligament (OPLL) syndrome. The characteristic dense bone within the ligament is depicted as a linear radiopaque strip of 1–5 mm thickness paralleling the posterior vertebral body margins (arrows). Note how it remains separate from the vertebral bodies. There is coexisting diffuse idiopathic skeletal hyperostosis (DISH) anteriorly (white arrow).

Comment: The length of this ossification may be only one vertebral body height or it may traverse a number of contiguous segments. Compression myelopathy can occur from the ossification. DISH may be present in up to 85% of OPLL patients.

posterior longitudinal ligament of the spine (Tsuki-moto, 1960; Terayama *et al.*, 1964). Known associations include diffuse idiopathic skeletal hyperostosis and an inherent predisposition for such to occur in the Japanese population (Japanese disease; Resnick *et al.*, 1978b). The most common location for OPLL to occur is in the cervical spine, followed by the thoracic and lumbar spines.

Many cases are asymptomatic although, when OPLL is present in the cervical spine, the incidence of symptoms is higher. Pain is conspicuously absent as progressive myelopathy develops with disturbed gait and increasing tactile disturbances. Clinical stigmata are usually manifest when the ossification occupies more than 60% of the spinal canal. Spinal cord changes in OPLL consist of compression-related abnormalities such as flattening, grey matter infarction and demyelination of the posterior and lateral white columns (Hirabayashi *et al.*, 1981).

On conventional lateral radiographs the characteristic dense bone within the ligament is depicted as a linear radiopaque strip of 1–5 mm thickness paralleling with the posterior vertebral body margins (Fig. 6.16). The length of this ossification may be only one vertebral body height or it may traverse a number of contiguous segments. Commonly, a radiolucent zone is interspaced between the ossified ligament and vertebral body corresponding to the unossified deeper ligamentous layers. Tomography is an excellent tool for demonstrating these features. Associated features of DISH may be apparent in up to 85% of patients with exuberant anterior hyperostosis, normal zygapophysial joints and normal intervertebral discs (Hakuda *et al.*, 1983).

On CT, the mineralized ligament is seen as a dense calcific opacity often with a distinct cortical surface surrounding a lucent core of cancellous bone. The zone of OPLL–vertebral body separation is seen clearly and the degree of spinal stenosis can be accurately assessed. MRI may show OPLL as a high-signal-intense (fatty marrow) or hypointense band (fibrous replacement of fatty marrow; Yoshino *et al.*, 1991) and spinal cord changes such as myelomalacia, atrophy and oedema are shown to greater advantage than by any other imaging modality (Yoshino *et al.*, 1991; Russell, 1995).

Calcific tendinitis of the longus colli

A self-limiting, transient, and acutely symptomatic hydroxyapatite deposition can occur at the supero-lateral group of longus colli tendons as they insert

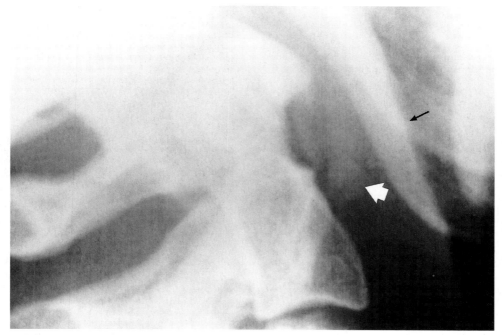

Fig. 6.17 Calcification of the longus colli. There is swelling of the retropharyngeal soft tissues anterior to the atlas (arrow). There is also very faint calcification within these soft tissues (white arrow).

Comment: The clinical syndrome of rapid onset over 2–5 days of a painful stiff neck, muscle spasm, painful dysphagia and a sense of globus hystericus is due to the deposition of hydroxyapatite crystals in the superolateral group of longus colli tendons as they insert anterior to the C2 and C3 vertebral bodies. Symptomatically, resolution occurs spontaneously over the next few weeks.

anterior to the C2 and C3 vertebral bodies (Haun, 1978; Newmark *et al.,* 1978). Symptomatically, the patient complains of a rapid onset over 2–5 days of a painful stiff neck, muscle spasm, painful dysphagia and a sense of globus hystericus (Bernstein, 1964) but recovery occurs spontaneously over the following 1–2 weeks.

A lateral radiograph or CT is diagnostic in the symptomatic phase, demonstrating an amorphous calcification up to 2 cm in diameter anterior and inferior to the anterior tubercle of the atlas within the retropharyngeal soft tissues (Haun, 1978; Newmark *et al.,* 1978; Fahlgren, 1988). The retropharyngeal interspace is often increased locally more than 7 mm (Fig. 6.17) and, on MRI T2-weighted imaging, the superior portion of the longus colli is of high signal intensity, corresponding to oedema (Artenian *et al.,* 1989). Symptoms subside in concert with resorption of the prevertebral calcification and swelling and no complications are expected (Hartley, 1964; Sutro, 1967).

References

Alengat, J., Hallet, M., Kido, D. (1982) Spinal cord compression in diffuse idiopathic skeletal hyperostosis. *Radiology* **142:** 119–132.

Artenian, D.J., Lipman, J.K., Scidmore, G.K., Brant-Zawadzki, M. (1989) Acute neck pain due to tendinitis of the longus colli: CT and MRI findings. *Neuroradiology* **31:** 166–174.

Baleriaux, D., Noterman, J., Ticket, L. (1983) Recognition of cervical soft disk herniation by contrast enhanced CT. *A.J.N.R.* **4:** 607–608.

Barucha, E.P., Dastur, H.M. (1964) Craniovertebral anomalies. A report on 40 cases. *Brain* **87:** 469–481.

Batzdorf, U., Batzdorf, A. (1988) Analysis of cervical spine curvature in patients with cervical spondylosis. *Neurosurgery* **22:** 827–836.

Bell, G.R., Ross, J.S. (1992) Diagnosis of nerve root compression. Myelography, computed tomography, and MRI. *Orthop. Clin. North Am.* **23:** 405–419.

Benitah, S., Raftopoulos, C., Baleriaux, D. *et al.* (1994) Upper cervical spinal cord compression due to bony stenosis of the spinal canal. *Neuroradiology* **36:** 231–233.

Bernado, K.L., Grubb, R.L., Coxe, W.S., Roper, C.L. (1988) Anterior cervical disc herniation. *J. Neurosurg.* **69:** 134–136.

Bernini, F.P., Elefante, R., Smaltino, F., Tedeschi, G. (1969) Angiographic study of the vertebral artery in cases of deformity of the occipito-cervical joint. *A.J.R.* **107:** 526–532.

Berns, D.H., Ross, J.S., Kormos, D., Modic, M.T. (1991) The spinal vacuum phenomenon: evaluation by gradient echo MR imaging. *J. Comput. Assist. Tomogr.* **15:** 233–236.

Bernstein, S.A. (1964) Acute cervical pain associated with soft-tissue calcium deposition anterior to the interspace of the first and second cervical vertebrae. *J. Bone Joint Surg. (Am.)* **37:** 426–432.

Bland, J., Boushey, D.R. (1990) Anatomy and physiology of the cervical spine. *Semin. Arthr. Rheum.* **20:** 1–20.

Boden, S.D., McCowin, P.R., Davis, D.O. *et al.* (1990a) Abnormal magnetic resonance scans of the cervical spine in asymptomatic subjects. *J. Bone Joint Surg. (Am.)* **72:** 1178–1184.

Boden, S.D., Davis, D.O., Dina, T.S. *et al.* (1990b) Abnormal magnetic resonance scans of the lumbar spine in asymptomatic subjects. A prospective investigation. *J Bone Joint Surg. (Am.)* **72:** 403–408.

Bogduk, N., Marsland, A. (1986) On the concept of third occipital headache. *J. Neurol. Neurosurg. Psychiatry* **49:** 775–780.

Bohrer, S.P., Chen, Y.M. (1988) Cervical spine annulus vacuum. *Skeletal Radiol.* **17:** 324–329.

Bolton, S.P. (1987) Elongated styloid process of the temporal bone. *J. Aust. Chir. Assoc.* **17:** 69–70.

Born, C.T., Petrik, M., Freed, M., Delong, W.G. (1988) Cerebrovascular accident complicating Klippel–Feil syndrome. *J. Bone Joint Surg. (Am.)* **70:** 1412–1415.

Brown, M.W., Templeton, A.W., Hodges, F.J. (1964) The incidence of acquired and congenital fusions in the cervical spine. *A.J.R.* **92:** 1255–1259.

Brown, B.M., Schwartz, R.H., Frank, E. *et al.* (1988) Preoperative evaluation of cervical radiculopathy and myelopathy by surface-coil MR imaging. *A.J.N.R.* **9:** 859–866.

Buna, M., Coghlan, W., deGruchy, M. *et al.* (1984) Ponticles of the atlas: a review and clinical perspective. *J. Manip. Physiol. Ther.* **7:** 261–269.

Busch, E., Wilson, P.R. (1989) Atlanto-occipital and atlanto-axial injections in the treatment of headache and neck pain. *Reg. Anesth.* **14:** 45.

Chiba, H., Annen, S., Shimada, T., Imura, S. (1992) Atlanto-axial subluxation complicated by diffuse idiopathic skeletal hyperostosis. *Spine* **17:** 1414–1417.

Curylo, L.J., Lindsey, R.W., Doherty, B.J., LeBlanc, A. (1996) Segmental variations of bone mineral density in the cervical spine. *Spine* **21:** 319–322.

Daffner, R.H., Deeb, Z.L., Rothfus, W.E. (1986) Pseudo-fractures of the cervical vertebral body. *Skeletal Radiol.* **15:** 295–298.

Davis, S.J., Teresi, L.M., Bradley, W.J. *et al.* (1991) Cervical spine hyperextension injuries: MR findings. *Radiology* **180:** 245–251.

Dillin, W., Booth, R., Cuckler, J. *et al.* (1986) Cervical radiculopathy: a review. *Spine* **11:** 988–991.

Dolan, K.D. (1977) Developmental abnormalities of the cervical spine below the axis. *Radiol. Clin. North Am.* **15:** 167–174.

Dreyfus, P., Michaelson, M., Fletcher, D. (1994) Atlanto-occipital and lateral atlanto-axial joint pain patterns. *Spine* **19:** 1125–1131.

Dunsker, S. (1981) *Cervical Spondylosis. Seminars in Neurosurgery.* New York: Raven Press.

Dussault, R.G., Kaye, J.J. (1977) Intervertebral disc calcification associated with spine fusion. *Radiology* **125:** 57–65.

Eagle, W.W. (1949) Symptomatic elongated styloid process. *Arch. Otolaryngol.* **49:** 490–503.

Edwards, W.C., LaRocca, H. (1985) The developmental sagittal diameter of the cervical spinal canal in patients with cervical spondylosis. *Spine* **10:** 42–49.

Eideken, J., Pitt, M. (1971) The radiologic diagnosis of disc disease. *Orthop. Clin. North Am.* **2:** 405–417.

Elster, A.D. (1984) Quadraplegia after minor trauma in the Klippel–Feil syndrome. *J. Bone Joint Surg. (Am.)* **66**: 1473–1474.

Elster, A.D., Jensen, K.M. (1984) Vacuum pheneomenon within the cervical spinal canal: CT demonstration of a herniated disc. *J. Comput. Assist. Tomogr.* **8**: 533–535.

Evans, W.A. (1932) Abnormalities of the vertebral body. *A.J.R.* **27**: 801–805.

Fahlgren, H. (1988) Retropharyngeal tendinitis: three probable cases with an unusually low epicentre. *Cephalgia* **8**: 105–112.

Fardon, D.F. (1978) Odontoid fracture complicating ankylosing hyperostosis of the spine. *Spine* **3**: 108–112.

Fielding, J.W., Hensinger, R.N., Hawkins, R.J. (1980) Os odontoideum. *J. Bone Joint Surg.* **62A**: 376.

Gatterman, M.I. (1981) Contraindications and complications of spinal manipulative technique. *ACA J. Chiro.* **15**: 75–82.

Geehr, R.B., Rothman, L.G., Kier, E.L. (1977) The role of computered tomography in the evaluation of the upper cervical spine pathology. *Comput. Tomogr.* **2**: 79–84.

Genez, B.M., Willis, J.J., Lowrey, C.E. *et al.* (1990) CT findings of degenerative arthritis of the atlanto-odontoid joint. *A.J.R.* **154**: 315–318.

Goldwin, R.L. (1979) Calcified plaque in the cervical spine with pain and paresthesia. *J.A.M.A.* **241**: 601–602.

Gore, D.R., Sepic, G.R., Garner, G.M. *et al.* (1986) Roentgenographic findings of the cervical spine in asymptomatic people. *Spine* **6**: 521–526.

Gore, D.R., Sepic, G.R., Garner, G.M. *et al.* (1987) Neck pain: a long term follow-up study of 205 patients. *Spine* **12**: 1–5.

Gray, S.W., Romaine, C.B., Skanaalakis, J.E. (1964) Congenital fusion of cervical vertebrae. *Surg. Gynecol. Obstet.* **118**: 373–385.

Gross, A. (1990) Traumatic basal subarachnoid haemmorhages: autopsy material analysis. *Forensic Sci. Int.* **45**: 53–68.

Grunshaw, N.D., Carey, B.M. (1994) Case report: gas within a cervical vertebral body. *Clin. Radiol.* **49**: 653–654.

Hakuda, S., Mochizuki, T., Ogata, M. *et al.* (1983) The pattern of spinal and extraspinal hyperostosis in patients with ossification of the longitudinal ligament and the ligamentum flavum causing myelopathy. *Skeletal Radiol.* **10**: 79–85.

Halla, J.T., Hardin, J.G. (1987) Atlantoaxial (C1–C2) facet joint osteoarthritis: a distinctive clinical syndrome. *Arthr. Rheum.* **30**: 577–582.

Harata, S., Tohno, S., Kawagishi, T. (1981) Osteoarthritis of the atlanto-axial joint. *Int. Orthop.* **5**: 277–282.

Harcourt, B.T., Mitchell, T.C. (1990) Occipitalization of the atlas. Review of the literature. *J. Manip. Physiol. Ther.* **13**: 532–538.

Hartley, J. (1964) Acute cervical pain associated with retropharyngeal calcium deposit. *J. Bone Joint Surg. (Am.)* **46**: 1753–1759.

Haughton, V.M. (1995) Anatomy of the cervical spine. *Neuroimag. Clin. North Am.* **5**: 309–327.

Haun, C.L. (1978) Retropharyngeal tendinitis. *A.J.R.* **130**: 1137–1143.

Heller, J.G. (1992) The syndromes of degenerative cervical disease. *Orthop. Clin. North Am.* **23**: 381–394.

Heller, A.C., Stanley, P., Lewis-Jones, B. *et al.* (1983) Value of x-ray examinations of the cervical spine. *Br. Med. J.* **287**: 1276–1278.

Hensinger, R.N. (1986) Osseous anomalies of the craniovertebral junction. *Spine* **11**: 323–327.

Hensinger, R.N. (1991) Congenital anomalies of the cervical spine. *Clin. Orthop. Rel. Res.* **264**: 16–38.

Hinck, V.C., Hopkins, C.E., Savara, B.S. (1961) Diagnostic criteria of basilar impression. *Radiology* **76**: 572–582.

Hirabayashi, K., Miyakawa, J., Satomi, K. *et al.* (1981) Operative results and post operative progression of ossification among patients with ossification of cervical posterior longitudinal ligament. *Spine* **6**: 354–360.

Hohl, M. (1974) Soft tissue injuries of the neck in automobile accidents. *J. Bone Joint Surg. (Am.)* **56**: 1675–1681.

Holmes, J.C., Hall, J.E. (1978) Fusion for instability and potential instability of the cervical spine in children and adolescents. *Orthop. Clin. North Am.* **9**: 923–930.

Holt, R.G., Helms, C.A., Munk, P.L., Gillespy, T. (1989) Hypertrophy of C1 anterior arch: useful sign to distinguish os odontoideum from acute dens fracture. *Radiology* **173**: 207–209.

Irvine, D.H., Forster, J.B., Newell, D.J. *et al.* (1965) Prevalence of cervical spondylosis in a general practice. *Lancet* **1**: 1089–1091.

Janeway, R., Toole, J.F., Leinbach, L.B., Miller, H.S. (1966) Vertebral artery obstruction with basilar impression. *Arch. Neurol.* **15**: 211–214.

Julkunen, H., Karava, R., Biljannen, V. (1966) Hyperostosis of the spine in diabetes mellitus and acromegaly. *Diabetologia* **2**: 123–126.

Julkunen, H., Heinonen, O., Pyorala, K. (1971) Hyperostosis of the spine in an adult population. Its relation to hyperglycemia and obesity. *Ann. Rheum. Dis.* **30**: 605–615.

Kelsey, J.L., Githens, P.B., Walter, S.D. *et al.* (1984) An epidemiological study of acute prolapsed cervical intervertebral disc. *J. Bone Joint Surg. (Am.)* **66**: 907–914.

Kohler, A., Zimmer, E.A. (1968) In: *Borderlands of the Normal and Early Pathologic in Skeletal Roentgenology,* 3rd edn (Wilk, S.P., ed.). New York: Grune & Stratton.

Kokubun, S., Sakurai, M., Tanaka, Y. (1996) Cartilaginous endplate in cervical disc herniation. *Spine* **21**: 190–195.

Kondo, K., Molgaard, C.A., Kurland, L.T., Onofrio, B.M. (1981) Protruded intervertebral cervical disc: incidence and affected cervical level in Rochester, Minnesota, 1950 through 1974. *Minn. Med.* **64**: 751–753.

Kopman, R., Weinstein, P., Gall, E. *et al.* (1982) Lumbar spinal stenosis in a patient with diffuse idiopathic skeletal hypertrophy syndrome. *Spine* **7**: 598–606.

Lambert, J.R., Tepperman, P.S., Jiminez, J., Newman, A. (1981) Cervical spine disease and dysphagia. Four new cases and a review of the literature. *Am. J. Gastroenterol.* **76**: 35–40.

Lang, P., Chafetz, N., Genant, H.K., Morris, J.M. (1990) Lumbar spinal fusion: assessment of functional stability with magnetic resonance imaging. *Spine* **15**: 581–588.

Larsson, E.M., Holtas, S., Cronqvist, S. *et al.* (1989) Comparison of myelography, CT myelography and magnetic resonance imaging in cervical spondylosis and disc herniation: pre- and postoperative findings. *Acta Radiol.* **30**: 233–239.

Laufer, L., Schulman, H., Hertzanu, Y. (1996) Vertebral pneumatocyst. A case report. *Spine* **21**: 389–391.

Lee, C., Woodring, J.H., Rogers, L.F., Kim, K.S. (1986) The radiographic distinction of degenerative slippage (spondylolisthesis and retrolisthesis) from traumatic slippage of the cervical spine. *Skeletal Radiol.* **15**: 439–443.

Lehto, I.J., Tertti, M.O., Komu, M.E. *et al.* (1994) Age-related MRI changes at 0.1T in cervical discs of asymptomatic subjects. *Neuroradiology* **36**: 49-53.

Leyson, S.M.D. (1988) The Klippel-Feil syndrome: a congenital abnormality of the cervical spine. *Eur. J. Chiro.* **36**: 32-39.

Lufkin, R.B., Vinueta, F., Bentson, J.R. *et al.* (1988) Magnetic resonance imaging of the craniocervical junction. *Comp. Med. Imag. Graph.* **12**: 281-289.

McManners, T. (1983) Odontoid hypoplasia. *Br. J. Radiol.* **56**: 907-910.

MacNab, I. (1975) Cervical spondylosis. *Clin. Orthop.* **109**: 69-77.

McRae, D.L. (1953) Bony abnormalities in the region of the foramen magnum: correlation of the anatomic and neurologic findings. *Acta Radiol.* **40**: 335-354.

McRae, D.L., Barnum, A.S. (1953) Occipitalization of the atlas. *A.J.R.* **70:** 23-26.

Maigne, J.Y., Deligne, L. (1994) Computed tomographic followup study of 21 cases of non operatively treated cervical intervertebral soft disc herniation. *Spine* **19**: 189-191.

Maimaris, C., Barnes, M.R., Allen, M.J. (1988) "Whiplash injuries" of the neck: a retrospective study. *Injury* **19**: 393-396.

Malghem, J., Maldague, B., Labaisse, M.A. *et al.* (1993) Intravertebral vacuum cleft: changes in content after supine positioning. *Radiology* **187**: 483-487.

Malhotra, V., Leeds, N.E. (1984) Case report 277: occipitalization of the atlas with severe cord compression. *Skeletal Radiol.* **12**: 55-57.

Mellstrom, A., Grepe, A., Levander, B. (1980) Atlantoaxial arthrography. A postmortem study. *Neuroradiology* **20**: 135-144.

Mercer, S., Bogduk, N. (1993) Intra-articular inclusions of the cervical synovial joints. *Br. J. Rheumatol.* **32**: 705-710.

Mercer, S.R., Jull, G.A. (1996) Morphology of the cervical intervertebral disc: implications for McKenzie's model of the disc derangement syndrome. *Manual Ther.* **2**: 76-81.

Modic, M.T., Masaryk, T.J., Ross, J.S., Carter, J.R. (1988b) Imaging of degenerative disk disease. *Radiology* **168**: 177-186.

Modic, M.T., Masaryk, T.J., Ross, J.S. *et al.* (1987) Cervical radiculopathy: value of oblique MR imaging. *Radiology* **163**: 227-231.

Modic, M.T., Ross, J.S., Masaryk, T.J. (1989) Imaging of degenerative diseases of the cervical spine. *Clin Orthop* **239**: 109-120.

Modic, M.T., Steinberg, P.M., Ross, J.S. *et al.* (1988a) Degenerative disk disease: assessment of changes in the vertebral body narrow with MR imaging. *Radiology* **166**: 193-199.

Mueller, N., Hamilton, S., Reid, G.D. (1983) Case report 248. *Skeletal Radio.l* **10**: 273-275.

Nagib, M.G., Maxwell, R.E., Chou, S.N. (1984) Identification and management of high risk patients with Klippel-Feil syndrome. *J. Neurosurg.* **61**: 525-530.

Newmark, H. III, Forrester, D.M., Brown, J.C. *et al.* (1978) Calcific tendinitis of the neck. *Radiology* **128**: 355-361.

Nguyen, V.D., Tyrrel, R. (1993) Klippel-Feil syndrome: patterns of bony fusion and wasp-waist sign. *Skeletal Radiol.* **22**: 519-523.

Nijensohn, E., Russell, E.J., Milan, M. *et al.* (1990) Calcified synovial cyst of the cervical spine: CT and MR evaluation. *J. Comput. Assist. Tomogr.* **14**: 473-476.

O'Connor, J.F., Cranley, W.R., McCarten, K.M., Radkowski, M.A. (1991) Radiographic manifestations of congential anomalies of the spine. *Radiol. Clin. North Am.* **29**: 407-414.

Oda, J., Tanaka, H., Tsuuki, N. (1988) Intervertebral disc changes associated with aging of human cervical vertebra. From the neonate to the eighties. *Spine* **13**: 1205-1211.

Oga, M.O., Yuge, I., Terada, K. *et al.* (1996) Tortuosity of the vertebral artery in patients with cervical spondylotic myelopathy. *Spine* **21**: 1085-1089.

Ono, K., Ota, H., Tada, K. *et al.* (1977) Ossified posterior longitudinal ligament. *Spine* **2**: 126-138.

Patel, S., Sanders, W. (1988) Synovial cyst of the cervical spine: case report and review of the literature. *A.J.N.R.* **9**: 602-603.

Penning, L., Wilmink, J.L., van Woerden, H.H. *et al.* (1986) CT myelographic findings in degenerative disorders of the cervical spine; clinical significance. *A.J.R.* **146**: 793-801.

Rahim, K.A., Stambough, J.L. (1992) Radiographic evaluation of the degenerative cervical spine. *Orthop. Clin. North Am.* **23**: 395-403.

Ramsey, J., Bliznak, J. (1971) Klippel-Feil syndrome with renal agenesis and other anomalies. *A.J.R.* **113**: 460-463.

Rao, K.C.V.G., Williams, J.P. (1994) Degenerative disk and vertebral disease. In: *MRI and CT of the Spine* (Rao, K.C.V.G., Williams, J.P., Lee, B.C.P., Sherman, J.L., eds). Baltimore: Williams & Wilkins.

Resnick, D. (1985) Degenerative diseases of the vertebral column. *Radiology* **156**: 3-14.

Resnick, D., Shaul, S.R., Robins, J.M. (1975) Diffuse idiopathic skeletal hyperostosis (DISH): Forrestier's disease with extraspinal manifestations. *Radiology* **115:** 513-524.

Resnick, D., Shapiro, R.F., Wiesner, K.B. *et al.* (1978a) Diffuse idiopathic skeletal hyperostosis (DISH). Ankylosing hyperostosis of Forrestier and Rotes-Querol. *Semin Arthritis Rheum* **7**: 153-187.

Resnick, D., Guerra, J., Robinson, C.A. *et al.* (1978b) Association of diffuse idiopathic skeletal hyperostosis (DISH) and calcification and ossification of the posterior longitudinal ligament. *A.J.R.* **131**: 1049-1056.

Reymond, R.D., Wheeler, P.S., Perovic, M., Block, B. (1972) The lucent cleft; a new radiographic sign of cervical disc injury or disease. *Clin. Radiol.* **23**: 188-192.

Ritterbusch, J.F., McGinty, L.D., Spar, J., Orrison, W.W. (1991) Magnetic resonance imaging for stenosis and subluxation in Klippel-Feil syndrome. *Spine* **16S**: 539-541.

Roach, J.W., Duncan, D., Wenger, D.R., Maravilla, A., Maravilla, K. (1984) Atlantoaxial instability and spinal cord compression in children - diagnosis by computerized tomography. *J. Bone Joint Surg. (Am.)* **66**: 708-715.

Robinson, R.A., Afeiche, N., Dunn, E.J., Northrop, B.E. (1977) Cervical spondylotic myelopathy: Etiology and treatment concepts. *Spine* **2**: 89.

Ross, J.S. (1991) Magnetic resonance assessment of the postoperative spine. Degenerative disc disease. *Radiol. Clin. North Am.* **29**: 793-808.

Ross, J.S., Ruggieri, J.P., Tkach, J.A. *et al.* (1992) Gd-DTPA enhanced 3D MR imaging of cervical degenerative disk disease: initial experience. *A.J.N.R.* **13**: 127-136.

Rowe, L.J. (1987) Clay shoveler's fracture. *ACA J. Chiro.* **21:** 83–86.

Rowe, L.J. (1988) Hemispherical spondylosclerosis. *J. Aust. Chiro. Assoc.* **18:** 55–56.

Rowe, L.J. (1990) The split vertebral body – a pseudo-fracture. *J. Aust. Chiro. Assoc.* **20:** 5–8.

Rowe, L.J., Yochum, T.R. (1996a) Traumatic injuries. In: *Essentials of Skeletal Radiology,* 2nd edn (Yochum, T.R., Rowe, L.J., eds). Baltimore: Williams & Wilkins.

Rowe, L.J., Yochum, T.R. (1996b) Arthritides. In: *Essentials of Skeletal Radiology,* 2nd edn (Yochum, T.R., Rowe, L.J., eds). Baltimore: Williams & Wilkins.

Ruggieri, P.M. (1995) Cervical radiculopathy. *Neuroimag. Clin. North Am.* **5:** 349–366.

Russell, E.J. (1990) Cervical disc disease. *Radiology* **177:** 313–325.

Russell, E.J. (1995) Computed tomography and myelography in the evaluation of cervical degenerative disease. *Neuroimag. Clin. North Am.* **5:** 329–348.

Russell, E.J., D'Angelo, C.M., Zimmerman, R.D. *et al.* (1984) Cervical disc herniation: CT demonstration after contrast enhancement. *Radiology* **152:** 703–712.

Schellas, K.P., Smith, M.D., Gundry, C.R., Pollei, S.R. (1996) Cervical discogenic pain. *Spine* **21:** 300–312.

Scher, A.T. (1979) Cervical spine fusion and the effects of injury. *S. Afr. Med. J.* **56:** 525–527.

Schmorl, G., Junghanns, H. (1971) *The Human Spine in Health and Disease,* 2nd edn. (Besemann, E.F., transl.). New York: Grune & Stratton.

Shore, L. (1935) On osteoarthritis in the dorsal inter-vertebral joint: a study in morbid anatomy. *Br. J. Surg.* **22:** 833–849.

Simon, J.E., Lukin, R.R. (1988) Diskogenic disease of the cervical spine. *Semin. Roentgenol.* **23:** 18–124.

Snow, R.D., Scott, W.R. (1994) Hypertrophic synovitis and osteoarthritis of the cervical facet joint. Report of two cases. *Clin. Imaging* **18:** 56–58.

Star, M.J., Curd, J.G., Thorne, R.P. (1992) Atlantoaxial lateral mass osteoarthritis. *Spine* **17**(suppl): S71–S76.

Stratford, J. (1957) Myelopathy caused by atlanto-axial dislocation. *J. Neurosurg.* **14:** 97–102.

Sutro, C.J. (1967) Calcification of the anterior atlanto-axial ligament as the cause for painful swallowing and for painful neck. *Bull. Hosp. Joint Dis.* **28:** 1–8.

Suzuki, K., Ishida, Y., Ohmori, K. (1991) Long term follow-up of diffuse idiopathic skeletal hyperostosis in the cervical spine. *Neuroradiology* **33:** 427–431.

Terayama, K., Maruyama, S., Miyashita, R. *et al.* (1964) Ossification of the posterior longitudinal ligament in the cervical spine. *Orthop. Surg.* **15:** 1083–1086.

Teresi, L.M., Lufkin, R.B., Reicher, M.A. *et al.* (1987) *Radiology* **164:** 83–88.

Torg, J.S., Pavlov, H., Genuario, S.E. *et al.* (1986) Neuropraxia of the cervical spinal cord with transient quadriplegia. *J. Bone Joint Surg. (Am.)* **68:** 1354–1370.

Toyone, T., Takahashi, K., Kitahara, H. *et al.* (1994) Vertebral bone-marrow changes in degenerative lumbar disc disease. *J. Bone Joint Surg. (Br.)* **76:** 757–764.

Tsukimoto, H. (1960) An autopsy report of syndrome of compression of spinal cord owing to ossification within the spinal canal of cervical spine. *Arch. Jpn Chir.* **29:** 1003–1009.

Underberg-Davis, S., Levine, M.S. (1991) Giant thoracic osteophyte causing oesophageal food impaction. *A.J.R.* **157:** 319–320.

von Luschka, H. (1850) *Die Nerven des menschlichen Wirbelkanales.* Tubingen: Laupp and Siebeck.

Von Torklus, D., Gehle, W. (1972) *The Upper Cervical Spine* (Michaelis, L.S., transl.). London: Butterworths, pp. 64–67.

Wackenheim, A. (1974) *Roentgen Diagnosis of the Craniovertebral Region.* New York: Springer-Verlag, p. 360.

Watkinson, A., Gargan, M.F., Bannister, G.C. (1991) Prognostic factors in soft tissue injuries of the cervical spine. *Injury* **22:** 307–310.

Whitecloud, T.S. III, Seago, R.A. (1987) Cervical discogenic syndrome: results of surgical intervention in patients with positive discography. *Spine* **12:** 313–316.

Wilson, D.W., Pezzuti, R.T., Place, J.N. (1991) Magnetic resonance imaging in the preoperative evaluation of cervical radiculopathy. *Neurosurgery* **28:** 175–179.

Yagan, R., Karlins, N. (1986) Quadriplegia in diffuse idiopathic skeletal hyperostosis after minor trauma. *A.J.R.* **147:** 858–859.

Yoshino, M.T., Seeger, J.F., Carmody, R.F. (1991) MRI diagnosis of thoracic ossification of posterior longitudinal ligament with concomitant disc herniation. *Neuroradiology* **33:** 455–458.

Yu, Y.L., Stevens, J.M., Kendall, B., du Boulay, G.H. (1983) Cord shape and measurements in cervical spondylotic myelopathy. *A.J.N.R.* **4:** 607–608.

Yu, S., Sether, L.A., Haughton, V.M. (1987) Facet joint menisci of the cervical spine: correlative MR imaging and cryomicrotomy study. *Radiology* **164:** 79–82.

7

Medical management of neck pain of mechanical origin

R. Cailliet

Examination

When a patient presents with a complaint of neck pain, or pain considered to evolve from the neck, a meaningful history and examination are mandatory.

The examination is the attempt of the examiner to determine the structural, physiological (neurological, orthopaedic, vascular and psychological) aspects of the impairment. The disability claimed must be ascertained by determining the impairment responsible.

Observation of the patient determines the limitations of motion in activities of daily living such as posture, movement, grimacing and restrictions. Observations also denote the malalignment of the body structures in stance, assuming sitting and lying. These are the major components elicited in evaluating the postural components of motion.

Active and passive methods of examination

Bony and soft-tissue palpation

The patient's neck can be palpated in the supine, seated or standing position. In the supine position the neck muscles and the effects of gravity are eliminated (McKeever, 1968). The following major bony structures are palpable:

1. Spinous processes: transverse and posterior.
2. Zygapophysial joints.
3. Mastoid processes.

The following soft tissues are palpable:

1. Muscles – accomplished by the active participation of the patient in initiating specific movements while the examiner palpates the involved muscles.
2. Ligaments.
3. Nerves.

Subjectivity of impaired nerve function is elicited from the history with symptoms such as tingling, pain and/or numbness alluding to their dermatomal area. Sensitivity is noted from direct pressure upon the precise nerve root dermatome.

Nerve function

1. *Motor:* testing by participation of the patient in performing specific motion and determining appropriate muscular activity, thereby ascertaining the muscles' appropriate nerve supply. The maximum effort expended by the patient must be ascertained.
2. *Sensory:* determining the dermatomal areas subjectively and confirming objectivity by various modalities such as touch, cotton swab, pinprick or scratch, tuning fork and position sense test. This is subjective and the examiner must determine its organic basis.
3. *Reflexes:* including the triceps, biceps, brachialis and brachioradialis. Hoffmann's test may indicate upper motor neuron pathology.

Range of motion

Range of motion testing reveals the integrity of anatomical joint structures and function; this is tested

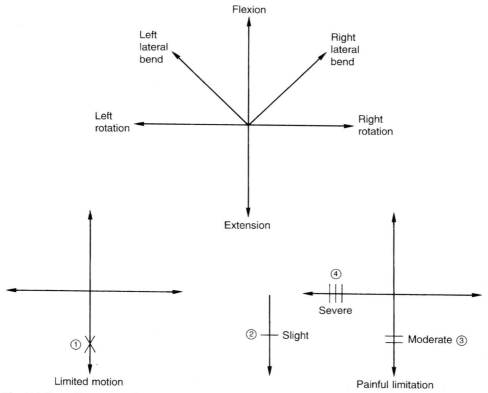

Fig. 7.1 Recording range of motion. The upper drawing is the composite record of range of motion. (1) × indicates mere limitation of range of motion in extension without pain; (2) slight pain and limitation in extension; (3) moderate pain and extension limitation; (4) severe pain and limitation in left rotation.

actively and passively. Actively implies testing motions performed actively by the patient upon observation and from instructions. In testing ranges of motion of the cervical spine the following motions are requested and observed (Fig. 7.1).

Passively testing range of motion measures motion performed by the examiner on the patient by movement of the head and neck involving each individual vertebral segment (Fig. 7.2).

Upper cervical examination

Upper cervical motion tests flexion of the head, extension, lateral flexion and rotation upon the cervical spine (occiput atlas–C1 axis–C2; Fig. 7.3).

Lower cervical examination

Lower cervical motion is tested by having the patient flex, extend, laterally flex and rotate the entire lower cervical spine (C3–7) without movement of the head

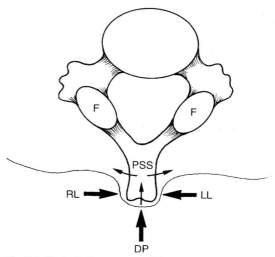

Fig. 7.2 Method of movement of the vertebral segment from direct pressure. Direct pressure (DP) upon the posterior superior spine localizes the specific vertebra. RL and LL is right and left lateral pressure upon the posterior superior spinous (PSS) process. (F) facet. From Cailliet (1995) with permission.

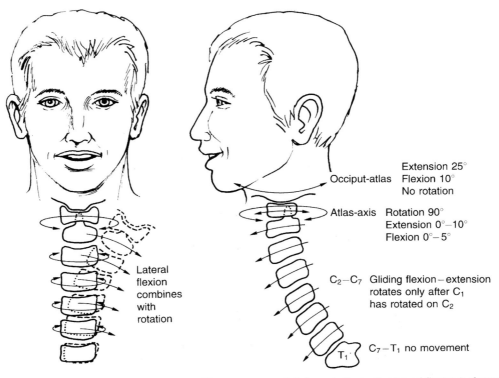

Extension 25°
Occiput-atlas   Flexion 10°
No rotation

Atlas-axis   Rotation 90°
Extension 0°–10°
Flexion 0°–5°

Lateral flexion combines with rotation

C_2–C_7 Gliding flexion–extension rotates only after C_1 has rotated on C_2

C_7–T_1 no movement

Fig. 7.3 Motion of cervical spine: upper and lower segments. Left figure indicates that lateral flexion is always accompanied by some rotation. The right figure indicates the degree of motion at each vertebral segment. From Cailliet (1995) with permission.

upon the spine. This is performed actively and passively.

Range of motion is estimated by noting the difference of the end-point of one direction versus the opposite end-point. Mechanical limitation is noted when motion stops, or when symptoms (unpleasant sensations) are produced. The site (segmental level) of sensation produced (i.e. local or referred) is determined.

As it is known through which foramen a specific nerve root emerges, and which foramina open and close upon specific motion (Fig. 7.4), the effects of specific neck movements are noted which determine the precise level of involvement.

As it has been generally accepted that the zygapophysial joints are a major source of neck pain, their identification is clinically tested using manual procedures. The accuracy has been confirmed (Jull *et al.*, 1988) as to location and source of pain. The techniques are numerous (Maigne, 1972; Maitland, 1977; Grieve, 1981; Bourdillon, 1982; Stoddard, 1983) and will not be elaborated on here. Whether the manual diagnosis as to site and source of pain is

accurate remains controversial but when compared to nerve root blocks they proved accurate (Jull *et al.*, 1988).

The neurological examination of the head and neck involves sensory, motor and autonomic testing. The upper cervical nerves (C1–3) are mostly sensory to the head. Motor testing of the upper cervical (occipital) nerve involves the muscles moving the head upon the neck. The neurological examination, sensory and motor, of the lower cervical spine (C3–8) involves the neurological examination of the upper extremities – musculoskeletal, axillary and median nerve (Fig. 7.5), ulnar nerve (Fig. 7.6) and radial nerve (Fig. 7.7).

The sensory (dermatomal) examination of the lower cervical segments is mostly limited to examination of the hand (Fig. 7.8). The details of the clinical examination are adequately summarized in the literature to which the reader is referred (Dwyer *et al.*, 1990; Cailliet, 1994b).

Confirmation is clinically possible with the performance of electromyography of nerve conduction velocity studies.

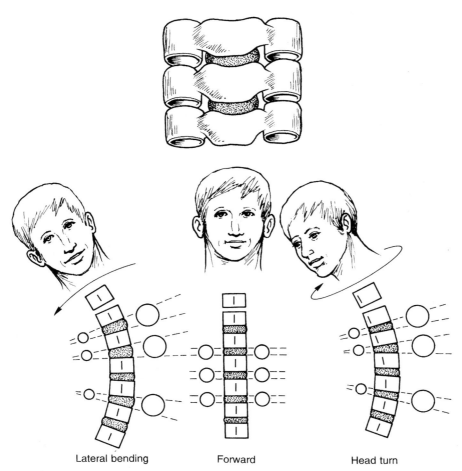

Lateral bending Forward Head turn

Fig. 7.4 Foraminal closure in lateral flexion and rotation of the head and neck. With the head in an erect posture (centre figure) the foramina are open equally. In right lateral flexion (left figure) the foramina are narrow on the concave side and open on the convex side. In rotation (right figure) the foramina are narrow on the side towards which the head turns and wider on the contralateral side. From Cailliet (1995) with permission.

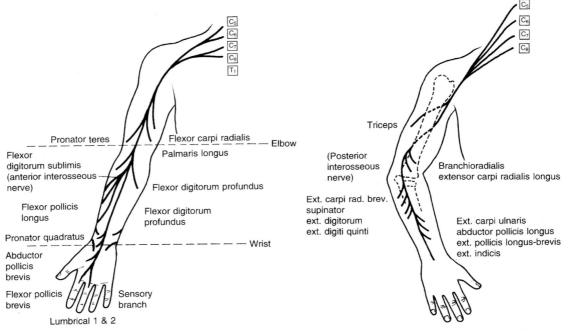

Fig. 7.5 Median nerve. From Cailliet (1995) with permission.

Fig. 7.7 Radial nerve. From Cailliet (1994b) with permission.

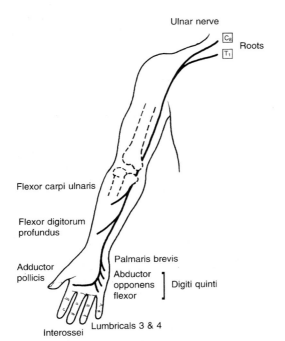

Fig. 7.6 Ulnar nerve. From Cailliet (1994b) with permission.

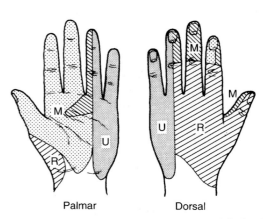

Fig. 7.8 Sensory mapping of peripheral nerves of the hand. The schematic areas of sensory innervation of the median nerve (M), radial nerve (R) and ulnar nerve (U). The dermatomes of the dorsum of the hand vary as the radial nerve may have no sensory area or merely a small area over the first dorsal interosseous. From Cailliet (1994b) with permission.

Clinical entities

Upper cervical segment (occiput–atlas–axis)

The symptoms are headache with hypersensitivity of the scalp in the Cl, C2 and C3 dermatomes. Tenderness with reproduction of the headache is determined by digital pressure upon the emergence site of the greater occipital nerve (Fig. 7.9). Diagnosis is confirmed by relief from local injection of an analgesic agent into the nerve or into the dorsal root ganglion of C2 (Fig. 7.10).

Lower cervical segment pain and impairment

Neck pain is a poorly understood symptom variously described as disc disease or soft-tissue injury pain (Bogduk and Marsland, 1988; Taylor and Finch, 1993). Pain is subjectively located in the neck, and motion is considered as causative or aggravating. Rest relieves pain.

Cervical zygapophysial joint pain

Distension of cervical zygapophysial joints with contrast medium can produce pain characteristic of

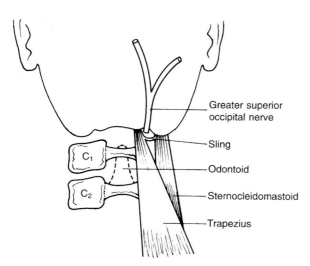

Fig. 7.9 Emergence of the greater superior occipital nerve. The greater superior occipital nerve, primarily C2 nerve root, emerges in a groove medial to the mastoid process of the occiput. It leaves in an opening between the insertion of the trapezius and the sternocleidomastoid muscles. A small fascial sling completes the opening. In some people the nerve emerges through the trapezius muscle. From Cailliet (1991) with permission.

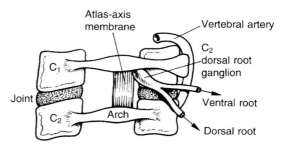

Fig. 7.10 Greater superior occipital nerve: its C2 root. The C2 dorsal root ganglion lies under the oblique inferior muscle (not shown), over the lateral atlantoaxial joint, being adherent to the capsule. It emerges lateral to the posterior atlas–axis membrane but does not penetrate it. It proceeds laterally to divide into a dorsal and ventral root. From Cailliet (1991) with permission.

the pattern complained of by the patient (Aprill *et al.*, 1990). Pain from the C2–3 joint is perceived in the upper neck and the occipital area (Fig. 7.11).

Pain from the C3–4 joint extends from the upper neck to the levator scapulae muscle. That from the C4–5 joint forms an angle between the lower neck and the upper shoulder girdle. From the C5–6 joint the pain extends from the lower neck over the supraspinatus area, and that from the C6–7 joint over the blade of the scapula. The areas are large and indistinct but reasonably consistent.

Compression upon the head with the head turned and laterally flexed causes radiation of pain down that extremity (Fig. 7.12). Traction of the head relieves radicular symptoms (Fig. 7.13).

Lesions of the cervical cord

Injuries of the cervical cord that result in paraplegia or quadriplegia are clinically discernible with upper motor neuron signs: Babinski, Hoffmann signs, hyperactive deep tendon reflexes, spasticity, clonus, etc.

For more subtle injuries of the cervical spine, clinical tests are less specific and thus often overlooked. For lesions from C4 caudally the nerve root levels are discernible with dermatomal and myotomal level testing. Above C4, there is a blind zone. The diagnosis of lesions within this zone is suggested from the Shimizu reflex (Fig. 7.14).

The Shimizu reflex is performed by having the patient seated with the elbow bent to 90° and the forearm supported (Shimizu *et al.*, 1993). The examiner taps the tip of the spine of the scapula in a caudal direction with a rubber reflex hammer. The reflex involves movement of the scapula from an abrupt stretching of the upper portion of the trapezius muscle. A positive test occurs with elevation of the scapula and/or abduction of the humerus: this indicates the possibility of a cord lesion between C2 and C4.

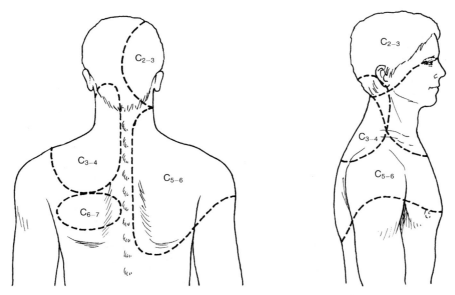

Fig. 7.11 Referred zones of cervical root levels (dermatomes). The graphic zones depict the dermatomal zones of cervical joints and roots C2–7. From Cailliet (1991) with permission.

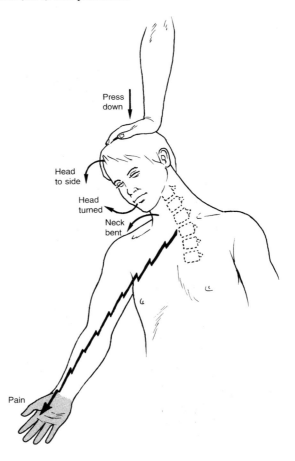

Fig. 7.12 Head compression causing radicular symptoms. Downwards compression upon the head (termed Spurling neck compression test) indicates probable nerve entrapment at the foramen. With the head turned and laterally flexed to the side of the symptoms, the head is forced downwards causing ipsilateral symptoms. Reproduction of radicular symptoms is considered a positive Spurling test. From Cailliet (1995) with permission.

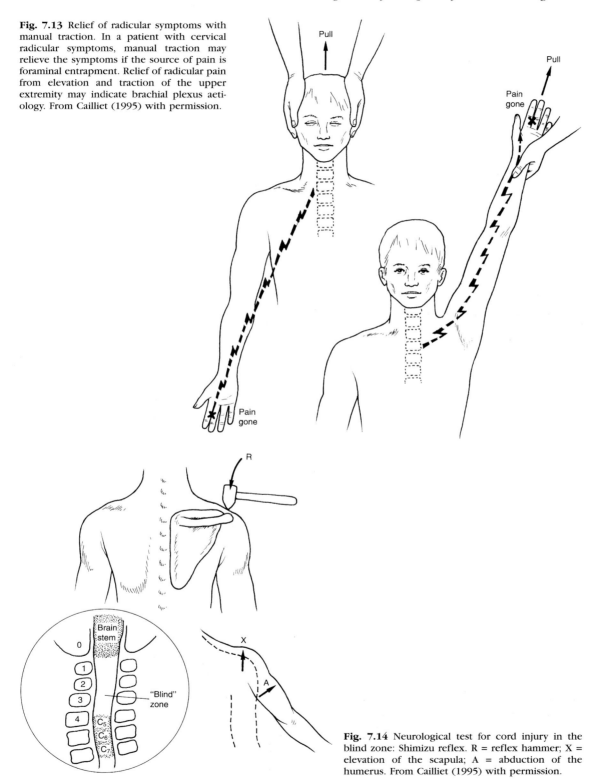

Fig. 7.13 Relief of radicular symptoms with manual traction. In a patient with cervical radicular symptoms, manual traction may relieve the symptoms if the source of pain is foraminal entrapment. Relief of radicular pain from elevation and traction of the upper extremity may indicate brachial plexus aetiology. From Cailliet (1995) with permission.

Fig. 7.14 Neurological test for cord injury in the blind zone: Shimizu reflex. R = reflex hammer; X = elevation of the scapula; A = abduction of the humerus. From Cailliet (1995) with permission.

Treatment protocols for cervical pain

Cervical pain may be related to an acute injury or be an exacerbation of a chronic process. Pain is vaguely localized in a general area and may be related to specific motions. As an example, radicular cervical pain can radiate to the top of the shoulder without necessarily being considered a radiculopathy if there is no radiation into the arm, hand or fingers.

In the acute phase of pain, rest, immobilization and local ice, followed by heat and gentle stretching, have benefits. Oral anti-inflammatory medication, if tolerated, is beneficial.

Reassurance is provided by a meaningful explanation and failure to use frightening words such as degenerative disc disease, arthritis or slipped disc. It is well-accepted that the significance of the symptoms assumed by the patient intensifies the severity of the pain and leads to possible chronicity and exaggeration of disability over impairment (Cailliet, 1994a).

Spasm is frequently initiated by localized pain from inflammation which can also become a tissue site of pain. This can be addressed by local ice, heat, massage, gentle stretching and isometric muscular contractions. Local injection of an analgesic agent into the painful muscle can be considered when local tenderness is significant.

Immobilization has been standard treatment for an acute musculoskeletal injury, but its value over early mobilization is being questioned (Mealy *et al.*, 1986). If immobilization is considered, a cervical collar or splint has been the traditional modality. The purpose of a collar is to hold the head in a comfortable gravity-aligned position and to prevent or minimize motion.

A standard collar (Fig. 7.15) is custom-made of felt that is 1–1.5 cm thick and cut to mould around the neck and jaw of the patient. No known orthosis or collar completely eliminates motion, so it must be assumed that it merely restricts motion, supports the head in a gravity-aligned posture and reminds the patient of excessive motion. By being under the chin

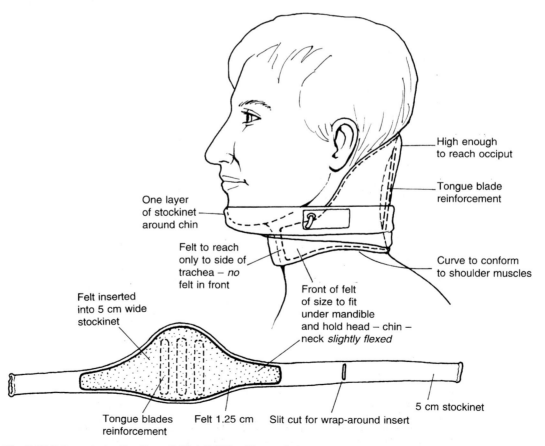

High enough
to reach occiput

Tongue blade
reinforcement

One layer
of stockinet
around chin

Felt to reach
only to side of
trachea – *no*
felt in front

Curve to conform
to shoulder muscles

Front of felt
of size to fit
under mandible
and hold head – chin –
neck *slightly flexed*

Felt inserted
into 5 cm wide
stockinet

5 cm stockinet

Tongue blades
reinforcement

Felt 1.25 cm

Slit cut for wrap-around insert

Fig. 7.15 Felt cervical collar. From Cailliet (1995) with permission.

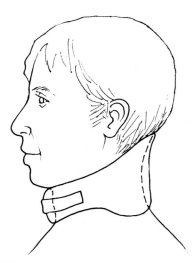

Fig. 7.16 Preformed plastic collars. A standard plexiglass cervical collar. The fibreglass preformed collar comes in several sizes that need to be fitted to the patient. They are held by a Velcro strap in the front. From Cailliet (1995) with permission.

it minimizes the need for muscular contraction to overcome the effects of gravity and also limits flexion. The elevation behind the head limits extension.

There are now available plastic collars that are easily applied, easy to keep clean and cosmetically acceptable (Fig. 7.16).

Only when there are neurological signs and symptoms, and a need for significant restriction of motion, should a brace be fitted (Fig. 7.17).

As a general rule, a collar should be worn constantly for the first week, then gradually decreased as tolerated. Most soft-tissue recovery occurs within 2 weeks. Prolonged immobilization encourages soft-tissue contracture, muscular atrophy and psychological dependence.

Traction has remained popular as a beneficial modality with varied medical opinions. Without subjective and objective radiculitis, the value of traction as compared to a cervical collar and analgesics produces no difference in outcomes (McKinney *et al.,* 1989).

In acute cervical injuries, continuous cervical traction for several days is valuable. In subacute or

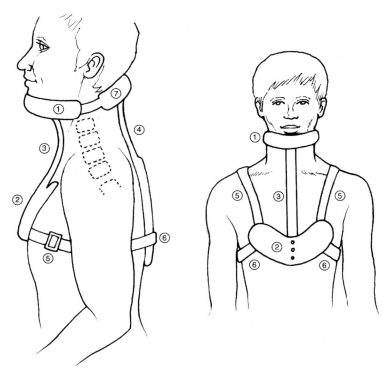

Fig. 7.17 Guildford cervical brace. This brace immobilizes the cervical spine with a rest positioned under the chin (1) and an occipital pad (7). A chest pad (2) is connected to an anterior bar (3) that elevates the chin and connects by a strap (6) to the thoracic portion which, by a vertical bar (4), attaches to the occipital pad. The shoulder straps (5) secure the chest pad. All parts adjust to make the brace customized to the specific patient. From Cailliet (1995) with permission.

chronic problems, traction for 20 min several times daily is beneficial. Manual traction before instituting mechanical traction will indicate the tolerance and benefit gained from that modality.

Manipulation or mobilization has been prevalent in today's society but its physiological benefit has not been proven nor have the indications for this approach been clarified.

There are several possible concepts as to the accomplishment of manipulation as follows:

1. Unlocking a 'jammed'; zygapophysial joint. This is based on the possible entrapment of a meniscus of a synovial fold. Restoration of movement to subluxed zygapophysial joint facets has also been postulated.
2. A neurogenic reaction from manipulation, in which the force alters the spindle systems' effect upon the muscle, alters the mechanoreceptors in the zygapophysial joints or has a central reaction on reflexes.
3. Elongation of the contracted zygapophysial joint capsule or periarticular ligaments which may have adhesions.
4. Recentralization of the nucleus within the intervertebral disc.

In standard procedures, force is applied in the direction that appears limited but the Maigne technique differs in that it is applied in the opposite unrestricted and painless direction (Maigne, 1973).

Modalities such as ice, heat, ultrasound, massage and electrical stimulation have their proponents but they should be considered as merely palliative and ancillary to a more active approach. None of these modalities are specific, curative or precise, and they extend the costs of treatments without benefit.

Exercise remains the most accepted modality. If there is limited range of motion, gentle gradual active exercise is indicated. Active is stressed, as exercises performed by the patient are preferable to those exercises being done to the patient. Strengthening exercises, addressing the muscles where a specific weakness is found from a meaningful clinical examination, are important.

Isometric exercises should be initiated initially, followed by kinetic exercises. Isometric contractions with no joint motion decrease spasm, pain and atrophy. Isometric exercises should be initiated early in the management of an acute cervical injury, in spite of pain, as there are few, if any, contraindications. Isometric exercises stretch the joint capsules to a slight but definite degree, beneficially compress the cartilage, strengthen the ligaments and tendons, and extrude toxic (ischaemic) materials from the muscles reflexly contracted by pain and inflammation. They are active and initiate the involvement of the patient towards recovery.

Isometric exercise should be followed by active assisted exercises that increase strength, endurance

and range of motion. Ultimately, resistance should be added to the exercise regime to increase strength and endurance.

Range of motion has been advocated but rarely defined or quantitated. A functional painfree increase in range of motion is desirable but to acquire complete and extreme range of motion, albeit physiological, is not necessary. In fact, it should be avoided, as many soft tissues that have been structurally damaged will not tolerate excessive elongation. Painfree and functionally adequate should be the guideline, with gradual restoration to greater range from normal daily use accepted at a later stage.

Restoration or institution of physiological posture is mandatory in all activities of daily living to minimize tissue stress and unphysiological muscular effort. A forwards head posture, ahead of the centre of gravity, places excessive stress upon all the cervical spine tissues (Fig. 7.18).

Physiological posture can be trained by a therapist and practised by the patient, at first with assistive

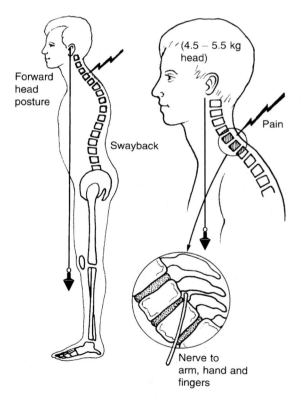

Fig. 7.18 Gravity effects of forwards head posture. With an erect posture the weight of the head (approximately 4.5–5.5 kg) is maintained directly above the centre of gravity. With the head forward, approximately 7.5 cm in front of the centre of gravity, it adds an estimated 13.5 kg of weight up on the cervical spine. From Cailliet (1995) with permission.

2.5 – 4.5 kg

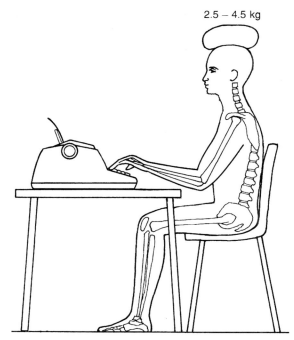

Fig. 7.19 Distraction exercise device. A device to assist in posture training. With a sandbag weighing 2.5–4.5 kg on the head, erect posture is maintained and the cervical lordosis decreased. This is a proprioceptive concept that is implemented as long as the device is worn during activities of daily living. From Cailliet (1995) with permission.

devices (Fig. 7.19) if necessary, until it becomes a normal way of life and ensures automatic unconscious implementation. All contributing factors such as occupational demands, emotional and physiological aspects, must be unearthed and addressed.

Hyperextension–hyperflexion cervical injuries: the whiplash syndrome

This syndrome is so common, and so controversial, that it merits separate mention (Barnsley *et al.*, 1993). By common definition, it is an injury that results from a motor vehicle accident causing acceleration forces to be imposed upon the head and neck.

At the time of impact the vehicle is accelerated forwards, followed immediately (100 ms) with forwards acceleration of the trunk and shoulders of the occupant (Fig. 7.20). The shoulders travel forwards under the head causing extension of the neck.

Assuming that the head is facing directly forwards, all forces are linear (sagittal); however, this rarely

occurs as some degree of rotation is usually present. This force causes rotation before extension takes place, resulting in stress upon the capsules of the zygapophysial joints, the intervertebral discs and the alar ligament complex of the upper cervical segment.

This force is applied first at the occipitocervical joint as the head is heavy (4.5–5.5 kg average weight). The force is then expended at the C6 joint. The head rotates forwards, followed by flexion of the neck which extends the posterior neck tissues which are elongated excessively, without muscular recoil, as the proprioceptors and spindle system do not react rapidly enough.

Clinically there are no external signs such as bruising, swelling or haemorrhage. Symptoms are subjective, with objective signs being minimal or non-specific. The most common lesions noted in the cervical spine after an acceleration–deceleration cervical injury are soft tissue: muscle, ligament, joint capsule and disc (Clemens and Burow, 1972; Dvorak *et al.*, 1987).

Cardinal symptoms of whiplash

The prominent symptom is neck pain which is consistent: a dull aching sensation initially noted at the base of the head which is aggravated by movement. Usually there is also an associated neck stiffness with restricted movement. Pain may radiate to the head, shoulder, arm and interscapular region.

Headaches frequently result from a whiplash injury and typically are occipital, radiating anteriorly into the temporal or occipital regions which are subserved by nerve roots C1–3.

The examination of the whiplash patient is as for any cervical injury. Treatment is also similar but with the exception that careful explanation and reassurance are mandatory because of all the lay publicity that has been given to this type of injury.

Conclusion

In 1995 a Quebec Task Force on Whiplash-Associated Disorders (Spitzer *et al.*, 1995) reached these conclusions:

> Pain . . . cannot be seen on radiographs, computer tomography or magnetic resonance imaging. Pain can be pursued using diagnostic blocks . . . it has been shown that zygapophysial joint pain is the most common basis for chronic neck pain after whiplash.

The task force studied thousands of medical articles regarding treatment and reached the following conclusions:

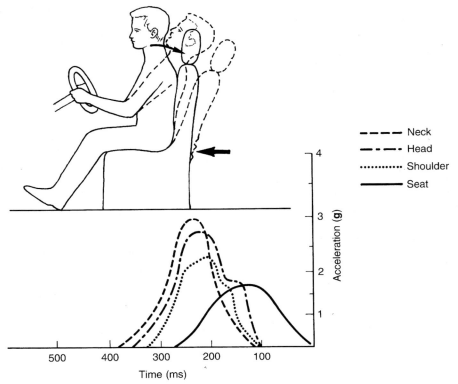

Fig. 7.20 Upper-body–neck deformations from rear-end collisions. From the effect of a linear force from the rear, the shoulder, head and neck deform at different times measured in milliseconds. The major forces (**g**) are expended within the time under 0.5 s. From Cailliet (1995) with permission.

1. Collars (immobilization): soft collars do not restrict the range of motion of the cervical spine yet may promote inactivity and delay recovery.
2. Rest: cumulative evidence suggests that prolonged periods of rest are detrimental to recovery.
3. Manipulation: equivalent immediate (less than 5 min) improvement in pain and mobility.
4. Mobilization: in combination with activating interventions appear to be beneficial in the short term but long-term benefit remains to be established.
5. Exercise: cumulative evidence suggests that active exercise may be beneficial in the short and long term.
6. Traction: there is no clinically significant benefit regarding range of motion or relief of pain.
7. Passive modalities, posture training and electrical therapy remain unproven.
8. Epidural or intrathecal steroid injections are of unproven long-term value.

Their conclusions are that time, sparing use of medication and regaining activities of daily living are remedial and all other modalities are placebo. Their studies, it must be stated, regarded cervical pain without objective radicular changes.

In the presence of nerve root impairment, more aggressive treatment must be undertaken – prolonged immobilization with a moulded orthosis for several weeks, during which time isometric muscle contractions are initiated. Traction, if subjectively beneficial, is acceptable. Manipulation, carefully monitored with repeated neurological examinations, may be valuable. Gradual isometric exercises, graduating to isokinetic exercises, should then be initiated. Ergonomic evaluation and correction of daily activities are a valid part of rehabilitation.

Chapter 5 is devoted to the effect of whiplash-type injuries on the neck and brain as this type of injury is an important and frequent cause of much suffering.

References

Aprill, C., Bogduk, N. (1992) The prevalence of cervical zygapophyseal joint pain: A first approximation. *Spine* **17**: 744–747.

Aprill, C., Dwyer, A., Bogduk, N. (1990) Cervical zygapophyseal joint pain patterns. II. A clinical evaluation. *Spine* **15:** 458–461.

Barnsley, L., Lord, S., Bogduk, N. (1993) The pathophysiology of whiplash. *Spine: State of the Art Reviews* **7:** 239–353.

Bogduk, N., Marsland, A. (1988) The cervical zygapophysial joints as a source of neck pain. *Spine* **13:** 610–617.

Bourdillon, J.F. (1982) *Spinal Manipulation,* 3rd edn. London: Heinemann.

Cailliet, R. (1991) *Neck and Arm Pain*, 3rd edn. Philadelphia: F.A. Davis.

Cailliet, R. (1995) *Soft Tissue Pain and Disability,* 3rd edn. Philadelphia: F.A. Davis.

Cailliet, R. (1994a) *Pain: Mechanisms and Management*, 1st edn. Philadelphia: F.A. Davis.

Cailliet, R. (1994b) Nerve control of the hand. In: *Hand Pain and Impairment,* 4th edn (Cailliet, R., ed.). Philadelphia: F.A. Davis, pp. 69–131.

Clemens, H.J., Burow, K. (1972) Experimental investigation of injury mechanisms of cervical spine at frontal and rear-frontal vehicle impacts. In: *Proceeding of the Sixteenth STAPP Car Crash Conference.* Warrendale: Society of Automotive Engineers, pp. 76–104.

Dvorak, J., Panjabi, M.M., Gerber, M., Wichman, W. (1987) CT-functional diagnostics of rotatory instability of upper cervical spine. I. An experimental study on cadavers. *Spine* **12:** 197–205.

Dwyer, A., Aprill, C., Bogduk, N. (1990) Cervical zygapophyseal joint patterns. I. A clinical evaluation. *Spine* **15:** 453–457.

Grieve, G.P. (1981) *Common Vertebral Joint Problems.* Edinburgh: Churchill Livingstone.

Jull, G., Bogduk, N., Marsland, A. (1988) The accuracy of manual diagnosis for cervical zygapophysial joint pain syndrome. *Med. J. Aust.* **148:** 233–236.

McKeever, F.A. (1968) Atlanto-axoid instability. *Surg. Clin. North Am.* **48:** 1375–1390.

McKinney, L.A., Dornan, J.O., Ryan, M. (1989) The role of physiotherapy in the management of acute neck sprains following road-traffic accidents. *Arch. Emerg. Med.* **6:** 27–33.

Maigne, R. (1972) *Douleurs d'Origine Vertébrale et Traitements par Manipulation,* 2nd edn. Paris: Expansion Scientific.

Maigne, R. (1973) *Orthopedic Medicine.* Springfield, IL: Charles C. Thomas.

Maitland, G.D. (1977) *Vertebral Manipulation,* 4th edn. London: Butterworth.

Mealy, K., Brennan, H., Fenelon, G.C. (1986) Early mobilization of acute whiplash injuries. *Br. Med. J.* **292:** 656–657.

Shimizu, T., Shimada, H., Shirakura, K. (1993) Scapulo-humeral reflex (shimizu). *Spine* **18:** 2182–2190.

Spitzer, W.A., Skovron, M.L., Salmi, L.R. *et al.* (1995) Scientific monograph of the Quebec task force on whiplash-associated disorders. *Spine* **20:** 8S–73S.

Stoddard, A. (1983) *Manual of Osteopathic Technique.* London: Hutchinson.

Taylor, J.R., Finch, P.M. (1993) Neck sprain. *Aust. Fam. Phys.* **22:** 1623–1629.

8

Surgical management of neck pain of mechanical origin

N. Jones

Introduction

Mechanical neck pain is extremely common, but only rarely is it improved by surgical intervention. The less common causes (trauma, tumours, rheumatoid arthritis) are more likely to respond to surgery than the single most important cause, degenerative disease. The usual indications for surgery in degenerative cervical spondylosis are nerve root or spinal cord involvement rather than neck pain.

Recent advances in spinal instrumentation have had a significant impact on cervical spine surgery, enabling immediate rigid fixation, usually without the requirement for external orthoses, but as yet this has not translated into an improvement in the surgical treatment of neck pain due to degenerative disease.

This chapter discusses the assessment and selection of patients for surgery and the various surgical techniques available.

History

Presenting history

The history is often skewed by medicolegal concerns when pain follows a motor vehicle accident or work injury, but it remains of paramount importance. The pain may be either axial or radicular and in many cases there are elements of both. From a surgeon's point of view it is the radicular component that is most useful in making a diagnosis and determining the place of surgery.

Axial pain

This is almost always present to some degree and the underlying pathology is debatable. Structures such as the disc, zygapophysial joints, ligaments and muscles probably all contribute. The resultant pain is fairly non-specific, but is most commonly worse on one side and tends to involve the muscles. This is often described as an ache in the shoulder, radiating to the interscapular area and often to the head, leading to tension-type headaches. The diffuse nature of this pain will usually distinguish it from an upper cervical radicular pain but in the absence of neurological abnormalities this is not always easy.

Axial pain that is worse at night, especially in an elderly patient, should arouse suspicions of an underlying malignancy.

Radicular pain

Cervical radicular pain is often equated with arm pain, and although this is usually the case, not all cervical radicular pain is felt in the arm and not all arm pain is radicular in nature.

Diffuse arm pain may be caused by such diverse problems as a Pancoast's tumour in the apex of the lung, reflex sympathetic dystrophy, local joint or muscle conditions and it is often a component of a functional problem.

True radicular arm pain is due to irritation or compression of a cervical nerve root. The most commonly affected are C6, C7 and C5, all of which cause arm pain. The third and fourth cervical nerve roots are associated with neck pain but are rarely involved in degenerative spondylosis. The eighth

Table 8.1 *Signs of cervical radiculopathy*

Nerve root	Sensory loss	Motor signs	Reflex
C5	Over deltoid	Shoulder abduction	None
C6	Thumb and index fingers	Elbow flexion	Biceps
C7	Middle finger	Elbow extension	Triceps
C8	Fourth and fifth fingers	Finger flexion and extension	Finger
T1	Axilla	Hand intrinsics	Horner's

cervical nerve root is also only rarely affected but does produce arm symptoms.

Radicular pain is felt in a myotomal as well as a dermatomal distribution. Often the pain is maximal in the myotome with paraesthesiae in the dermatome. A C5 radiculopathy produces pain in the shoulder and in the deltoid muscle. Compression of C6 causes pain which radiates into the biceps muscle and into the thumb and index finger; C7 pain involves the triceps muscle and the middle finger, and C8 involves the medial aspect of the forearm and the fifth finger (Table 8.1).

Myelopathy

With severe degenerative disease there may be compression of the spinal cord from osteophytes or disc material. The pain associated with myelopathy is usually more chronic and less severe than that associated with radiculopathy. Cervical myelopathy often causes quite vague symptoms. The spasticity and weakness it produces in the lower limbs may be reflected in mild gait disturbances, a decrease in exercise tolerance or frequent tripping due to mild dorsiflexion weakness. Upper cervical cord compression may produce the syndrome of 'numb, clumsy hands', manifested by diffuse numbness in the hands and an inability to perform fine motor tasks, such as doing up buttons or picking up coins. Any of these symptoms should alert the practitioner to the possibility of spinal cord compromise, a condition which may progress rapidly to quadriplegia after minor trauma or manipulation.

Past history

Most patients with neck pain will be able to recall some injury, often dating back to childhood falls or school sporting injuries. It is often difficult to determine the significance of these compared with the normal effects of day-to-day life. Occasionally, a patient will present with severe degenerative changes

at one level with little or no evidence of generalized spondylosis, suggesting that previous trauma may have been relevant.

Other medical conditions

One of the most important conditions associated with mechanical neck pain is rheumatoid arthritis. This chronic inflammatory disorder has a predilection for the upper cervical spine, particularly the atlantoaxial level. Atlantoaxial subluxation is found in almost 50% of rheumatoid patients at postmortem (Lipson, 1984). Ankylosing spondylitis and osteoporosis are also important general medical problems to be considered. A full history and systems review may reveal symptoms consistent with other significant underlying conditions, particularly malignancy. An elderly person presenting for the first time with neck pain should be assumed to have metastatic disease until proven otherwise (Fig. 8.1).

Examination

General physical examination

A complete general physical examination is important in the assessment of the patient presenting with neck pain. One should look for signs of conditions with a known association with neck pain, such as osteoarthritis or rheumatoid arthritis. Signs of weight loss, organomegaly or lymphadenopathy should make one suspicious of underlying malignancy. Patients with diabetes mellitus are more prone to infections and brachial neuritis.

Cervical spine examination

Inspection

The patient is observed while at rest during the taking of the history. The range and freedom of neck movements are noted. The neck is then inspected after removal of the upper clothing. The webbed neck and low hairline of Klippel–Feil syndrome are indicators of an underlying congenital cervical spine abnormality. Similarly, the tilted head and ocular imbalance resulting from atlantoaxial rotatory subluxation are obvious.

Active movement

The patient is asked to flex, extend, rotate and laterally flex the neck while attention is paid to the

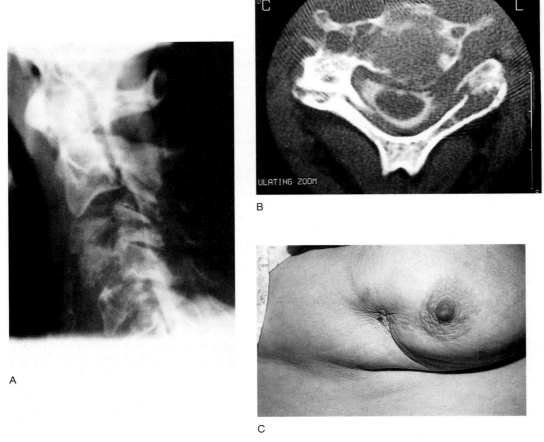

Fig. 8.1 (A) A cervical myelogram and (B) computed tomographic scan showing metastases from (C) a breast primary.

range of each movement, the rhythm of the movement and any apparent discomfort.

Palpation

The cervical spine is palpated gently, starting from the craniocervical junction and progressing caudally, one segment at a time. It is rare to elicit any sign other than local tenderness. Marked superficial tenderness may be an indicator of a functional component to the illness (Waddell *et al.*, 1980). The spine is then palpated more firmly if the gentle palpation did not produce any tenderness. The muscles are then palpated, starting with the insertions of the trapezius muscles, which is a common site for focal tenderness. This is continued across the shoulder and along the medial border of the scapula.

Passive movement

The passive range of neck movements can be assessed but generally adds little to the information already gleaned from active movements.

Other manoeuvres

Compression or traction can be applied to the cervical spine with consequent worsening or alleviation of nerve root compression symptoms respectively. Spurling's manoeuvre involves hyperextension of the neck and rotation away from the painful arm. This is said to narrow the intervertebral foramen on the side and reproduce radicular arm pain.

L'Hermitte's sign is pain shooting down the legs after flexion of the neck. This is an indicator of either cervical spinal cord compression or demyelination.

Neurological examination

Radiculopathy

Usually the history will have given a strong indication of which signs to expect on examination. Pain, paraesthesiae, numbness or weakness in the distribution of a particular nerve root should be supported by the appropriate motor and sensory signs. Given time, the weakness will be accompanied by wasting and fasciculations and there may even be trophic changes in the areas of numbness.

Involvement of C5 will cause weakness of the deltoid and supraspinatus muscles which abduct the shoulder and the infraspinatus which externally rotates the shoulder. There is some C5 input to the biceps reflex which may be reduced but should still be present. Numbness is found over the upper lateral arm.

Compression of C6 causes weakness of elbow flexion and supination and depression or absence of the biceps reflex. Numbness affects the lateral forearm and the thumb and index finger.

A C7 radiculopathy will produce weakness of elbow extension and wrist flexion and extension. The triceps reflex is depressed or absent. There is sensory loss affecting the middle finger, and often the posterior forearm.

Weakness of finger flexion and extension and a loss of the finger jerk follow C8 nerve root compression. There is associated numbness in the fifth finger and medial forearm.

Although T1 lesions are rare, they may imply sinister pathology yet be mistaken for a functional problem. When severe, they will cause weakness of the intrinsic muscles of the hand. A useful sign to look for is a Horner's syndrome, comprising ptosis, meiosis and anhidrosis, due to involvement of the sympathetic chain. There is no accompanying reflex, and sensory loss is in the axilla.

Myelopathy

Neurological examination of the patient with neck pain is not limited to the upper limbs. If the cord is involved there will be abnormalities at and below the level of involvement. Lower motor neuron signs predominate at the level of compression and these will be similar to those described under radiculopathy, though often bilateral. Below this level there will be upper motor neuron signs. The tone is increased and there may be clonus in the knees or ankles. Reflexes are brisk and there may be abnormal reflexes (Hoffmann's sign in the hand and Babinski's sign in the foot). The abdominal reflexes are lost in cases of spinal cord compression.

Other

A complete neurological examination may reveal rarer causes of neck pain. Cranial nerve abnormalities may point to a lesion of the skull base or an intrinsic brainstem abnormality. Supratentorial neurological abnormalities might suggest disseminated malignancy.

Investigation

Blood tests

Blood tests are most useful in the search for associated pathology. A raised erythrocyte sedimentation rate may suggest infection or rheumatoid arthritis; anaemia or hypercalcaemia may be associated with myeloma and elevated prostate-specific antigen with prostatic carcinoma.

Plain radiographs

Considerable diagnostic information can be gleaned from plain radiographs. These should include lateral and anteroposterior projections, as well as an open-mouth view of the craniocervical junction. Oblique views are sometimes helpful but foraminal stenosis is much better appreciated with computed tomography (CT). If instability is suspected, careful flexion and extension views can be obtained. In rheumatoid arthritis, particular attention should be paid to the C1-2 level for atlantoaxial subluxation.

Degenerative changes on plain radiographs are almost universal and their presence does not necessarily explain symptoms. Clinical correlation is of paramount importance.

Plain radiographs may also detect changes of rheumatoid arthritis, metastases, trauma, osteoporosis and infection. Congenital anomalies such as os odontoideum and Klippel-Feil syndrome will also be apparent.

CT scan

CT gives the best detail of the bony structures in the cervical spine. The resolution of the cord is usually inadequate and shoulder artefacts often obscure the lower levels (C6-7 and C7-T1). Particularly in thin individuals at levels above C6-7, plain CT can be sufficient to confirm a diagnosis of disc prolapse or foraminal stenosis (Fig. 8.2), although the degree of confidence is usually less than in the lumbar spine.

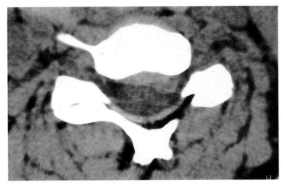

A

(MRI), although it is still the best investigation for degenerative disease when MRI is unavailable or is not tolerated by the patient. Occasionally CT–myelography is still used when MRI gives equivocal results and is particularly useful when there are large or widespread osteophytes. In such cases, the superior bone resolution of the CT and the presence or absence of nerve root sheath opacification with dye can provide strong evidence for or against nerve root compression (Fig. 8.3).

MRI

MRI has rapidly become the investigation of choice for most problems in the neck. It is non-invasive and produces images of the cervical spine unobtainable with any other modality. Shoulder artefact is not a problem, allowing excellent visualization of the cervicothoracic junction. The soft tissues of the neck, the spinal cord and the nerve roots are seen particularly well (Fig. 8.2b). Images can be obtained in a variety of formats.

Disadvantages of MRI include claustrophobia, which is a common cause of failed examination, movement artefacts during the relatively long examination times and metal artefacts due to even tiny metallic fragments. Cost and availability also need to be considered.

Nuclear bone scan

This is a relatively simple investigation with reasonable sensitivity but poor specificity. It is usually used

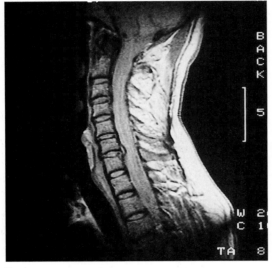

B

Fig. 8.2 (A) Plain computed tomographic scan showing a left posterolateral disc prolapse at C5–6. (B) A C6–7 disc prolapse demonstrated with magnetic resonance imaging.

In metastatic disease, the degree of bone destruction will be more obvious than on plain radiographs. Soft-tissue abnormalities may also be seen and some appreciation of the incursion into the spinal canal can be made.

The addition of reconstruction techniques, particularly with spiral CT scanning, can add considerably to the definition and diagnostic capability of this investigation.

Myelography

Myelography with concomitant CT has now been largely replaced by magnetic resonance imaging

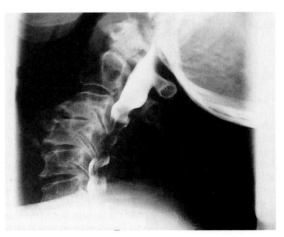

Fig. 8.3 A cervical myelogram of a patient with myel-oradiculopathy.

as a screening test for metastatic disease or infection, but it has largely been supplanted by computerized imaging techniques.

Nerve conduction studies

Electromyography and nerve conduction studies are rarely used in Australia for the investigation of radiculopathy. Overlap of myotomes and delay in the development of changes make the results relatively non-specific in most cases. Some authors advocate electromyographic examination of the paraspinal muscles as a way of increasing specificity (Johnson and Melvin, 1971), but the combination of clinical assessment and imaging is easier and gives superior results.

Treatment

Indications for surgery

Atlantoaxial instability

In an adult, a gap of greater then 3 mm between the arch of C1 and the odontoid process is indicative of instability. Anterior subluxation of greater than 10–12 mm implies destruction of the entire ligamentous complex (Fielding *et al.,* 1974). A gap of 6 mm or more is considered an indication for surgery. In rheumatoid disease, subluxation is often associated with cranial settling. The degree of brainstem compression arising from this can be determined most effectively with MRI.

Unlike subaxial degenerative disease, the most common indication for surgery at C1–2 is neck pain, which is present in the majority of rheumatoid patients with atlantoaxial subluxation (Pellici *et al.,* 1981; Menezes and VanGilder, 1988). A prime consideration is also prevention of neurological compromise due to progressive slip.

Subaxial instability

This may be severe in trauma and rheumatoid arthritis, but in degenerative spondylosis there is usually only a relative instability. Loss of disc space height will allow some movement but significant displacement implies damage to the anulus and/or facet joints. Some movement is normal in flexion–extension radiographs but this should not exceed 3.5 mm (White *et al.,* 1975). Surgery for rheumatoid subaxial subluxation involves either anterior or posterior fusion. Zygapophysial joint injuries are usually treated posteriorly and vertebral body injuries

anteriorly. Fusion for degenerative disease is more commonly carried out anteriorly (Fig. 8.4d).

Radiculopathy

This is the most common indication for cervical spine surgery. There is almost always an element of mechanical neck pain but the arm symptoms and signs are the reasons for surgery. In a younger patient it is usually due to an acute disc prolapse but in an elderly patient the nerve root is frequently injured in a stenotic foramen, often after a minor injury or repetitive or unusual neck movements (painting the ceiling is a common antecedent to such a radiculopathy). Most often, a bout of radiculopathy will settle with conservative treatment alone and surgery will not be required. The indications for surgery are essentially threefold and are described below. In all cases it is imperative that the pain, numbness, weakness and radiological abnormalities are consistent with each other. There is no point removing a C7–T1 disc for a C6 radiculopathy.

1. If there is significant neurological compromise in the form of weakness or numbness, surgical decompression is indicated as a matter of urgency. The definition of significant is relative and the degree of deficit that worries one individual may not concern another. Reflex changes alone are unimportant, other than as an indicator to the affected nerve root. Sensory changes, including paraesthesiae, vary in significance with their location or intensity. Numbness of the thumb and index finger of the dominant hand is more serious then numbness over the deltoid. The most important neurological deficit is weakness and again the relevance varies with the individual, the particular muscles involved and the degree of weakness. A global weakness is often seen in someone with arm pain and this needs to be distinguished from a true radicular weakness due to nerve root compression. Reflex changes can help in this regard.
2. If the pain is in the distribution of a nerve root but there are no neurological signs and, despite conservative treatment, it persists beyond a reasonable period (usually 6 weeks), surgery may be indicated. This is referred to as irritative brachalgia (as opposed to compressive brachalgia, described above, where there is a neurological deficit).
3. In cases of irritative brachalgia, surgery may sometimes be indicated prior to 6 weeks when the pain is severe and unremitting with usual conservative measures.

Myelopathy

Surgical decompression is almost always indicated in cervical myelopathy. This is a slowly progressive

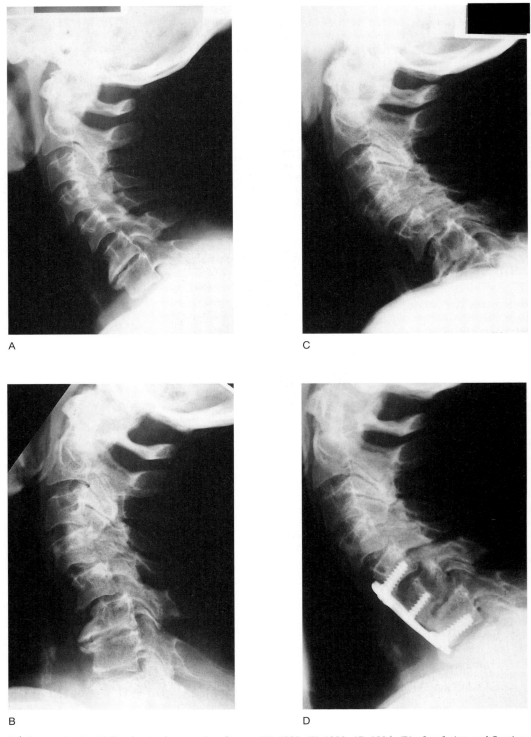

A

C

B

D

Fig. 8.4 Progressive instability due to degenerative disease. (A) 1988; (B) 1993; (C) 1994; (D) after fusion and fixation with an anterior plate.

disorder which can usually be stabilized by surgery but significant improvement is uncommon. The longer surgery is delayed, the greater the long-term deficit is likely to be.

Tumour

Metastatic tumours are a relatively frequent cause of mechanical instability and neck pain, often without neurological deficit. They may also cause neck pain without instability. Treatment depends to a large extent on the clinical state and prognosis of the individual patient. If there is no neurological deficit and the spine is stable, radiotherapy is the treatment

of choice. Surgery is indicated when radiotherapy has failed or if there is bony compression of the spinal cord. Surgical excision of a single affected vertebral body with fixation and stabilization will usually improve pain control significantly. When metastases are widespread in the spine, surgery becomes much more difficult and is rarely indicated.

Benign tumours such as schwannoma are much rarer and cause radicular pain rather than mechanical neck pain (Fig. 8.5).

Trauma

Although acute spinal injury is an important cause of instability and mechanical neck pain, the indications

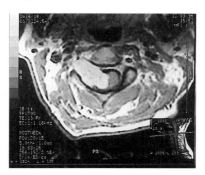

A

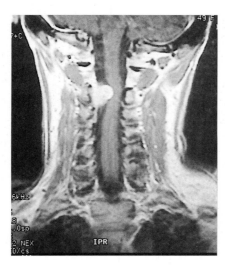

B

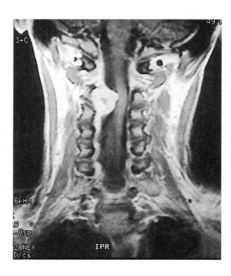

Fig. 8.5 (A) Axial and (B) coronal magnetic resonance images of a right C2 schwannoma presenting with neck and occipital pain.

for surgery are quite controversial and beyond the scope of this chapter.

Non-surgical treatment

A variety of non-surgical treatment options are available for mechanical neck pain and these are covered in greater detail elsewhere in this book. In most cases, non-surgical treatment will be the most appropriate form of treatment, with surgery reserved for the minority of patients with the specific indications discussed above.

Surgical treatment

Cervical spine surgery can be divided into operations done from an anterior approach and those done from a posterior approach. In many centres there is a historical preference for one over the other but, in general, the spine surgeon should be familiar with both and tailor the operation to the individual circumstances.

Anterior cervical spine surgery

C1-2

The most common indication for anterior surgery at this level is rheumatoid arthritis with cranial settling. Although this is associated with mechanical neck pain, the greater concern is usually neurological compromise. The odontoid process may be removed transorally to decompress the cervicomedullary junction. This is then followed by a posterior stabilization procedure.

Subaxial cervical spine

Anterior cervical discectomy is a common neurosurgical operation, done for either radiculopathy or myelopathy. The same approach can be used for fusion in trauma or vertebral body excision in tumour.

The approach is usually from the right side with a skin crease incision at the affected level. The platysma is divided and the plane medial to the sternocleidomastoid muscle is entered. The carotid sheath is retracted laterally and the trachea and oesophagus medially. This leads directly to the anterior surface of the cervical spine. The level is checked radiographically and self-retaining retractors are inserted beneath the longus colli muscles. The disc is then excised. There are several variations of this operation.

Smith–Robinson

This technique involves excision of the disc and any osteophytes through the disc space, usually using a disc space spreader to widen the gap. A bone graft is taken from the iliac crest and impacted into the disc space to effect a fusion of the level. Some surgeons perform the discectomy but do not fuse the level; this would be considered the exception rather than the rule.

Cloward

The Cloward technique involves drilling a circular hole centred on the disc space. This is carried down to the posterior cortex which is removed with curettes and punches. Any osteophytes are also removed. The posterior longitudinal ligament may also be removed to expose the dura and allow access to any disc fragments that may have penetrated this ligament. A bone dowel slightly larger than the hole drilled is taken from the iliac crest and impacted into the hole (Fig. 8.6). Rather than autogenous bone, some surgeons use allograft, xenograft or artificial bone substitutes.

Corpectomy (Fig. 8.7)

This is particularly useful when there are degenerative changes causing spinal cord compression at

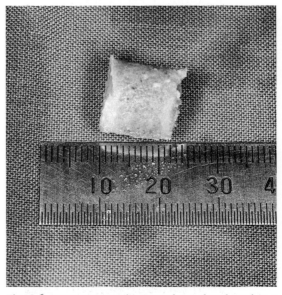

Fig. 8.6 An autogenous iliac crest bone dowel used in a Cloward anterior cervical fusion.

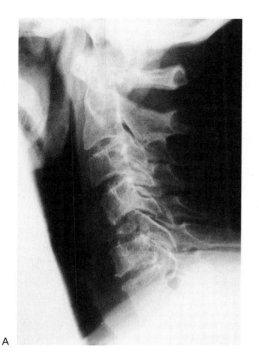

A

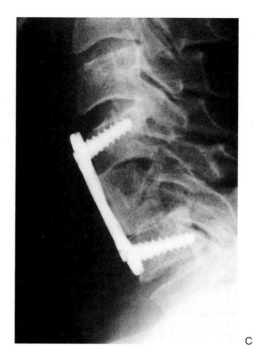

C

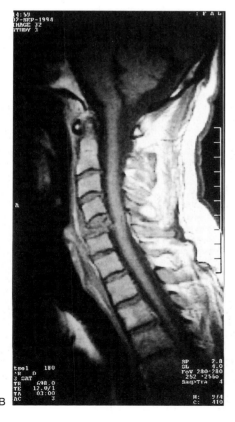

B

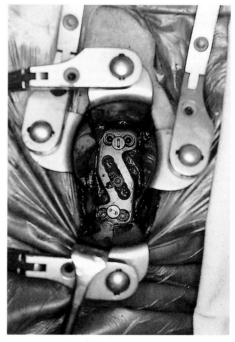

D

Fig. 8.7 (A) Plain radiograph showing a C5 vertebral body metastasis; (B) magnetic resonance imaging of the same case; (C) a corpectomy has been performed and the body replaced with autogenous iliac crest. Internal fixation has been achieved with an anterior Orion plate; (D) an operative photograph of a similar case.

two adjacent levels. Rather than making two separate holes at the disc levels, the intervening vertebral body is drilled away, exposing the posterior longitudinal ligament which is usually also removed to expose the dura. The decompression is completed by removing the anterior part of the inferior margin of the upper vertebral body and the superior margin of the lower vertebral body. This allows for a very thorough decompression of the cord in cases of cervical myelopathy and is also useful in isolated metastases in a single vertebral body.

The most common graft material is autogenous iliac crest but substitutes may be used. Vertebral body replacements can be made from titanium and other materials.

Corpectomy can be used over longer lengths but it then becomes impossible to maintain the normal cervical lordosis and there is considerable stress on the two ends of a long strut graft (usually fibula).

Internal fixation

A wide variety of anterior plating devices is now available to supplement anterior fusion. The most commonly used are made of titanium, which allows postoperative MRI. The screws are usually of a type that locks into the plate, allowing adequate rigidity without having to penetrate the posterior cortex of the vertebral body. These plates are extremely useful in surgery for trauma and also provide immediate stability in multilevel fusions. The fusion rate for single-level anterior cervical fusion is very good without fixation (Robinson *et al.*, 1962), and in nontraumatic cases the use of a plate at one level may not add significant benefit.

Posterior cervical spine surgery

C1–2

Various methods of fusion at the C1–2 level have been devised. Gallie and Brook's fusions involve wiring the posterior arch of the atlas to the axis with interposing bone graft. Halifax interlaminar clamps are also used to achieve the same result. Magerl's technique of direct screw fixation provides excellent results, including stability in rotation which is somewhat lacking with the other techniques. This can be combined with wiring techniques and braided cables are now often used in place of wires (Fig. 8.8).

Subaxial cervical spine

Myelopathy

Cervical laminectomy is frequently used for the treatment of myelopathy, particularly when the com-

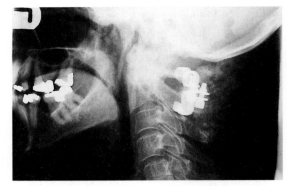

A

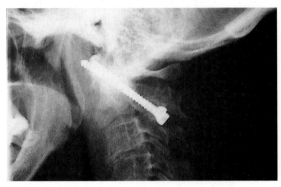

B

Fig. 8.8 Two methods used to treat rheumatoid atlantoaxial instability. (A) Halifax clamps and bone graft; (B) titanium transfacet C1–2 screws

pression extends over several levels in a patient who still has a lordotic cervical spine. This is much simpler than an anterior approach over multiple segments and, with due care being taken to preserve the zygapophysial joints, fusion is not necessary.

The operation is done through a midline incision posteriorly over the spinous processes. The paraspinal muscles are stripped from the bone and retracted laterally. The spinous processes are then removed and the laminae drilled away or removed with bone nibblers and punch rongeurs. Great care must be taken when removing the inner cortex as the cord is compromised within a narrow canal and anything else inserted into the canal will further reduce the space available for the spinal cord. It is usually not necessary to remove the laminae of C2 and the strong muscular attachments to the C2 spinous process can be left intact.

When sufficient bone has been removed the dura will bulge out of the defect and, unless there is a kyphosis, this will allow the cord to move posteriorly.

Radiculopathy

Single- or multiple-level nerve root compression can be treated from a posterior approach. This is most suited to laterally placed soft disc protrusions or foraminal narrowing, particularly if it is due to posterior osteophytes (Fig. 8.9).

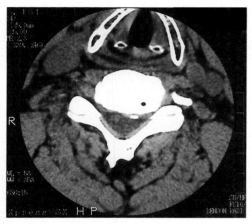

A

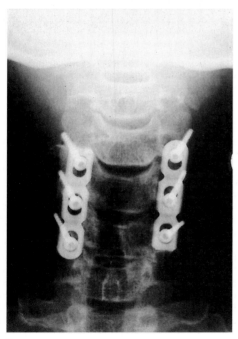

B

Fig. 8.9 (A) Computed tomographic scan showing severe bilateral foraminal stenosis at C5–6. The appearances at C4–5 were similar. (B) Lateral mass plates were used for stability after bilateral foraminotomies at C4–5 and C5–6.

A foraminotomy can be performed through a small incision placed in the midline or more laterally at the affected level. By using the same retractors as for a lumbar microdiscectomy, the exposure is adequate with a 2-cm skin incision. The operating microscope provides superior visualization and illumination. The medial part of the zygapophysial joint is drilled away to reveal the nerve root. This is then followed laterally using a drill and a small punch rongeur to undercut the bone laterally, leaving the joint intact.

Posterior fixation

The most common indication for posterior fixation of the subaxial cervical spine is trauma, particularly when posterior elements are involved, as in zygapophysial joint facet dislocations.

Posterior fixation can also be used to improve stability after extensive or wide laminectomy or multiple-level foraminotomies (Fig. 8.9). It is possible to perform a much wider decompression of a nerve root if the zygapophysial joint can be compromised but, if this is done bilaterally or at multiple levels, the consequent instability may be problematic.

There are various wiring techniques which are quite suitable for trauma. Wires can be passed through holes drilled in spinous processes, around spinous processes, under laminae, or combinations of these. Cables can be substituted for wire and Halifax clamps can also be used.

After laminectomy, wiring becomes impractical and posterior fixation is best achieved with lateral mass plates. These plates are fixed to the spine with screws passed into the lateral masses and provide excellent stability. The lateral mass at C7 is quite thin and a screw may be placed in the pedicle at this level instead. At C2, a longer screw is used to penetrate the pedicle.

References

Fielding, J.W., Cochran, G.V.B., Lawsing, J.F. III *et al.* (1974) Tears of the transverse ligament of the atlas: a clinical and biomechanical study. *J. Bone Joint Surg. Am.* **56A**: 1683–1691.

Johnson, E.W., Melvin, J.L. (1971) Value of electromyography in lumbar radiculopathy. *Arch. Phys. Med. Rehabil.* **52**: 239–243.

Lipson, S.J. (1984) Rheumatoid arthritis of the cervical spine. *Clin. Orthop.* **182**: 143–149.

Menezes, A.H., VanGilder, J.C. (1988) Transoral-transpharyngeal approach to the anterior craniocervical junction: ten-year experience with 72 patients. *J. Neurosurg.* **69**: 895–903.

Pellici, P.M., Ranawat, C.S., Tsairis, P. *et al.* (1981) A prospective study of the progression of rheumatoid arthritis of the cervical spine. *J. Bone Joint Surg. Am.* **63A**: 342–350.

Robinson, R.A., Walker, A.E., Ferlic, D.C., Wiecking, D.K. (1962) The results of anterior interbody fusion of the cervical spine. *J. Bone Joint Surg.* **44A:** 1569–1587.

Waddell, G., McCulloch, J.A., Kummel, E., Venner, R.M. (1980) Non-organic physical signs in low back pain. *Spine* **5:** 117–125.

White, A.A. III, Johnson, R.M., Panjabi, M.M., Southwick, W.O. (1975) Biomechanical analysis of clinical stability in the cervical spine. *Clin Orthop.* **109**: 85–95.

9

Chiropractic management of neck pain of mechanical origin

M. I. Gatterman

Introduction

Once a diagnosis has been made using conventional approaches such as taking a careful history, performing a thorough physical examination including orthopaedic and neurological tests, followed by imaging and laboratory tests as indicated (Chapter 7), a diagnosis of mechanical spinal pain can be made.

The mechanical lesion treated by chiropractors is referred to as a spinal functional lesion - a subluxation. This has been defined as a motion segment in which alignment, movement integrity and/or physiological function are altered (Gatterman and Hansen, 1994). Motion segments are the functional units of the body characterized by articulating surfaces and their connecting structures. The spinal motion segment of Junghanns is made up of two adjacent vertebra and the connecting tissues binding them to each other (Schmorl and Junghanns, 1971). The typical motion segment (or functional spinal unit) of the spine is a complex of three joints, the two zygapophysial (posterior) joints and the intervertebral disc. Movement at any one of these joints has a significant effect on the other two joints in the three-joint complex with degenerative changes affecting the quality and quantity of movement of the motion segment as a whole (Gatterman, 1990). In the cervical spine the two most cephalad vertebrae form atypical motion segments with no discs separating the anterior portions of these segments. The occipitoatlantal articulation has two paired condyles on the occiput that fit into the concave articular surfaces of the atlas. The body of the atlas in the atlantoaxial (C1-2) segment is replaced by the peg-like odontoid process of the axis which is bounded anteriorly by the arch of the atlas and posteriorly by the transverse cruciate ligament. These two atypical motion segments allow for a considerable range of movement in the upper cervical region. The primary motion at occiput-C1 is flexion and extension, while C1-2 allows for 50% of the total cervical rotation. Motion in the mid and lower cervical motion segments includes flexion and extension, and coupled lateral flexion and rotation. Consistent with spinal motion in general, movement in the cervical spine is guided by the morphology and plane of the zygapophysial articular surfaces.

The exact mechanisms that cause subluxation of the zygapophysial articulations have not been established. Biomechanical models that have been proposed are listed in Table 9.1 (Mootz, 1995). Cervical subluxation syndromes affecting the cervical motion segments are commonly accompanied by neck pain and restriction of range of motion and may be localized to a spinal level by palpation for painful zygapophysial joints and muscle spasm, and possibly by functional radiography (Dvorak *et al.*, 1988).

Table 9.1 *Models of chiropractic subluxation*

Biomechanical models

Vertebral malposition
Fixation caused by adhesion
Fixation caused by synovial fold entrapment
Fixation caused by nuclear fragmentation
Disc deformation caused by tissue creep
Hypermobility and ligamentous laxity
Mechanical joint locking

Modified from Mootz (1995).

Aetiology of mechanical disorders

The aetiology of cervical spine subluxation is thought to include progressive degeneration, trauma and aberrant neurological reflex patterns (Mootz, 1995). In addition to degenerative changes that occur with the ageing process, it has been speculated that frank trauma such as injury from a whiplash mechanism, or microtrauma produced by faulty sleeping posture and other habitual positions that produce repetitive strain can cause subluxations. Differentiation of subluxations must include the recognition of subluxation due to overt pathology and the non-manipulable subluxation. A non-manipulable subluxation is a vertebral motion segment with radiological or clinical features indicating that an adjustive force or osseous manipulation to this motion segment would be harmful or dangerous and is therefore contraindicated (Peterson, 1995). This extreme form of subluxation has been referred to as a medical subluxation or surgical subluxation (Sandoz, 1971) and it is imperative that the distinction be made on the basis of the magnitude of damage to supporting structures and clinical findings.

Chiropractic treatment for mechanical pain of the cervical spine is primarily manipulation but this should only be used when it is considered safe in a particular case. Manipulation is a manual procedure that involves a carefully directed thrust to move a joint past the physiological range of motion without exceeding the anatomical limit (Sandoz, 1976, 1981).

In contrast to the non-manipulable subluxation, the subluxation chiropractors treat with manipulation is not commonly diagnosed by radiographic findings but rather is determined by palpatory indications (Haas and Panzer, 1995) of localized pain and muscle spasm (Bryner, 1989). A manipulable subluxation is one in which restricted function can be improved by manual thrust procedures (Gatterman and Hansen, 1994).

The process and mechanics of spinal degeneration

The intrinsic forces that make the healthy spine a comparatively stable and mobile mechanical unit are vested in the elastic properties of some structures of the spine. Forces acting on the typical cervical motion segment include the axial pressure of the head on the nuclei pulposi and the tension exerted by ligaments holding each segment together, thus forming an intrinsic equilibrium. Relatively little muscular force is required from the contractile elements to maintain erect posture when this intrinsic equilibrium is preserved. When the intervertebral disc degenerates, this intrinsic balance mechanism is disrupted. With reduced turgidity, as the nucleus pulposus loses its hydrophilic properties, segmental instability occurs because the inelastic ligaments cannot shorten to compensate for the loss of disc height. The resultant increase in muscle activity required to stabilize the degenerating spine leads to the familiar pain–spasm–pain cycle.

Hall (1965) reviewed the pattern of degeneration of the cervical spine. In the early stages, he noted cavities at the lateral margin of the anular fibres of the intervertebral disc that spread from one side to the other with accompanying loss of disc height and ligamentous laxity. In the final stage, the intervertebral distance is greatly reduced and the bone structure becomes distorted by osteophyte formation that results in stabilization of the excess mobility allowed by intersegmental ligaments.

In the following decade Kirkaldy-Willis *et al.* (1978) documented similar changes in the lumbar spine that provide a working model for the diagnosis and management of mechanical low back pain (Kirkaldy-Willis, 1984; Kirkaldy-Willis and Hill, 1979). In this model, following the initial stage of dysfunction, loss of the intrinsic equilibrium creates an unstable phase of kinesiopathology during which subluxation occurs (Keim and Kirkaldy-Willis, 1980). In the final stage, stabilization occurs, when motion in the zygapophysial joints and disc becomes restricted by osteophytic proliferation; this stage is characterized by cartilage degeneration, loss of disc substance, soft-tissue fibrosis and the formation of osteophytes (Keim and Kirkaldy-Willis, 1980).

In the cervical spine the joints of Luschka also exhibit degenerative changes, with the joint between the bodies of the vertebrae altered from a fibrocartilaginous amphiarthrosis to a ball-and-socket-shaped diarthrosis (Hall, 1965). Sandoz (1989) described an intermediate phase prior to stabilization during which reversible joint fixations (manipulable subluxations) occur. He noted that the restricted motion typically occurs at the extremes of segmental range of motion and may produce acute pain of mechanical origin. In contrast, he noted that chronic segmental joint fixations encountered in the final stage of stabilization most commonly occur at, or near, the neutral position and are not reversible (Sandoz, 1989).

The mechanics of cervical spine injury

Injuries to the cervical spine may be classified according to the structures involved and by the mechanism of injury (Whitley and Forsyth, 1960; Babcock, 1976). Stability is dependent on ligamentous integrity and the absence of neurological insult. Instability has been defined as:

> Loss of the ability of the spine under physiologic loads to maintain relationships between vertebrae in such a way that there is neither damage nor subsequent irritation to the spinal cord or nerve roots and, in addition, there is no development of incapacitating deformities or pain due to structural changes (White and Panjabi, 1978).

If severe instability is suspected based on severe pain, signs of neurological compromise or radiographic findings (McGregor and Mior, 1990), the patient should be referred for a surgical opinion.

Cervical spine injuries

In general, spinal injuries are classified according to the mechanism of injury (Table 9.2). Hyperflexion injuries most commonly result from blows to the back of the head and forceful decelerations, for example produced by motor vehicle accidents (MVA). Pure flexion trauma may result in wedge fracture of the vertebral body with ligamentous

Table 9.2 *Classification of spinal injuries by mechanism of injury*

Hyperflexion injuries
Anterior subluxation syndrome
Bilateral zygapophysial joint facet subluxation
Wedge compression fracture
Flexion teardrop fracture

Lateral flexion and rotation injuries
Rotational subluxation syndrome
Unilateral zygapophysial joint facet subluxation

Hyperextension injuries
Posterior subluxation syndrome
Hyperextension fracture–dislocation
Fracture of the posterior arch of the atlas
Traumatic spondylolisthesis
Laminar fracture

Vertical compression injuries
Compression fracture
Burst fracture
Jefferson burst fracture (C1)

Mixed mechanism injuries
Atlanto-occipital dislocation
Odontoid fracture
Total ligamentous disruption

Modified from Fitz-Ritson (1995).

damage, loss of stability and neurological damage. With severe injuries, the anterior longitudinal ligament and intervertebral disc may be disrupted, with bilateral zygapophysial joint dislocation. Obviously such cases require referral for appropriate surgical intervention (Chapter 8).

Hyperextension injuries to the cervical spine are most likely to occur from a blow to the forehead or from whiplash injury produced by sudden acceleration and are more common than hyperflexion injuries. Hyperextension injuries frequently involve the atlantoaxial joint; hyperextension combined with compressive forces, such as occur with diving accidents, may result in fractures and dislocations leading to instability and cord damage. Violent hyperextension with the fracture of the pedicles of C2 and forwards movement of C2 on C3, produces the hangman's fracture. Burst fractures from compressive forces are rare and may involve explosion of compressed disc material as well as disruption of the vertebral body. Displaced fragments can produce cord injury in otherwise stable segments (Fitz-Ritson, 1995). All these conditions require referral for appropriate surgical intervention (Chapter 8).

Whiplash injuries

Whiplash is not a diagnostic term, but rather a descriptive label that implies a mechanism of injury whereby the body comes to a sudden stop followed by a sudden snap of the unsupported neck and head. By far the most common cause of whiplash injury is the MVA. The high incidence, litigious nature of personal injury and the frequency of ongoing complaints following low-speed impact make this a highly controversial subject which is dealt with in detail in Chapter 5.

The vulnerability of the neck is created by the 3.5–5.5 kg head (Jackson, 1977) sitting on top of the cervical spine with its multitude of joints, 50 pairs of muscles and a complex ligamentous/capsular network. From this perspective we have a ball (the head), a flexible chain (the neck) and a rigid base (the upper back). It is not surprising that this structure is subject to subluxation syndromes accompanied by soft-tissue damage (Hohl, 1983) when a sudden motion whips the head and neck (most commonly in flexion and extension).

Athletic injuries to the cervical spine

Injuries to the cervical spine include those from athletic activities such as football, soccer, skiing, diving, boxing, hockey and gymnastics. The mechanical vulnerability of the head–neck coupling increases the risk of severe disruption of the motion segments. Bony elements, ligaments, discs and muscular supporting structures as well as neurovascular structures can be affected.

Occupational and lifestyle trauma to the cervical spine

A variety of occupational risk factors have been suggested for mechanical disorders of the neck. The introduction of modern technology has resulted in monotonous tasks that impose static and repetitive loads. These tasks affect the joints and muscles which, in turn, can contribute to subluxation syndromes. Consequently, a relationship has been found between time spent working with office machines, including visual display units, and the occurrence of musculoskeletal symptoms. Other factors contributing to these disorders are mental strain, lack of situational control and low job satisfaction. A study of 420 medical secretaries found that 63% had neck pain at some time during the previous year due to working with office machines for 5 h or more per day (Kamwendo *et al.,* 1991).

Clinical features of mechanical neck pain

The clinical presentation of neck pain depends on the underlying anatomical and functional disturbance. Neck pain and restriction of motion are the most common presenting complaints and 45% of the general population are afflicted at some time during their lives (Kelsey, 1982). Furthermore, as many as one-third of these individuals will continue with chronic moderate to severe pain 15 years after the initial onset (Gore *et al.,* 1986).

History

Patients who present with mechanical neck pain give varied histories as to the onset of their affliction. Most frequent presentations indicate a history of recent trauma from MVA, falls or sports injuries, or cumulative trauma from habitual occupational postures. Less frequently there will be a history of, for example, antecedent viral illness or exposure to blasts of cold air causing neck stiffness.

Table 9.3 *Static and motion palpation procedures used in the manual therapy*

STATIC PALPATION	MOTION PALPATION
Soft tissue	*Active/passive segmental range of motion*
Tenderness	
Oedema	Tenderness
Temperature	Quality
Moisture	Quantity
Muscle tone	
Hyperaemic response	*Accessory motions*
Motility	
Trophic changes	Joint play
	End play or end feel
Bony	Joint challenge/tenderness
Tenderness	
Malposition	
Anomalies	

Modified from Haas and Panzer (1995).

Examination

Palpation remains the primary diagnostic procedure to localize pain in amenable structures, for example muscles and zygapophysial joints, by clinicians whose disciplines practise the art of manual therapy. Chiropractors (Schafer and Faye, 1989; Faye and Wiles, 1992; Haas and Panzer, 1995) along with medical practitioners (Mennel, 1965), osteopaths (Beal, 1989; Greenman, 1989), and physical therapists (Magee, 1987) who utilize manipulative therapy acknowledge this essential skill. Haas and Panzer (1995) recorded the static and motion palpation procedures used in the manual therapy decision-making process (Table 9.3).

Joint play assessment and motion palpation are commonly taught chiropractic procedures (Bryner and Bruin, 1991); however, reliability of palpatory procedures has not demonstrated consistent inter-examiner reliability for motion palpation, muscle tension and malposition (Haas and Panzer, 1995). Pain provocation, however, has been shown to have fair to good reliability among palpators. Motion palpators have demonstrated moderate to good intraexaminer reliability, indicating their ability to be consistent with themselves (Haas and Panzer, 1995).

One remarkable study (Jull *et al.,* 1988) demonstrated a high level of accuracy for the diagnosis of symptomatic cervical zygapophysial joint dysfunction correlating manual diagnosis with radiologically controlled diagnostic blocks. Three palpatory criteria were used to test the mechanical properties of all the cervical joints: abnormal end feel; abnormal quality of resistance to movement; and local pain on palpation. Because some patients could not tolerate a full examination of every joint movement because of the high irritability of the pain, it was established that, at a minimum, passive, accessory intervertebral movement would be assessed in all subjects. All symptomatic subjects in this study had experienced chronic cervical spine pain for at least 12 months. Nerve blocks were used to determine the specific cervical zygapophysial sites of pain and dysfunction. The blinded examiner examined the patients 1–4 weeks after the initial diagnostic block procedure to ensure that the effects of the block had worn off and no trace of any needle-puncture site remained. This examiner was able to identify correctly 15 of 20 patients with confirmed zygapophysial joint pain or dysfunction, determine the correct segmental level in all 15 patients, and identify the 5 patients with non zygapophysial joint pain. This study concluded that 'manual diagnosis by a trained manipulative therapist can be as accurate as can radiologically-controlled diagnostic nerve blocks in the diagnosis of cervical zygapophysial syndrome' and that the three diagnostic indicators chosen were 'highly specific for symptomatic zygapophysial joints'. The study demonstrates that, when symptomatic subjects are examined and compared to a known gold standard for comparison, palpatory evaluation is an accurate tool for manual diagnosis of mechanical lesions of the cervical spine.

Functional tests

In addition to palpatory examination, several functional tests may help to differentiate between pain of mechanical origin arising from the anterior or posterior elements and this may provide useful information for the examiner.

Distraction

Traction of the neck with the patient seated or supine may relieve mechanical pressure on joints and nerve roots. One hand is placed under the patient's chin and the other hand around the occiput. The examiner slowly applies traction to the patient's head to determine whether there is relief or a decrease in the patient's pain.

Foraminal compression

Conversely, with the patient seated and the neck extended and laterally flexed, axial compression to the neck will compress the zygapophysial joints and compromise the lateral canal, possibly increasing mechanical neck pain. With nerve root involvement, pain will radiate into the arm on the side to which the neck is laterally flexed. The distribution of the pain and altered sensation can give some indication as to which nerve root is involved.

Cervical extension and rotation

The usefulness of screening the patient for risk of cerebrovascular injury by placing the neck in extension and rotation prior to manipulation has recently been questioned (Cote *et al.*, 1996). None the less, the predictive value of this test has not been established and, given that some patients will show signs of discomfort when placed in this position, the prudent manipulator will gently place the patient's neck in extension and rotation, looking for signs of blanching, nystagmus or cyanosis around the mouth before deciding whether it is safe to use spinal manipulation. These signs, or complaints of dizziness or nausea, suggest that the patient does not tolerate this position and may be at risk of a cerebrovascular accident. Cervical spine manipulation using extension and rotation on such a patient should be avoided (see also Chapter 12).

Radiographic evaluation

The primary use of radiography in the evaluation of mechanical disorders of the cervical spine is to identify conditions that contraindicate or require modification of spinal manipulation (Gatterman, 1992). At least 31 conditions have been identified that suggest modification of manipulative therapy and, in at least 20 of these conditions, radiography is part of the standard practice for establishing the diagnosis (Gatterman, 1991).

Flexion and extension views of the cervical spine are included in the Davis series (Davis, 1945), the standard views taken following cervical spine trauma. The flexion–extension examination is useful in determining motion and instability. Atlantoaxial instability is recognized radiographically as an increase in the atlantodental interval measuring more than 3 mm in adults and 5 mm in children on the neutral lateral and flexion views (Yochum and Rowe, 1987). Similarly, hypermobility, hypomobility and aberrant and paradoxical motion (Fig. 9.1 A–C) have been described by chiropractic authors (Grice, 1977; Mannen, 1980; Henderson and Dorman, 1985). Overlay studies (Fig. 9.1D and E) are useful to identify abnormalities of cervical flexion–extension motion. This procedure is performed most frequently in patients after spine trauma and is used to indicate the presence of any excessive or abnormal segmental motion (White and Panjabi, 1978; Vernon, 1982; McGregor and Mior, 1990). Outlines of the vertebral bodies from flexion, neutral and extension radiographs are superimposed and traced on acetate transparencies with coloured fine-tip pens. Segmental motion between flexion, neutral and extension can then be depicted. Excessive lateral translation of the atlas lateral masses in relation to the axis, showing atlantoaxial instability

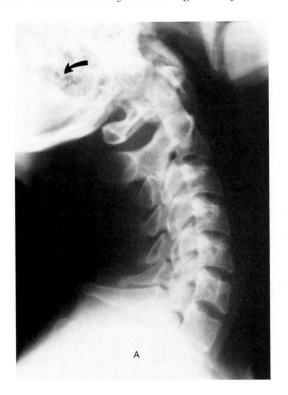

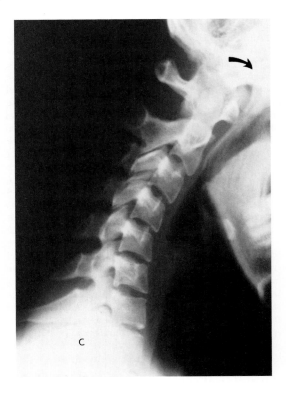

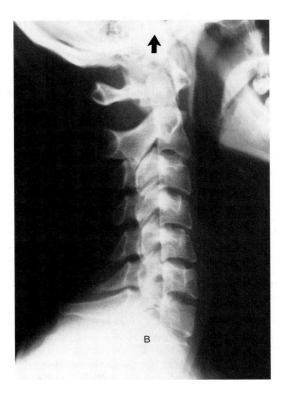

Fig. 9.1 Cervical spine lateral flexion–extension overlay study. (A) Extension; (B) neutral and (C) flexion (C) radiographs can be analysed for intersegmental motion by tracing the anatomical outlines from the neutral radiograph (solid line in D and E). These are compared with the extension (D) and flexion (E) tracings (dotted lines in D and E), which are superimposed on the neutral tracings. The procedure is performed most frequently in patients after spinal trauma and can be used to detect excessive or abnormal motion. From Taylor (1995) with permission.

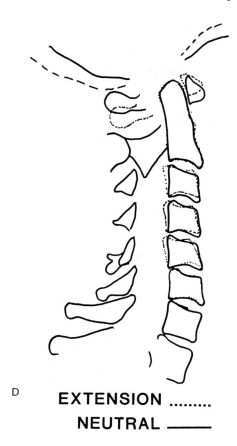

D
EXTENSION ....
NEUTRAL _____

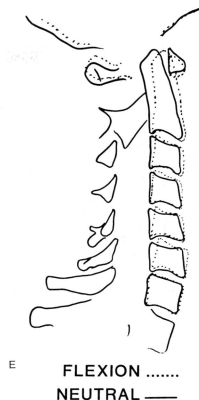

E
FLEXION ....
NEUTRAL _____

and abnormal motion in rotary atlantoaxial subluxation, can be shown with lateral flexion views taken with an open mouth (Reich and Dvorak, 1986).

Differential diagnosis

The history and physical examination, with appropriate imaging and laboratory procedures as indicated, help to determine whether the neck pain is mechanical in origin or whether there are other pathological changes requiring non-manipulative additional therapeutic procedures. It should be remembered that mechanical neck pain rarely occurs without accompanying soft-tissue pathology (Chapter 1).

In addition to subluxation of cervical motion segments producing mechanical neck pain, among the conditions that must be ruled out or confirmed are muscle syndromes, ligamentous sprain, degenerative joint disease, cervical disc herniation, torticollis, myofascial pain syndromes and inflammatory

disease. Table 9.4 outlines some of the more common mechanical and pathological disorders of the cervical spine encountered in chiropractic practice.

Management

The first consideration in the treatment of mechanical neck pain is manipulation when no contra-indication is present (Table 9.4). Indications for the type and location of manipulation are primarily dependent on palpatory findings of segmental muscle and/or zygapophysial tenderness and motion restriction. Chiropractic manipulation (commonly called the adjustment) tends to be applied specifically to a single vertebra with a short-lever, high-velocity, low-magnitude thrust or impulse. Long-lever arm procedures have the mechanical advantage of developing greater force at the expense of specificity and control. The direction of applied force is along the plane lines of zygapophy-

Table 9.4 *Differential diagnosis of some common disorders of the cervical spine*

Condition	History and symptoms	Diagnosis indicators	Management
Muscle syndromes			
Cervical strain	History of trauma (whiplash); neck pain radiating into the head, shoulders and arms	Spasm and trigger points in neck muscles; pain on active ROM ± pain on passive ROM	Trigger point therapy (manual), electrotherapy and exercise
Postural strain	History of forwards head with static loading of neck extension muscles; pain radiating into neck, head, shoulders and arms	Trigger points in extensor muscles of the neck	Trigger point therapy (manual), electrotherapy, exercise and postural retraining
Acute torticollis	History of viral infection, synovial fold pinching or exposure to a cold draught	Wry neck from spasm in the sternocleidomastoid muscle	Trigger point therapy (manual), electrotherapy and manipulation when indicated
Biomechanical disorders			
Zygapophysial joint subluxation	History of unguarded movement or trauma; pain in neck, head or arm	Palpation may reveal restricted segmental motion and tenderness	Manipulation
Cervical zygapophysial joint sprain	History of trauma; pain and stiffness of neck, protective muscle spasm: pain may radiate to occiput and into shoulders	Motion palpation may reveal absence of segmental restriction; stress radiographs may reveal hypermobile vertebral motion once muscle spasm reduces	Restrict excess motion with cervical collar when acute; exercise
Spondylosis and spondyloarthrosis	Neck pain and stiffness; decrease in range of motion; pain may refer to cervico-shoulder, occipital and interscapular regions, dizziness	Radiographs reveal decreased disc height, osteophytes, sclerosis of vertebral body end-plates, decreased zygapophysial facet joint and uncovertebral joint spaces with osteophytes and sclerosis	Gentle manipulation depending on degree of degenerative changes; traction, exercise; restriction of excess motion by cervical collar may benefit when acute
Cervical disc herniation	History of trauma; neck and shoulder pain radiating down the arm in the distribution of involved nerve root; paraesthesia: numbness, tingling; sensory and reflex deficits	Possible loss of appropriate reflex and sensation, ± muscle weakness and wasting; advanced imaging necessary (MRI, CT scan)	Refer severe cases for surgical evaluation; moderate cases may respond to a trial of specific gentle manipulation; restrict excess motion, electrotherapy and exercise
Inflammatory disease			
Rheumatoid arthritis	Neck pain, progressive pain of myelopathy, neurological manifestation that may be subtle (i.e. easy fatigability or difficulty in walking, with sensory loss or gross paralysis)	Radiographs may reveal osteoporosis, hypermobility, dislocations and subluxations of the cervical spine; atlantoaxial dislocation may occur with lysis of transverse ligaments; flexion–extension views necessary for accurate evaluation (3 mm gap between odontoid and atlas anteriorly; 4–5 mm forward subluxation is significant). Positive rheumatoid factor may be found	Manipulation contraindicated in cases of vertebral segmental instability; restriction of excess motion and referral for medicinal treatment ± surgical stabilization
Ankylosing spondylitis	Predominantly seen in males: stiffness, spinal pain, muscle pain and loss of chest expansion	Possibly high ESR and positive HLA-B27 during active phase; radiographs demonstrate a progressive loss of segmental motion with ossification of ligaments – 'bamboo spine'; disc spaces are not narrowed as in degenerative joint disease; ligamentous laxity above rigid segments may be seen with atlantoaxial occipital dislocation	Gentle mobilization, heat, mild exercise, manipulation considered when acute phase is past; refer for anti-inflammatory medication when necessary

ROM = Range of motion; MRI = magnetic resonance imaging; CT = computed tomographic; ESR = erythrocyte sedimentation rate; HLA = human leukocyte antigen.

Note: In all cases, the clinician *must* consider the possible risk factors of a cerebrovascular accident occurring due to injury of the vertebral or carotid arteries. If in doubt regarding risk factors, *do not* treat by manual therapy.

Modified and updated from Gatterman (1990).

sial joint facets, with the objective of gapping the joint. As the articular surfaces suddenly move apart an audible release may be heard, possibly from a sudden liberation of dissolved synovial fluid gases. The typical chiropractic manipulation is forceful enough to produce the articular cracking noise but not so great as to separate the joint beyond the limits of its anatomical integrity. Prior to the thrust the joint must be tractioned to the point of tension so as to prevent the applied force from being absorbed by the surrounding soft tissues (Haas, 1990).

Complications from cervical manipulation

The benefits of cervical manipulation have been overshadowed by association of manipulation of the cervical spine with serious cerebrovascular accidents. Complications have occurred in patients who have received manipulation uneventfully in the past and without obvious risk factors for a cerebrovascular accident, such as arteriosclerosis, hypertension, heavy smoking or oral contraceptive use. In general, cervical manipulation is a relatively safe form of therapy in the hands of skilled practitioners but, like other precise manual skills, requires prolonged and specific training followed by persistent practice. Both benefit and risk are important considerations in the evaluation of treatment options as, although the exact incidence of cerebrovascular accidents following manipulation is unknown, it has been estimated to occur in 1 per million to 1 per three million manipulations (Guttman, 1983; Dvorak and Orelli, 1985; Carey, 1993). This indicates that carefully performed cervical spine manipulation is probably safer than complications from medical treatment for mechanical neck pain. The incidence of serious gastrointestinal bleeding from prescription non-steroidal anti-inflammatory drugs has been estimated at 1 per 1000 patients and 3.2 per 1000 patients age 65 and over (Gabriel *et al.,* 1991).

While mobilization is considered safer than manipulation, it has been suggested that manipulation is more effective in the treatment of mechanical neck pain than non-thrust mobilization (Cassidy *et al.,* 1992). Most complications of spinal manipulation can be avoided by careful evaluation of each patient based on a good working knowledge of the relevant anatomy, physiology and kinesiology. Excess force should always be avoided, preferably using specific short-lever thrusts as opposed to high-force, long-lever rotational manoeuvres. Soft-tissue and mobilizing techniques may also prove beneficial.

There is no substitution for skill, knowledge and finesse. Like any other skilled procedure, the expected results and number of complications depend on the ability of the clinician. Lack of diagnostic and manipulative skills should be considered a definite contraindication to cervical manipulation.

Contraindications to cervical manipulation

This topic is dealt with in detail in Chapter 12 so will only be summarized here.

Contraindications to cervical manipulation range from non-indication to lack of a clear indication and from relative contraindication to absolute contraindication. Frequently, manipulation is contraindicated in one area of the spine, yet beneficial in another region (Gatterman, 1981; Stoddard, 1983). Unstable fractures or ligamentous instability from traumatic injuries or pathological conditions are absolute contraindications for the involved area. A relative contraindication is osteopenia, whether from osteoporosis or osteomalacia. While osteopenia precludes forceful manipulation, light mobilization techniques and non-thrust adjustments may prove beneficial. Lower-extremity symptoms accompanying neck pain may indicate disc protrusion with cord involvement requiring medical referral. Early recognition of these conditions and immediate referral for neurological decompression are essential to prevent permanent neurological deficits. The contraindications to manipulation are for the most part common sense and require modification of treatment based on presentation.

Supporting evidence for manipulation of mechanical neck pain

While the evidence supporting manipulation for the treatment of mechanical neck pain is not as conclusive as that for the treatment of acute low back problems (Bigos *et al.,* 1994), there is convincing evidence that manipulation of the cervical spine is more effective than either mobilization or muscle relaxants. In patients with minor cervical spondylosis or non-specific neck pain, manipulation with pain medication has been shown to be more effective than drugs alone (Sloop *et al.,* 1982). In subjects with neck, arm or hand pain from cervical spine lesion with reduced range of motion, increased range of motion following manipulation with medication was maintained at 1 week and 3 weeks when compared to those receiving medication alone (Sloop *et al.,* 1982). In subjects with chronic neck pain, the manipulated group demonstrated a 40–50% rise in pain threshold around the manipulated joint compared to no change in the group that received mobilization (Vernon *et al.,* 1990). Patients with unilateral neck pain showed a greater mean decrease in pain intensity following rotational manipulation than those receiving mobilization without a thrust (Cassidy *et al.,* 1992). Greater mean improvement in physical functioning, and pain improvement in patients with non-specific neck complaints with limited range of motion, was demonstrated in a group receiving manipulation and/or mobilization compared to groups receiving exercise, massage and other forms of physical therapy, and a control group receiving detuned short-wave diathermy and those continuing treatment with general practitioners (Koes *et al.,* 1992a,b, 1993).

Management of neck pain by chiropractors involves more than simple manipulation of cervical joint dysfunction. Adjustments include a variety of osseous manual thrust (Bartol, 1995) and reflex (Bergmann, 1995) techniques. Traditional chiropractic care involves the whole patient (Gatterman, 1995), with spine and nervous system function viewed as integral components (Troyanovich and Harrison, 1996). The chiropractor approaches the spine as a multilinked mechanical system that combines weight-bearing with physiological movement (Gatterman, 1990). Restoration of mobility and a reduction in pain are the primary goals of chiropractic management of mechanical neck pain, along with the overall objective of improved posture and general well-being. Modification of precipitating factors in the workplace and other activities of daily living are equally important in the management and prevention of neck pain of mechanical origin.

References

Babcock, J.L. (1976) Cervical spine injuries. *Arch. Surg.* **11:** 646–651.

Bartol, K. (1995) Osseous manual thrust techniques. In: *Foundation of Chiropractic: Subluxation* (Gatterman, M.I., ed.). St Louis: Mosby, pp. 88–104.

Beal, M.C. (1989) Perception through palpation. *J. Am. Osteopath. Assoc.* **89:** 1334–1352.

Bergmann, T.F. (1995) Chiropractic reflex techniques. In: *Foundation of Chiropractic: Subluxation* (Gatterman, M.I., ed.). St Louis: Mosby, pp. 106–122.

Bigos, S., Bowyer, O., Breen, G. *et al.* (1994) *Acute Low-back Problems in Adults. Clinical Practice Guideline.* Quick reference guide number 14. AHCPR publication no. 95–0643. Rockville, MD: US Department of Health and Human Services, Public Health Service, Agency of Health Care Policy and Research.

Bryner, P. (1989) A survey of indications: knee manipulation. *Chiro. Tech.* **1:** 140–145.

Bryner, P., Bruin, J. (1991) Survey of the status of technique teaching in chiropractic colleges. *Chiro. Tech.* **3:** 30–32.

Carey, P.F. (1993) A suggested protocol for the examination and treatment of the cervical spine: managing the risk. *J. Can. Chiro. Assoc.* **37:** 104–106.

Cassidy, J.D., Lopes, A.A., Yong-Hing, J. (1992) The immediate effect of manipulation versus mobilization of pain and range of motion in the cervical spine: a randomized controlled trial. *J. Manip. Physiol. Ther.* **15:** 570–575.

Cote, P., Kreitz, B., Cassidy, J.D., Theil, H. (1996) The validity of the extension-rotation test as a clinical screening procedure before neck manipulation: a secondary analysis. *J. Manip. Physiol. Ther.* **19:** 159–164.

Davis, A.G. (1945) Injuries of the cervical spine. *J.A.M.A.* **127:** 149–156.

Dvorak, J., Orelli, F. (1985) How dangerous is manipulation to the cervical spine? *Man. Med.* **2:** 1–4.

Dvorak, J., Froehlich, D., Penning, L. *et al.* (1988) Functional radiographic diagnosis of the cervical spine: flexion/extension. *Spine* **13:** 748–755.

Faye, L.J., Wiles, M.R. (1992) Manual examination of the spine. In: *Principles and Practice of Chiropractic,* 2nd edn (Haldeman, S., ed.). San Mateo, CA: Appleton & Lange, pp. 301–318.

Fitz-Ritson, D. (1995) Cervicogenic sympathetic syndromes: etiology, treatment, and rehabilitation. In: *Foundations of Chiropractic: Subluxation* (Gatterman, M. I., ed.). St Louis: Mosby, pp. 318–339.

Gabriel, S.E., Jaakkimainen, L., Bombardier, C. (1991) Risk for serious gastrointestinal complications related to use of nonsteroidal anti-inflammatory drugs: a meta-analysis. *Ann. Intern. Med.* **115:** 787–796.

Gatterman, M.I. (1981) Contraindications and complication of spinal manipulative therapy. *ACA J. Chiro.* **15:** 575–586.

Gatterman, M.I. (1990) *Chiropractic Management of Spine Related Disorders.* Baltimore: Williams & Wilkins, pp. 22–36.

Gatterman, M.I. (1991) Standards of practice relative to complications of and contraindications to spinal manipulative therapy. *J. Can. Chiro. Assoc.* **35:** 232–236.

Gatterman, M.I. (1992) Standards of contraindications to spinal manipulative therapy. In: *Chiropractic Standards of Practice and Quality Care* (Vear, J.H., ed.). Aspen: Gaithersburg, pp. 221–236.

Gatterman, M.I. (1995) A patient-centered paradigm: a model for chiropractic education and research. *J. Altern. Complement. Med.* **1:** 371–386.

Gatterman, M.I., Hansen, D. (1994) The development of chiropractic nomenclature through consensus. *J. Manip. Physiol. Ther.* **17:** 302–309.

Gore, D.R., Sepic, S.B., Gardner, G.M., Murray, M.P. (1986) Neck pain: a long-term follow-up of 205 patients. *Spine* **12:** 1–5.

Greenman, P.E. (1989) *Principles of Manual Medicine.* Baltimore: Williams & Wilkins, pp. 61–70.

Grice, A.S. (1977) Preliminary evaluation of 50 sagittal cervical motion radiographic examinations. *J. Can. Chiro. Assoc.* **21:** 3–4.

Guttman, G. (1983) Injuries to the vertebral artery caused by manual therapy. *Man. Med.* **21:** 2–14.

Haas, M. (1990) The physics of spinal manipulation. Part IV. Theoretical consideration of the physician impact force and energy requirements needed to produce synovial joint cavitation. *J. Manip. Physiol. Ther.* **13:** 378–383.

Haas, M., Panzer, D.M. (1995) Palpatory diagnosis of subluxation. In: *Foundations of Chiropractic: Subluxation* (Gatterman, M.I., ed.) St Louis: Mosby, pp. 53–67.

Hall, M.C. (1965) *Luschka's Joint.* Springfield, IL: Charles C Thomas, p. 44.

Henderson, D.J., Dorman, T.M. (1985) Functional roentgeno-metric evaluation of the cervical spine in the sagittal plane. *J. Manip. Physiol. Ther.* **8:** 219–227.

Hohl, M. (1983) Soft tissue neck injuries. In: *The Cervical Spine* (Baily, R.W., ed.). Philadelphia: JB Lippincott, pp. 282–287.

Jackson, R. (1977) *The Cervical Syndrome*, 4th edn. Spingfield, IL: Charles C. Thomas.

Jull, G., Bogduk, N., Marsland, A. (1988) The accuracy of manual diagnosis for cervical zygapophyseal joint pain syndromes. *Med. J. Aust.* **148:** 233–236.

Kamwendo, K., Liton, S.J., Moritz, U. (1991) Neck and shoulder disorders in medical secretaries. Part 1: pain prevalence and risk factors. *Scand. J. Rehabil. Med.* **23:** 141–152.

Keim, H.A., Kirkaldy-Willis, W.H. (1980) Low back pain. *CIBA Clinical Symposia*, pp. 32–36.

Kelsey, J.L. (1982) *Epidemiology of Musculoskeletal Disorders*. New York: Oxford University Press, p. 146.

Kirkaldy-Willis, W.H. (1984) *Managing Low Back Pain*. New York: Churchill Livingstone.

Kirkaldy-Willis, W.H., Hill, R.J. (1979) A more precise diagnosis for low back pain. *Spine* **4:** 102–109.

Kirkaldy-Willis, W.H., Wedge, J., Yong-Hing, K., Reilly, J. (1978) Pathogenesis of lumbar spondylosis and stenosis. *Spine* **4:** 293–294.

Koes, B.W., Bouter, L.M., van Mameren, H., Essers, A.H.M. (1992a) The effectiveness of manual therapy, physio-therapy, and treatment by the general practitioner for nonspecific back and neck complaints: a randomized clinical trail. *Spine* **17:** 28–35.

Koes, B.W., Bouter, L.M., van Mameren, H. *et al.* (1992b) Randomized clinical trail of manipulative phsyiotherapy for persistent back and neck complaints: results of one year follow up. *Br. Med. J.* **304:** 601–605.

Koes, B.W., Bouter, L.M., van Mameren, H. *et al.* (1993) A randomized clinical trial of manual therapy and physio-therapy for persistent back and neck complaints: sub-group analysis and relationship between outcome measures. *J. Manip. Physiol. Ther.* **16:** 211–219.

McGregor, M., Mior, S. (1990) Anatomical and functional perspectives of the cervical spine. Part III: the "unstable" cervical spine. *J. Can. Chiro. Assoc.* **34:** 145–152.

Magee, D.J. (1987) *Orthopedic Physical Assessment.* Phil-adelphia: WB Saunders.

Mannen, E.M. (1980) The use of cervical radiographic overlays to assess response to manipulation. A case report. *J. Can. Chiro. Assoc.* **24:** 108–109.

Mennel, J.M. (1965) *Joint Pain: Diagnosis and Treatment Using Manipulative Techniques.* Boston: Little Brown, pp. 3–5.

Mootz, R.O. (1995) Theoretical models of chiropractic subluxation. In: *Foundations of Chiropractic: Subluxa-tion* (Gatterman, M.I., ed.) St Louis: Mosby, pp. 175–189.

Peterson, C.K. (1995) The nonmanipulable subluxation. In: *Foundations of Chiropractic: Subluxation* (Gatterman, M.I., ed.). St Louis: Mosby, p. 124.

Reich, C., Dvorack, J. (1986) The functional evaluation of craniocervical ligaments in sidebending using x-rays. *Man. Med.* **2:** 108–113.

Sandoz, R. (1971) Newer trends in the pathogenesis of spinal disorders. *Ann. Swiss Chiro. Assoc.* **5:** 112.

Sandoz, R. (1976) Some physical mechanisms and effects of spinal adjustments. *Ann. Swiss Chiro. Assoc.* **6:** 91.

Sandoz, R. (1981) Some reflex phenomena associated with spinal derangements and adjustments. *Ann. Swiss Chiro. Assoc.* **7:** 45.

Sandoz, R. (1989) The natural history of a spinal degen-erative lesion. *Ann. Swiss Chiro. Assoc.* **9:** 149–192.

Schafer, R.C., Faye, L.J. (1989) *Motion Palpation and Chiropractic Technique: Principles of Dynamic Chiro-practic.* Huntington Beach, CA: Motion Palpation Institute.

Schmorl, G., Junghanns, H. (1971) *The Human Spine in Health and Disease,* 2nd edn. New York: Grune & Stratton.

Sloop, P.R., Smith, D.S., Goldenberg, E., Dore, C. (1982) Manipulation for chronic neck pain. A double blind controlled study. *Spine* **7:** 532–535.

Stoddard, A. (1983) *Manual of Osteopathic Medicine,* 2nd edn. London: Hutchinson, pp. 290–291.

Taylor, J.A.M. (1995) The role of radiography in evaluating subluxation. In: *Foundations of Chiropractic: Subluxa-tion* (Gatterman, M.I., ed.). St. Louis: Mosby.

Troyanovich, S., Harrison, D. (1996) Chiropractic biophysics (CBP) technique. *Chiro. Tech.* **8:** 1–6.

Vernon, H. (1982) Static and dynamic roentgenography in the diagnosis of degenerative disc disease: a review and comparative assessment. *J. Manip. Physiol. Ther.* **5:** 163–169.

Vernon, H.T., Aker, P., Burns, S., Vijakaanen, S., Short, L. (1990) Pressure pain threshold evaluation of the effect of spinal manipulation in the treatment of chronic neck pain: a pilot study. *J. Manip. Physiol. Ther.* **13:** 13–16.

White, A.A., Panjabi, M.M. (1978) *Clinical Biomechanics of the Spine.* Philadelphia: JB Lippincott, p. 192.

Whitley, J.E., Forsyth, H.F. (1960) The classification of cervical spine injuries. *A.J.R.* **83:** 633–644.

Yochum, T.R., Rowe, L.J. (1987) Radiographic positioning and normal anatomy. In: *Essentials of Skeletal Radiology* (Yochum, T.R., Rowe, L. J., eds). Baltimore: Williams & Wilkins, pp. 1–94.

10

Osteopathic management of cervical pain

T. McClune, R. Clarke, C. Walker and R. Burtt

Introduction

Cervical spine disorders are a common source of discomfort and disability. The previous chapters in this book have attempted to unravel the current knowledge surrounding pathology, biomechanics and the like, in order to provide a useful framework for clinical management. This chapter aims to set out an approach to management adopted by the osteopath. However, as with the other manipulative professions (and arguably most of clinical medicine), osteopaths vary dramatically in their beliefs and methods, so what follows is distilled from a mixture of traditional practice and contemporary research findings; the intention is to provide a rational framework for the assessment, treatment and rehabilitation of patients with cervical syndromes, within the setting of an osteopathic clinic. Inevitably there will be considerable overlap with the chapters from the other therapies which use physical modes of therapy, and doubtless there will be osteopaths (and scientists) who will disagree with what follows.

Clinicians traditionally use three main sources for their choice of treatment (Weber and Burton, 1986): their own experience, what they learn from colleagues, and reports from investigations. The first two are empirical and unreliable, but are the most frequently used sources; the third, whilst being the most rational basis of the three, suffers from the problem of dissemination – it follows that, at best, the resultant therapy will be suboptimal. In describing the osteopathic approach we are aware that we only offer a part of an overall management strategy, a part that is underdeveloped yet offers the possibility of considerable help for a proportion of the patients. Demands for strict scientific proof of the efficacy of any treatment, though absolutely essential, must not be confused with the duty to comfort the patient (Weber and Burton, 1986), always bearing in mind the need to avoid iatrogenic effects or disastrous consequences of inappropriate intervention.

In common with low back trouble, cervical syndromes are experienced by most people, at some stage in their lives, to some extent. Chronicity is not uncommon, and the clinical challenge is arguably not just the resolution of immediate symptoms (the natural history is considered benign in many cases); rather it is the reduction of recurrence rates and the prevention of persistent pain and disability.

The literature in respect of cervical spine syndromes is more fragmented than for lumbar disorders, and there are no structured clinical guidelines available (at least in the UK). Nevertheless, there are sufficient clinical similarities between lumbar and cervical syndromes to indicate that the principles set out in the American and British guidelines for low back pain (Bigos *et al.,* 1994) are appropriate, in general terms, for cervical or neck trouble. The essential message, once serious pathology has been ruled out, is that the approach should be one of early positive management promoting early return to normal activity (including work) along with a reduction of passive (rest and avoidance) approaches. However, it would be a mistake to equate cervical and lumbar problems; they are distinct spinal areas with discrete possibilities for referral of symptoms, for concomitant disease, or for serious pathology; careful initial assessment is of particular importance in cases of cervical symptoms.

Cervical pain is a common presenting symptom in osteopathic practice; figures vary between 20% (Burton, 1981) and 25% (Burns and Lyttelton, 1994). This compares with approximately 40–50% of patients presenting with low back pain (Burton, 1981; Burns and Lyttelton, 1994). The symptom of headache, which can frequently be related to cervical disorders, may represent around 10% of consultations to osteopaths (Burton, 1981; Burns and Lyttelton, 1994). The most frequent presentation will be for what can be considered mechanical dysfunction where assessment and treatment approaches based on mechanical principles will be appropriate. It is these disorders, and the possibility for their management by osteopaths, which are the focus of this chapter, but other diagnoses will be given the attention they deserve. Although issues such as work-relatedness and psychosocial factors are important and will be mentioned, their detailed consideration will be left to other authors in this book.

So far as efficacy of osteopathic (or other manipulative) management is concerned, relatively few rigorous randomized controlled trials have been performed. Nevertheless, what evidence there is (Howe *et al.*, 1983; Vernon *et al.*, 1990; Koes *et al.*, 1992) is generally supportive. Disasters seem to be rare, and are probably confined to situations where there has been a failure to diagnose complicating pathology.

Assessment

Interview

The first stage in the diagnostic process is the interview. This is a series of structured questions with the purpose of finding the answers necessary to form a differential diagnosis. It is also the starting point for developing a therapeutic relationship with the patient, obtaining mutual trust and confidence.

The main objectives are:

1. To identify the presenting symptoms.
2. To identify any possible cause.
3. To establish the start point and progression of the presenting symptoms.
4. To obtain details of any previous history of a cervical spine condition.
5. To determine the symptom-modifying factors (aggravating and relieving factors).
6. To identify any diurnal pattern of symptoms.
7. To obtain information on any other relevant medical problems.
8. To permit some insight into occupational, general lifestyle and relevant psychosocial issues.

Presenting symptoms

An osteopath will first determine the site and nature of pain and associated symptoms. From these the clinician is able to identify the area of concern and the tissues involved. Injury to and subsequent inflammation of the joint capsule, muscles and ligaments is said to produce a dull deep ache, nagging ache or burning ache. A throbbing, beating, pounding pain suggests inflammation with vascular congestion. An extreme, unremitting, throbbing pain is more indicative of a serious pathology. A transient catch may be due to a functional defect of a joint segment, resulting in a disturbance of joint mechanics. The above must be considered as traditional concepts as in general they have not been confirmed by scientific research. Any involvement of a spinal nerve root can produce a severe, sickening toothache type of pain, which may also be described as shooting and associated with paraesthesia or anaesthesia.

Cervical spine pain can present with or without radicular pain. In general the upper cervical complex (occiput to C2) refers pain from the occiput, superolaterally to the temporal area and into the orbit of the eye. The middle and lower cervical spine refers pain into the shoulder and arm, to the hand. The presence of anaesthesia/paraesthesia or motor weakness in a dermatomal/myotomal distribution can indicate nerve root irritation. A more generalized distribution may be an accompaniment of non-radicular pain.

Onset and temporal pattern

The causation is important to determine, as fully as possible. Combined with a knowledge of subsequent events, one can form a diagnosis and begin to develop a management plan. The nature, extent and fluctuations in disability, any relationship with work, response to past treatment and any relevant past history can help direct overall management. With regards to temporal pattern, a distinguishing feature of inflammation is early-morning irritability and stiffness. Symptoms worsening as the day progresses indicate muscular fatigue, and an increase of pain at night should be investigated more fully, as serious pathology needs to be eliminated.

Previous history

Previous history of low back pain is significant in the prognosis of an episode of low back pain. The same could arguably be true for cervical pain of musculoskeletal origin. Obvious trauma to the cervical spine, e.g. whiplash injury, can have long-lasting effects, with episodes of remission and recurrence. Previous medical history may guide the diagnosis. Previous malignancy is a 'red flag' which warrants further investigation in a patient presenting with neck pain and/or associated symptoms. Previous history of anticoagulant medication would preclude high-velocity thrust (HVT) treatment techniques. Response to previous treatment to the cervical spine would also help in the management process.

Symptom-modifying factors

In low back pain, symptom-modifying factors may function as discriminating factors (Burton, 1987; Langworthy and Breen, 1992) and can give an indication of disability and loss of function and hence the degree of severity. It seems reasonable to assume that this is also true of the cervical spine. General questions are asked as to which factors, if any, increase or decrease the presenting symptom. The answers to such questions will both guide treatment as well as aid diagnosis. For example, neck extension increasing neck pain, which is relieved by neck flexion, may indicate zygapophysial joint inflammation.

Lifestyle and psychological influences

An osteopath will question the patient on general health and lifestyle to gain a more comprehensive understanding of the patient's condition, as well as ensuring that there are no underlying conditions separate to or causing the present problem that either need further referral or are contraindicated to osteopathic manipulation. When asking questions about the patient's occupation, an osteopath is searching for factors which may predispose, cause or maintain the patient's problems. Work practices and daily activities often influence the spinal mechanics; advice given often needs to address these issues. The patient's general psychological status, including attitudes to pain and treatment, should be assessed.

Clinical examination

Table 10.1 is a summary of a protocol used by osteopaths to exclude instability/pathology prior to high velocity thrust (HVT) manipulation of the upper cervical segments. Parts of the protocol will be

Table 10.1 *Osteopathic screening protocol for upper cervical high-velocity thrust (HVT) manipulation*

Rapid osteopathic screening examination for the cephalocervical region prior to HVT

Neurological elements
Tendon reflexes upper and lower limbs, bilateral plantar responses

Exclude organic neck stiffness, neck flexion test (Kernig's sign)

If the patient complains of sensory changes or weakness of the limbs, assessment of sensation and motor power is necessary

Intracranial contents
Pupils should be equal, central, regular and react to light. Unilaterally dilated pupil – if pupils are asymmetrical, the larger may be associated with a Hutchinson's pupil. Unilaterally constricted pupil – exclude Horner's syndrome

Note that both neck and upper limb pain can be referred from dysfunction of the heart and subdiaphragmatic organs such as the gallbladder. If symptoms cannot be produced by musculoskeletal examination, the possibility of visceral referral from these areas must be considered. Consider also the possibility of lung apex involvement, and percuss and auscultate these areas if necessary

Try to elicit oculomotor ataxia (nystagmus). Vertical nystagmus (jerky/bobbing up and down) is pathognomonic of brainstem compromise, and a contraindication for HVT

Skeletal elements
Passive examination of cervical column, with patient supine, neck in neutral position (a pillow helps prevent extension)

Note any persistent paravertebral spasm or tenderness

Brief palpation of surface of skull, for bumps, holes, deformities, local areas of tenderness

Palpate extracranial circulation – exclude arteritis (hard, tender, pulseless cord), superficial temporal artery

Vascular elements
Auscultate and palpate (separately) the transcervical portion of the common carotid arteries. HVT is contraindicated in the presence of an intrinsic bruit/audible flow murmur, asymmetry of pulse volume, with asymmetrical conduction of ordinary heart sounds, i.e. one side muffled compared to the other. Auscultate the vertebral artery in the vertebral triangle, at the apex of the posterior triangle of the neck where it arises from the first part of the subclavian artery

Trial leverage
Passively put the cervical spine into a minimum leverage position and sustain for 30 s. Instruct the patient to report any disturbance of feelings or perceptions: vertigo (sense of internal instability), anxiety, subjective distress, nausea, epigastric discomfort, any visual disturbance, i.e. diplopia (double vision) or amblyopia or paraesthesia anywhere in the body, especially the face. The patient may superficially cooperate but you palpate an increasing involuntary muscular resistance. In the case of any of the above, HVT techniques should be avoided

---

performed routinely during a clinical examination, other parts will be used prior to HVT only.

Observation

Observation begins with general surface anatomy, then more specific regions are assessed, followed by palpation, to confirm or rule out visual impressions.

Spinous processes can be palpated for any deviation from the midline in the frontal plane, and depression or prominence in the sagittal plane. Deviation of the skull and cervical or thoracolumbar spinal curves from the normal position can be assessed. A rotational or lateral displacement of the thoracic spine, ribcage or scapulae indicates the presence of a scoliosis.

Observation is made regarding pelvic tilt, unilateral erector spinae or limb girdle muscle hypertonicity/hypertrophy. This assessment of the symmetry to posture can guide the clinician to possible areas of overuse or biomechanical dysfunction. The transition from the cervical lordosis to thoracic kyphosis should be a smooth minimal curve, although a prominence at the C7 spinous process is expected. Note the presence of any lateral deviation within the cervical spine (e.g. torticollis) which often results from protective muscular spasm associated with trauma, or the possibility of bony pathology. If the patient needs to support the upper limb, this may indicate nerve root compromise. In advanced stages of bony pathology or soft-tissue infection the head may be supported by the hands. Inspect for colour changes. Erythema may indicate infection, inflammation or acute somatic dysfunction.

Specific muscle bulk, signifying atrophy or hypertrophy, is possible to detect with observation, often confirmed with palpation. Noting signs of trauma (scars, bruises, lacerations, abrasions and swelling) is important, and may help identify cause and extent of injury. A brief inspection of supraclavicular fossae would indicate if any lymph node enlargement is present, which would require further investigation.

If the symptoms are aggravated by sitting, observation would continue with the patient in a sitting position. Again, alteration of surface anatomy and morphology from the expected may help in the identification of areas of dysfunction.

Musculoskeletal assessment

The assessment of spinal somatic dysfunction is the central issue of our clinical practice. Neumann (1989) suggests that diagnostic signs of somatic dysfunction are:

1. Joint movement restriction.
2. Neuroreflexive disturbance manifesting as:
   (a) local segmental tissue irritation and/or
   (b) peripheral segmental irritation (segmentally related dermatomes).

The evaluation of the biomechanical function of the musculoskeletal system will include examining symmetry of motion, movement of complete sections of the spine (regional motion testing) and of single spinal functional units (intersegmental motion testing). The quantitative value given to a range of movement is subject to error; the judgement is made based on the recognized physiological normal values, which will alter depending primarily on age, disc degeneration, previous injury and sport participation. Instrumentation such as a goniometer can be used, which would arguably be more accurate (Alaranta *et al.,* 1994); however, in a clinical setting this accuracy is not necessary for the evaluation of dysfunction. The qualitative value given to the range of movement is as important, and a combination of the two is our aim.

Active motion

The overall motion of both cervical and thoracolumbar regions may be assessed whilst standing. However, active movements of the cervical spine may be tested in the seated position to stabilize the trunk, and in elderly patients or those prone to dizziness. The expected range of motion in the cervical spine is set out below (Kahn and Monod, 1989; McRae, 1990).

1. Ask the patient to bend the head forwards – about 70° should be expected.
2. Ask the patient to tilt the head backwards, into extension (exercising care if the patient is elderly, or there is a history of vertigo or dizziness) – about 70° should be expected.
3. Ask the patient to tilt the head towards each shoulder in turn, without shrugging the shoulders – 45° is the normal range.
4. Instruct the patient to look over each shoulder in turn. Normally the chin stops just short of the coronal plane at the shoulders – about 90° should be expected.

A note is made of overall range of movement and at which spinal segments that movement occur. The next stage is to identify any limitation of movement, and the likely cause. The possibilities are muscle guarding, ligament shortening, bony apposition or presence of pain. The quality of movement and the reproduction or exacerbation of symptoms, the presence of protective deformity, deviation, abnormal contours, loss of normal curvature on movement may help identify tissues contributing to dysfunction (Corrigan and Maitland, 1991). A note is made of any paraesthesia and concomitant symptoms, and which movement or position affects them.

To demonstrate the cervical origin of arm pain, the neck is moved into extension, rotation and then lateral flexion towards the painful side together with gentle but gradually increasing pressure (Spurling manoeuvre). Pain and/or paraesthesia down the arm indicates nerve compromise, rather than a thoracic outlet syndrome. This also exerts maximum load on the intervertebral joints and can reproduce musculoskeletal referred pain of non-root origin, which tends to be of a more vague distribution, not normally below the elbow, and without paraesthesia.

Palpation

Palpation will include the neck, scapula, mid/upper thoracic areas and ribcage. Muscular state (resting tone, bulk, temperature, abnormal mass) and muscular symmetry are noted, as is tenderness to pressure. Symmetry of the ribcage and bony landmarks are noted. Variation from the expected normal is the purpose of such examination. When estimating the normal, bear in mind work activities, sports participation, previous injury and personality type.

Local segmental irritation

Facet joint somatic dysfunction is said to be usually associated with tissue changes around the involved joint, segmental irritation points (Neumann, 1989), tender nodular areas resulting from increased tension in the deep musculature of the neck and swelling of connective tissues.

These points change with the direction and extent of passive joint movement, becoming more tender and easier to palpate as the restricted joint approaches its end-point.

Peripheral segmental irritation

Patients commonly experience neck pain which radiates to one or both shoulders, elbows or hands. Radicular and peripheral joint pathology as the cause of these symptoms should be excluded. Neurological and clinical examination of the relevant peripheral joints will be necessary for this purpose. Referred pain or hyperalgesia of musculoskeletal origin from a vertebral segment, without root involvement by mechanical irritation or compression, is often found in zones related to, but not always confined to, the associated dermatomal areas. This so-called sclerotome distribution is less distinct than the dermatome, and is subject to considerable individual variation. However, musculoskeletal referred pain in the neck, trunk and limb may not be a matter of somatic neurons alone. Pain is often referred from spinal segments to body parts which have no nerve connections other than autonomic nerves (Grieve, 1991). The sympathetic nerve distribution may be an important factor in patterns of referred pain of musculoskeletal origin. Pain conveyed by autonomic nerves is diffuse and poorly localized. Accompanying the spread of pain is often referred tenderness, muscle hypertonus and sometimes vasoconstriction, manifesting as flushing or sweating. The effects of segmental somatic dysfunction are listed in Table 10.2 and the effects of cervical musculoskeletal dysfunction are listed in Table 10.3.

In order to identify surface anatomical landmarks on the cervical and upper thoracic spine and shoulder girdle, palpate for bony prominence including the inion, mastoid processes, spinous processes of C2-7 and zygapophysial joints below C2 (for

Table 10.2 *Effects of specific segmental somatic dysfunction*

Segmental level of somatic dysfunction	Distribution of pain	Musculature affected	Possible concomitant involvement
Occipitoatlanto Atlantoaxial	Suboccipital, occiput temporal region, orbit	Rectus capitis posterior (major and minor), oblique capitis (inferior and superior)	Temporomandibular joint dysfunction
C3-4 and C4-5	From anterior aspect of shoulder to elbow crease	Deltoid, supraspinatus, infraspinatus, teres minor	Periarthritis of shoulder
C5-6	Anterior shoulder, lateral side of the arm and thumb	Biceps, brachioradialis	Lateral epicondylitis, radial styloiditis, bicipital tendinitis, radial tunnel syndrome
C6-7	Posterior aspect of shoulder and arm; index, middle and ring fingers	Triceps brachii	Medial epicondylitis, extensor or flexor tendinitis
C7-8	Medial aspect of arm, ring and little finger	Hypothenar muscles	

osteophytic lipping and tenderness). In the unimpaired person, C6 moves anteriorly with respect to C7 with cervical spine extension, allowing localization of C7, which is not always the most prominent vertebra. Palpate the neck for altered bony alignment, cervical rib or muscular spasm (Corrigan and Maitland, 1991). The information gained from this palpation helps to identify alteration from the expected normals. After general identification of surface landmarks, using the pads of fingers, palpate for subtle changes in the texture of skin, fascia, muscle, ligaments and tendons, by gradually increasing pressure of fingertips to examine structures layer by layer. Feel for abnormal tensions which may indicate contracture or fibrous changes of the fascia. Follow the directions of muscle fibres to their insertions, noting their tone, level of contraction, presence of contracture or spasm, bogginess (fluid) or ropiness/fibrosis (chronic contraction), and diffuse or localized tenderness.

Soft-tissue texture varies according to chronicity. Acute somatic dysfunction gives rise to increased temperature, bogginess and oedema, increased moisture, tension, tenderness and a rigid end feel. Chronic dysfunction generally does not give rise to increased temperature or oedema; there is a 'ropiness' feel to the myofascial structures. Palpate the supraclavicular fossae for cervical rib with local tenderness, tumour masses and enlarged cervical lymph nodes. Palpate the axilla for enlarged lymph nodes. Examine anterior neck structures (thyroid gland). Assess the patient's hands, forearm and upper arm for intrinsic muscle wasting and temperature changes.

Passive motion testing

The objective in assessing joint movement passively is to identify the range of movement, and the reason for any limitation of movement. In order to examine a group of spinal segments, the patient is asked to lie supine and, using both hands to support the head and neck, the clinician guides the patient passively through flexion, extension, lateral flexion and rotation. Observe range and quality of movement, end feel and reproduction or exacerbation of symptoms. The next stage is to identify the precise location of the spinal segment(s) involved, and determine whether they are hypo- or hypermobile. Hypomobility can result from ruptured disc, trauma, degenerative change, inflammatory or destructive processes. Hypermobility can exist in the early stages of disc degeneration/spondylosis, before any compensatory mechanism to stabilize the segment occurs. Determine the direction and extent of motion restriction and any change in joint play and end feel. Evaluate also whether the hypomobile segment is accompanied by local segmental irritation. The presence of hypomobility and segmental irritation indicates joint disturbance, but is not pathognomonic of somatic dysfunction. Peripheral segmental irritation is also clinically useful as an indicator of disturbance in the related cervical joint (Neumann, 1989).

Occipitoatlantal, atlantoaxial and lower cervical joints are tested separately in the supine position. Whilst guiding the patient's movements passively, evaluate quality and end feel range of motion in all planes of movement at each joint, in addition to any soft-tissue changes. The main physiological movement is a nodding action (flexion and extension) with a potential for a small amount of rotation and lateral flexion.

To examine flexion and extension, hold the occiput in both hands and place the tips of both index fingers behind the transverse processes of C1. Rock the occiput to produce a nodding movement and assess the movement between the mastoid processes and transverse processes of C1. With remaining fingertips, palpate depth and tissue texture changes in the occipitoatlantal sulcus as you flex and extend the occiput. Normal range of motion is 10° of flexion and 25° of extension.

To assess lateral flexion, place the tip of the left index finger between the left transverse process of C1 and adjacent mastoid processes. Cradle the occiput in both hands. Tilt the head on the upper cervical area fully back and forth and palpate the opening and closing of the gap between the transverse process of C1 and the mastoid process, noting changes in tissue tension.

To assess rotation, use the same positions as with lateral flexion, and rotate the head back and forth. As maximum rotation is approached, the transverse process of C1 is felt to draw nearer to the mastoid process on the contralateral side. Zygapophysial joint crepitis is common in arthrosis. Most somatic dysfunction involves the minor motions of side flexion and rotation.

Segments C1-2

The movement affected by somatic dysfunction is rotation. The normal is 25° to each side. Palpating the spinous process of C2, rotate the head until the spinous process is felt to move. Normally C2 does not begin to rotate until the head has rotated 20–30°. However, in the case of somatic dysfunction, the spinous process starts to move much earlier (Neumann, 1989). Note the degree of freedom of rotation, and changes in symmetry and tissue texture.

Segments C2-7

Support the occiput with one hand, and flex and extend whilst palpating with the index fingers of the other hand between spinous processes for the amount of separation. To assess lateral flexion, support the occiput and neck in both palms, whilst palpating the lateral aspect of the lateral masses with the pads of index fingers. Assess the extent of gapping.

To assess rotation, place the pad of both index fingers on the posterolateral aspect of the lateral masses. Pivot the head away from the joint being assessed, rotating the neck down to, but not beyond, this joint. Assess the extent of opening between two articular processes.

Cervicothoracic junction C6–T3

This is a transitional area between two distinct areas of the spinal column (cervical and thoracic) and, because of the presence of the first rib, this region should be examined as a separate unit, with the patient in the side-lying position. Face the patient and rest your sternum on the deltoid area of the patient's uppermost folded arm to stabilize the trunk. Support the head with your cranial forearm, with fingers curling around the patient's lower neck. Flexion, extension, rotation and lateral flexion are all tested in this position, whilst one finger of the caudal hand palpates movement between adjacent spinous processes. Lateral flexion and rotation are repeated to the opposite side. Palpate also first rib movement with respiration.

Other tests

Brachial plexus/upper limb tension test

Broadly analogous to the straight leg raising test, this is carried out to assess the involvement of nerve root tension. Fix the shoulder girdle with the glenohumeral joint abducted to 90°, with elbow extended and the forearm supinated. Superimpose wrist and finger extension. Normal subjects may experience stretching over the anterior shoulder, cubital fossa and lateral forearm, often accompanied by tingling in the lateral three digits. To cause maximum nerve root tension, superimpose contralateral cervical lateral flexion and depress the shoulder girdle (Elvey, 1994).

The arm abduction stresses both cervical nerve roots and subclavian artery and vein. Addition of contralateral cervical lateral flexion puts additional tension on nerve roots, but not on vessels, allowing differentiation between neural and vascular tissues. To differentiate between muscular and neural tension, flex the elbow and reduce shoulder abduction. This reduces tension in peripheral nerves but not in cervical and shoulder girdle musculature (e.g. scalenes). Hence, if pain reduces, nerve root tension is indicated. This test may indicate the presence or absence of nerve root tension, but not the nature or site of the pathology. The response may be the same, even for different conditions. For example,

carpal tunnel syndrome, ulnar nerve entrapment at the elbow, proximal radicular syndrome suprascapular nerve problems, thoracic outlet syndromes, space-occupying masses like Pancoast tumour, extraneural tissue adhesions (e.g. after trauma or surgery) may all give a positive brachial nerve root tension test.

Therefore, the real benefit of the test is to differentiate between muscular and nerve root irritability. A sensitized cervical nerve root can mimic an intrinsic shoulder joint condition. To differentiate between these, assess the range of shoulder abduction, with the shoulder girdle fixed. Repeat this with the neck laterally flexed to the opposite side, which applies tension to the upper roots of the brachial plexus. If the range of active abduction is now decreased, this suggests nerve root pathology as the limiting factor. Likewise, if contralateral cervical rotation is reduced with the arm abducted compared to that with the shoulder in neutral, this suggests that cervical nerve roots on the tested side are sensitive to tension.

Peripheral joints

When examining the neck and upper limb, always check the scapulothoracic, acromioclavicular, sternoclavicular, glenohumeral and upper rib joints as faults may occur at any of these sites. With distal upper-extremity pain, check the integrity of the elbow, forearm, wrist and hand – again a possible site of musculoskeletal dysfunction.

Cervical rib

Look for evidence of ischaemia in one hand (coldness, discoloration, trophic changes). Palpate the radial pulse and apply traction to the arm. Obliteration of pulse is not diagnostic, but is suggestive if there is no change on the other side. Ask the patient to turn the head to the affected side and take a deep breath (and hold it). Obliteration of the radial pulse is suggestive of a cervical rib causing the vascular changes, as is a murmur heard over the subclavian artery.

Resisted isometric muscle contraction

This may be used to identify weakness in muscles and attachments, and to determine if the motor component of nerve function is normal.

General medical screening

The initial interview may raise doubt that the presenting condition is of musculoskeletal origin. See Table 10.1 for a clinical screening protocol designed to identify underlying pathology which would preclude manipulative treatment. Medical screening is important because self-referred patients give only a one-off history; they are already symptomatic and impatient for treatment. There are two sources of clinical error – to miss a detectable pathology and to hurt the patient by treating a surgically unstable body.

Classification of musculoskeletal dysfunction

The upper cervical complex (occiput to C2)

Both these joints possess articular nociceptors and sensory afferents and hence have the potential to produce upper neck pain. The tissues causing pain production are the suboccipital muscles, C1 and C2 nerve roots, the upper cervical ligaments and zygapophysial joints. Referred pain from the occipitoatlantal joint is variable and diffuse but tends to be suboccipital, temporal or radiating from C5 to the vertex. The atlantoaxial joints produce more localized pain, lateral and posterior at the C1–2 segmental level (Grieve, 1981a; Ehni and Brenner, 1984; Star and Thorne, 1992; Dreyfuss and Fletcher, 1994).

The occipitoatlantal joint can become problematic as a result of a primary trauma or due to chronic postural dysfunction. A sudden or excessive movement of the head will cause the zygapophysial joints to move beyond their normal range of movement, resulting in excessive stretching of the capsule and ligaments with impingement and 'jamming' of the facet surfaces. Pain occurs due to the subsequent synovial irritation and inflammation. The swelling may cause encroachment of the nerve root and other tissues. A protective muscle spasm also occurs, giving ischaemic pain. These will all result in restricted joint mobility. Altered neuromuscular activity may contribute to a chronic pain situation resulting from an acute condition, which has no obvious reason for persistent symptoms.

Irritation of local myofascial–periosteal attachments as a result of acute or sustained muscle contraction also produces local pain or tenderness, especially at the base of the occiput. The hypertonic suboccipital muscles may cause irritation of the superior occipital nerve in this area, causing pain in the top and side of the scalp, radiating to the frontal area. There are various positions in which the occipitoatlantal joint can become restricted: either anteriorly or posteriorly, unilaterally producing ipsilateral pain and resistance of movement, with increased movement contralaterally (torsion), either anteriorly or posteriorly bilaterally, giving bilateral pain and resistance (flexion or extension) laterally, unilaterally with ipsilateral pain and resistance (side-

bending). If anterior one side, and posterior on the other, bilateral pain may occur due to rotation.

Trauma to the head or neck, e.g. from a fall, or during contact sport or a knock to the vertex, can result in a restriction of the occipitoatlantal joint and associated pain. The patient is typically a young adult presenting with ipsilateral suboccipital pain, often spreading to the frontal and supraorbital area. He or she will have an accentuated cervical lordosis due to upper cervical muscle spasm. Rotation and side-bending towards the affected side will be painful and restricted, and away from that side will elicit a pulling sensation in the symptomatic side. The overlying tissues will feel thickened and tender. Any neurological symptoms, such as occipital paraesthesia or numbness with weakness on active resisted chin movements, may indicate a tearing of the craniovertebral ligaments with subsequent instability and trespass on the C2 nerve root. In this case care should be taken and mobilization/manipulation contraindicated.

Postural strain develops over a period of time, often with insidious onset. The individual may be asymptomatic for a period of time, with pain only experienced when there is an increased load placed on the tissues and a subsequent tissue response provoking muscular ischaemia or fatigue. This may result from activities such as desk work, producing flexion injuries of the occipitoatlantal joint, or from jobs involving sustained extension of the occipitoatlantal joint, such as decorators or car mechanics. The atlantoaxial joint tends to become restricted in rotation. This can occur, for example, as a result of an uncoordinated movement during sleep or due to working in confined spaces. There may be an acute or chronic history. The patient can present with a variety of symptoms, including occipital and hemicranial pain, face pain and occasionally paraesthesiae and stiffness of the upper neck with diffuse headache. Side-bending and rotation are painful and restricted on the symptomatic side. The head and neck may be in a normal position or in some cases side-bent to one side and rotated to the other, with hypertonia of the contralateral sternocleidomastoid muscle. Caution is necessary if the onset is traumatic because excessive rotation can also be associated with anterior shift of the atlas, especially if there is a transverse ligament deficiency, e.g. in rheumatoid arthritis, which can lead to a compromise of the vertebral arteries with brainstem and cerebellar infarction (Chapter 12).

Arthrotic changes occur most commonly at the anterior atlantoaxial joint and also at the occipitoatlantal and lateral atlantoaxial joints. Patients are commonly mature or middle-aged with a history of symptoms for months or years, often initiated by a traumatic stress. They may complain of a nagging headache in the forehead and eyes, with a feeling of retro-orbital pressure. The pain tends to get worse as the day goes on. It is aggravated by prolonged flexion or extension, which can also cause dizziness. Nuchal crepitus is commonly present. On palpation there is thickening and tenderness of the suboccipital soft tissues. There is often a variety of accompanying symptoms, including vertigo, momentary vagueness, nausea, dysphasia, dysphonia, blurred vision, vaso- and sudomotor changes and miosis.

The upper cervical spine is involved in 40% of rheumatoid arthritis cases (Sharp and Purser, 1961), with atlantoaxial subluxation occurring in 25% (Conlon *et al.,* 1966) due to softening and weakening of the transverse ligament. Symptoms are commonly upper cervical and suboccipital pain, spreading to mastoid, temporal or frontal areas. Great care must be taken in all cases of suspected rheumatoid arthritis, with spinal manipulation absolutely contraindicated and referral to a rheumatologist necessary.

Headaches

Headache is a common symptom and its causes are too numerous to be discussed fully here. We will comment on those which relate to the musculoskeletal system. Approximately 10% of consultations to an osteopath are for headaches (Burton, 1981; Burns and Lyttelton, 1994).

Tension headache

This is characterized by a persistent low-intensity, non-pulsatile ache, typically in the forehead, temples, suboccipital area and neck. There is often a feeling of pressure at the vertex or a tight band-like sensation. There is usually a history of problems over a few years. The problem is more common in females (3 : 1; Jerrett, 1979) and tends to occur between the ages of 30 and 40.

Pain occurs as a result of sustained muscular contraction, which is brought about by various local, cortical and thalamic reflexes.

Pain may result from:

1. Irritation of the periostium due to traction exerted by the contracted muscle at its site of insertion.
2. A build-up of metabolites with subsequent ischaemia, and increased intramuscular pressure in the muscle belly.
3. Irritation of the superior occipital nerve as it passes through the contracted suboccipital muscles, which refers pain to the top and side of scalp and frontal area. Also its connections with the fifth, ninth and tenth cranial nerves result in pain perception in the cranial vault.
4. Emotional factors: somatization of anxiety in the form of increased skeletal muscle contraction; musculoskeletal-type headaches are often worse during times of stress.

Cervicogenic headache

This presents as a unilateral deep, dull pain starting in the neck or occiput and radiating to frontal, temporal and supraorbital areas. There is often referred pain into the ipsilateral upper extremity. Associated symptoms can include nausea, dizziness/vertigo, blurred vision and dysphasia. The duration of pain varies greatly, from hours to weeks, but usually lasts a few days. Symptoms are frequently brought on by awkward neck movements or uncomfortable positions during sleep. There may be history of a recent neck trauma. Patients are commonly young or middle-aged females (sex ratio 3 : 1; Merskey and Bogduk, 1994a). These headaches are thought to be strongly associated with musculoskeletal dysfunction and arthrosis of the upper cervical spine, and less frequently with spondylosis of the lower cervical segments (Grieve, 1981b).

The associated symptoms are probably initiated due to irritation of the sympathetic nerve component in the upper cervical nerve roots (Merskey and Bogduk, 1994b) via the superior cervical ganglion, and due to links with the spinal tract of cranial nerve V, which is accompanied by parasympathetic and sympathetic neurons. Dizziness and vertigo are likely to be initiated by distorted afferent impulses from mechanoreceptors in the upper cervical zygapophysial joints, which are involved in equilibrium.

Vascular headache

Although migraine is thought to be due to a vascular disturbance, notably dilation of the arteries of the scalp and increased cerebral blood flow, it can be accentuated by musculoskeletal problems, especially at the occipitoatlantal joint, due to vasomotor effects via the sympathetic nervous system. It is often found to occur in conjunction with tension headaches – defined as a mixed headache.

It is a problem frequently encountered, although exact prevalence still remains unclear, probably due to the fact that there are several different types of migraine and hence diagnostic criteria vary considerably between studies (Mounstephen and Harrison, 1995).

1. *Classical migraine.* This is a throbbing headache associated with a prodromal state and preceded by an aura usually with visual symptoms. It accounts for about 10% of all cases of migraine (Grieve, 1981b). It is more common in females (2 : 1; Jerrett, 1979) and tends to occur from childhood to about 35 years of age. There is a premonitory phase, lasting from hours to a few days. Pain then starts, usually in the unilateral frontotemporal area and may spread to the whole hemicranium, lasting from 4 to 72 h. It is aggravated by stooping or exercise. Often the patient also experiences nausea, vomiting and photophobia. Attacks usually occur about 1–4 times a month.

2. *Common migraine.* This occurs more often than the classic type (2/3 : 1; Merskey and Bogduk, 1994b). They both have the same characteristics, except that the common type has no premonitory stage or aura but instead is only accompanied by nausea, vomiting and photophobia. Attacks also tend to last for longer – from 4 h up to 2 days or more. These two forms of migraine are traditionally explained in terms of vascular changes. We would however suggest that a musculoskeletal component is invariably present, which does respond to manipulative treatment (Parker *et al.,* 1978).

3. *Cluster headache.* These occur as 1–3 attacks per day in bouts of 4–12-week duration, with remission lasting for 6–18 months. They are characterized by severe unilateral stabbing, burning, throbbing pain in the ocular, frontal and temporal areas which can spread to the whole hemicranium, neck and shoulder. There is associated ipsilateral lacrimation, photophobia and rhinorrhoea, with nausea in severe cases. They start between the ages of 18 and 40 and are more common in males (9 : 1), especially in heavy drinkers and smokers.

4. *Temporal arteritis.* This is a vasculitis of the temporal arteries. It is included here because in one-third of cases it is associated with polymyalgia rheumatica, a connective tissue disorder presenting as pain and stiffness in the cervical spine and shoulder girdle muscles and therefore could be confused with a simple musculoskeletal problem. The patient is commonly a female of over 50 years of age, complaining of a constant unilateral or bilateral throbbing or aching pain and tenderness in the temporal area. Patients may also report pain on prolonged chewing (due to intermittent claudication of temporalis muscles) and various systemic symptoms such as malaise, low-grade fever and weight loss.

5. *Headache of organic aetiology.* This is important to bear in mind as it often presents with symptoms similar to that of migraine and therefore must be included in the differential diagnosis.
   (a) Meningitis.
   (b) Subarachnoid haemorrhage.
   (c) Chronic subdural haematoma.
   (d) Post-concussion syndrome.
   (e) Intracranial tumour.

Typical cervical spine

This can be classified as segments C3–7. Joint structure at these segments consists of a symphysis type at the intervertebral discs and synovial type at the zygapophysial surfaces. The detailed anatomy of soft-tissue attachments has been described elsewhere in this book. The biomechanical properties which osteopaths are interested in relate to the plane of joint movement and the expected range of movement. The cervical facets are oriented at a 45° angle to the transverse plane. There is a large degree of variation amongst individuals with regards to the amount of movement in the cervical spine. Approximately 90° of axial rotation takes place in C3–7 (45° each side of neutral). Lateral flexion is about 49° each side, flexion about 40° and extension 24°. The distribution of movement is fairly equal throughout the segments (Kahn and Monod, 1989). Assessment of the mid cervical spine should not be limited to the local tissues; adjacent structures have a direct influence on the biomechanical function of the mid-neck. The upper thoracic and shoulder girdle structures are included in this assessment.

In cervical somatic dysfunction (hypomobility syndrome), the typical pattern of restriction is painful limitation of extension with restriction of lateral flexion and rotation towards the painful side, producing ipsilateral suprascapular pain. This is a regular compressive pattern which is generally eased by flexion. Less commonly, the pattern is restricted movement in one direction only. Regular stretching patterns include restriction of movement (rotation and lateral flexion) away from the painful side, the pain being aggravated by flexion and relieved by extension. Non-traumatic disorders tend to exhibit these regular patterns, whereas traumatic conditions do not, as do conditions involving more than one component, e.g. zygapophysial joint, foraminal tissues, disc. Within this section it is assumed that all pathological conditions which preclude spinal manipulation have been rejected. Pain originating from mid cervical structures (zygapophysial joints, muscle, interspinal ligaments) is a common symptom in clinical practice. The cause of presenting condition is variable:

1. Direct muscle strain.
2. Repetitive/cumulative muscle strain.
3. Direct joint/ligament strain.
4. Repetitive/cumulative joint or ligament strain.
5. Complex tissue strain (whiplash).

Degenerative change within the intervertebral discs of the cervical spine is generally a natural process of ageing, which is caused by the mechanical forces exerted on the tissue during daily activities. The degenerative change will result in narrowing of the intervertebral space, which in turn will cause the zygapophysial joint and the uncovertebral joint surfaces to approximate. The increased loading of these joint surfaces will result in degenerative changes accelerating (Barnsley *et al.,* 1993). The osteoarthrosis at the uncovertebral joints may result in osteophyte formation, with the effect of protrusion into the intervertebral foramen. This may compromise the cervical nerve roots (Jackson, 1977). A decrease in disc height will initially result in segmental instability (Grieve, 1991). There will be relative hypermobility at the affected segment. There may be hypomobility at adjacent segments. The surrounding tissue will then compensate for the hypermobility and the interspinal ligaments, joint capsule and adjacent musculature will shorten and fibrosis will occur (collagen infiltration). The net effect will be a stabilization. The shortening of the interspinal tissue and the formation of osteophytes is the natural response to the disc thinning. However, failure of such a mechanism to exist, which results from demands exceeding capabilities, may result in the symptomatic picture we associate with cervical spondylosis. The change in biomechanical function of the mid cervical spine as a result of the degenerative process causes identifiable clinical changes. On examination, muscle tone often changes, chronic thickening of the cervical erector spinae muscles results, and nodules or fibrous tissue are palpable. Zygapophysial joint movement reduces. The cervical spine often increases its lordosis; this may be associated with an increase in the upper thoracic kyphosis. The changes at segmental level may cause nerve root compromise. Osteophyte formation or a reduction in the size of the intervertebral foramen will be the cause of such nerve root irritation. Pain and other neurological symptoms (paraesthesia, anaesthesia or paresis) may result. The distribution of such symptoms will depend on the spinal level affected (Table 10.2).

Cervicothoracic region

This is the transitional area between the mobile cervical spine and relatively immobile thorax. The area is vulnerable to overstrain/overload, in particular in the C7–T1 apophyseal joint and adjacent connective tissues, which can have direct effects on the integrity of related structures (brachial plexus, sternoclavicular and acromioclavicular) (see also Chapter 3).

Thoracic outlet syndrome

This describes a variety of signs and symptoms resulting from compression of the neuromuscular bundle as it passes through the thoracic outlet. Symptoms radiate across the shoulder girdle and axilla and into the arm. There are three sites where the neurovascular bundle is most vulnerable to compression, hence a classification of three syndromes has been proposed:

1. A triangle formed by the anterior and medial scalene muscles and the first rib, on to which they insert – *anterior scalene syndrome*.
2. Between the clavicle and first rib – *claviculocostal syndrome*.
3. Between pectoralis minor, near its attachment to the coracoid process and the ribcage – *pectoralis minor syndrome*.

A reduction in size of any of these already narrow passageways will lead to compression. The compression can result from:

1. *Cervical rib.* This is a congenital bony or fibrous overdevelopment of the transverse process of C7. It is usually bilateral and varies in size from a small protrusion to complete rib. There may also be a fibrous band attaching to the first thoracic rib. Consequently, the neurovascular bundle must pass over this higher barrier, which may cause it to become stretched. It may also be compressed by the fibrous band.
2. Abnormal fibrous bands in scalenius medius may cause a kinking of the lower brachial plexus.
3. Fracture of the clavicle or first rib with subsequent malunion or callus formation can reduce the claviculocostal space.
4. Altered rib mechanics, e.g. elevation of the first and second ribs due to trauma or hypertonia of the scalenes, can result in chronic pressure on the structures in this area.
5. Poor posture, with sagging, protracted shoulders, may place increased tension on the scalenes and shoulder girdle muscles.
6. Overuse with resultant hypertrophy or hypertonia of the scalenes or pectoralis minor may occur in asthmatics and in occupations requiring prolonged work in hyperabduction, e.g. painters, car mechanics.
7. Sleeping postures with the arm hyperabducted can cause a stretch of pectoralis minor.
8. Reflex contraction and spasm of the scalenes may result from whiplash trauma, nerve root irritation or inflammation of the lower cervical zygapophysial joints.

Thoracic outlet syndrome tends to be more common in middle-aged females. Symptoms vary depending on whether there is neural or vascular compression or a combination. The lower trunk of the brachial plexus is most vulnerable to compression, hence affecting the C8 and T1 nerve roots.

Neurological signs and symptoms

These tend to be the most frequent, occurring in 90% of cases:

1. Pain, paraesthesia or numbness starting in the root of the neck or shoulder, radiating down the medial aspect of the arm, forearm and hand.
2. Subjective weakness with occasional wasting of the intrinsic muscles of the hand.
3. Cramping of the finger flexor muscles.

4. Horner's syndrome – ptosis, enophthalmos, anhydrous facial flushing and miosis (ipsilateral to the lesion).

Vascular signs and symptoms

These occur in about 10% of cases:

1. Diminished radial and ulnar pulses, especially on activity.
2. Raynaud's phenomenon.
3. Oedema of the hand.
4. Heavy feeling of the upper extremity.
5. Pallor or bluish discoloration of the hand.
6. Coldness and cramping of the hands and fingers.

There are various clinical tests that can be carried out to aid evaluation. The onset of symptoms or a reduction of the radial pulse denotes a positive test:

1. *Adison's test.* This places increased compression on all sites. The radial pulse is palpated. The patient extends and rotates the head towards the affected side. The arm is abducted and extended. The patient takes a deep breath.
2. *Costoclavicular test.* The radial pulse is palpated whilst the patient sits in a military position – chest out, shoulders back and down, thus approximating the clavicle and ribs.
3. *Hyperabduction test.* This implicates pectoralis minor. The radial pulse is palpated and the arm elevated to 180°.
4. *Intermittent claudication test.* This exercises the forearm muscles in the presence of impaired arterial blood flow. Both arms are elevated, abducted and externally rotated. The fingers are then rapidly flexed. In this case a positive test occurs, with onset of paraesthesia and pain in the forearm after a few seconds.
5. *Spurling manoeuvre.* This aids differential diagnosis from pure nerve root compression. With the patient seated, the head is compressed downwards. If pain occurs down the arm, this is probably due to nerve root compression.

In addition to these, a full evaluation of mobility of the clavicular, lower cervical, upper thoracic and costovertebral joints is carried out and muscle tone is assessed. Treatment is aimed at restoring appropriate joint mobility, reducing hypertonicity in the scalenes and pectoralis minor, improving strength of the shoulder girdle muscles, advice on improvement of posture and reduction of any emotional tension. This is achieved through direct joint manipulative techniques, various soft-tissue stretching/massage techniques and remedial exercises.

There are other conditions producing similar signs and symptoms which must always be considered in the differential diagnoses. These include:

1. Pancoast tumour at the apex of the lung.
2. Syringomyelia and other tumours of the spinal cord.
3. Cervical spondylosis or disc prolapse.
4. Carpal tunnel syndrome.
5. Thrombosis of the subclavian vein.
6. Friction neuritis of the ulnar nerve.
7. Peripheral artery disease.

Specific presentation

Whiplash

An increasing number of patients are presenting to osteopaths with neck pain following a road traffic accident. There is an increasing likelihood of litigation, so that a clearer understanding of the condition and a well-defined management plan are necessary. This section discusses a particular type of trauma which affects primarily the cervical spine; the thoracic spine is also involved with this type of injury. It can be termed a whiplash-associated disorder. The Quebec Task Force classified whiplash-associated disorder as follows (Spitzer *et al.*, 1995):

- *Grade 0*: No complaint about the neck; no physical signs.
- *Grade I*: Neck complaint of pain, stiffness or tenderness only; no physical signs.
- *Grade II*: Neck complaint and musculoskeletal signs (including decreased range of motion and tenderness).
- *Grade III*: Neck complaint and neurological signs (decreased or absent tendon reflexes, weakness, sensory deficit).
- *Grade IV*: Neck complaint and fracture or dislocation.

The trauma occurs primarily during a road traffic accident. A similar type of injury could occur during boxing or motor racing, and also in what would normally be classed as non-traumatic – flopping into a chair (Allen *et al.*, 1994). The majority (90%) of reported whiplash injuries occur with a rear-end shunt, the patient being in the stationary front car.

Anatomical effects

The biomechanics of the injury result in a primary movement of extension followed by flexion. Relative to the trunk the head acceleration can be as high as 12 **g** in the extension phase and 16 **g** in the flexion phase (Martinez and Garcia, 1968). The mandible and brain are two structures that are independent of the skull. In the extension phase the mandible will stay stationary, with the mouth opening and the brain,

Table 10.3 *Cervical musculoskeletal dysfunction*

Cause	Significant disc degeneration	Muscle tone	Active joint mobility	Passive joint mobility	Neurological changes
Acute muscle strain	Possible shortening of tissue with advanced degeneration	Hypertonic cervical tissue	↓ Mobility, often all directions	↓ Mobility of joints adjacent to tissue injury	Possible subjective symptoms in the arm
Chronic muscle pain	Possible shortening of muscle tissue, predisposing to recurrent microtrauma	Hypertonic and/ or fibrotic cervical tissue, and often periscapular muscles	↓ Mobility if affected tissues stretched	↓ Mobility of joints adjacent to the muscle fibrosis	Unusual, except if disc degeneration is advanced
Acute joint/ ligament strain	Approximation of zygapophysial joints, increasing degenerative changes, therefore shortened capsule/ ligaments and ↑ potential of strain	Hypertonic, protective guarding of cervical muscles	↓ Mobility, particularly if injured tissue is stretched	↓ Mobility of affected segments, often unilateral	Possible subjective symptoms in the arm
Chronic joint/ ligament dysfunction	Approximation of zygapophysial joints, increasing degenerative changes, therefore shortened capsule/ ligaments and ↑ potential to strain	Fibrotic changes adjacent to affected segments, often fibrotic changes in periscapular muscles	↓ Mobility of affected segments, particularly when affected segments are moved	↓ Mobility of affected segments	If disc degeneration is advanced, possible nerve root compression
Acute complex tissue injury, e.g. whiplash	Soft-tissue shortening, zygapophysial joints approximated, i.e. vulnerable to strain/ inflammation	Hypertonic, protective guarding/direct trauma of cervical muscles and often hypertonic periscapular muscles	↓ Mobility in most planes of movement, particularly in the acute phase	↓ Mobility at affected segments, often involving many cervical segments	Nerve root compression possible if disc herniation present or advanced disc degeneration present prior to injury
Chronic complex tissue injury	Possible increase in disc degeneration; degeneration may be accompanied by herniation, particularly if trauma affected the intervertebral disc	Chronic hypertonic/ fibrotic cervical and periscapular muscles	↓ Mobility often involving > one plane of movement	↓ Mobility often involving > one segmental level	Nerve root compression possible if there is unresolved disc herniation or advanced disc degeneration

which lies free in the skull, impacted as the skull ends its extension phase (Bogduk, 1986). During the extension phase of whiplash the anterior structures of the cervical vertebral column are strained and the posterior structures are compressed. Anterior structures subject to strain are intervertebral discs, anterior longitudinal ligament, prevertebral muscles, oesophagus and pharynx. Posterior structures subject to compression are the cervical zygapophysial joints and the spinous processes. The force transmitted at the craniocervical junction will cause the odontoid process to compress the anterior arch of the atlas; the forwards movement of the atlas will be transmitted to the head through the atlanto-occipital joints. The dropping of the mandible would cause the anterior capsule to be strained (Bogduk, 1986). During the flexion phase the posterior longitudinal ligament, the interspinal ligaments, the ligamentum nuchae, the posterior neck muscles and the capsules of the zygapophysial joints would be subject to strain. The compressed anterior structures would be the intervertebral discs and the vertebral bodies.

The liability to injury would be greater in the extension strain because there is nothing to prevent the head extending beyond the natural range. In flexion the chin will make contact with the sternum and thus prevent excessive flexion (Bogduk, 1986).

Pathophysiological effects

The most likely pathological effects of whiplash, as demonstrated from clinical and experimental studies, include strain of the longitudinal ligament, disc herniation, vertebral end-plate avulsion, muscular strain or rupture (particularly the sternocleidomastoid and longus colli), zygapophysial joint fractures and capsular damage, and a variety of brain injuries (Bogduk, 1986). Odontoid fractures are more common than vertebral body fractures. Zygapophysial joint pain is the single most common basis for persistent pain after whiplash (Barnsley *et al.*, 1995). The clinical implication of the musculoskeletal effects is that somatic dysfunction will result. This will present as hypertonic musculature, reduced joint mobility, pain experienced at the affected spinal segments, and pain experienced in associated dermatomes or sclerotomes.

Guidelines

Guidelines, based on the Quebec Task Force and its recommendations, which have implications for practising osteopaths are given below.

The Quebec Task Force studied the literature regarding whiplash injuries, and produced guidelines for clinical practice. Manipulation was recommended in the early stages of a whiplash-associated disorder grades I–III. Early return to usual activities should be emphasized, soft collars should be avoided, medica-

tion should be used in a limited way, rest is seldom necessary and reassurance of a good prognosis is encouraged. Failure to resolve within approximately 3 months, progressive neurological signs or persistent severe arm pain should initiate further referral (Spitzer *et al.*, 1995)

Management of cervical pain

Aims

The principal aim of osteopathic treatment when applied to mechanical neck pain is the restoration of optimal function to the cervical spine and its surrounding tissues for that individual. This is achieved with a variety of manual techniques directed at joints and surrounding soft tissue.

There is much discussion in osteopathic circles regarding natural healing mechanisms within the body, though traditionally treatment is applied with the intention of enhancing such repair and recovery. All human bodily functions rely on a homeostatic balance within the physiology of the tissues; if this situation alters then pathological change may take place in the tissues. It therefore follows that abnormal function is a step towards pathological change within tissues, such as fibrotic infiltration of muscle, ligament, fascia, synovium and joint capsules or degenerative changes in hyaline cartilage. Medication and surgery will often be incompatible with such changes, leaving physical approaches as an alternative; manipulative treatment is one such approach. If no treatment is offered in these circumstances, does the functional state of cervical spine continue to deteriorate, leading to irreversible structural changes and chronic pain and disability? The answer is: probably – sometimes. It may depend on the individual's make-up (both physical and psychological).

Tissues which may influence neck movement are the target for treatment; attempts may be made to reduce muscle tone, stretch fibrotic areas and increase elasticity of joint capsules and intersegmental ligaments. If movement, and therefore function, is improved, then normal repair mechanisms should ensue. The notion proposed by osteopaths is that the correction of subtle impairments of movement at a segmental level is of paramount importance for correct function.

The osteopath's approach will go beyond the mechanical consequences of impaired mobility. It is suggested that fear of pain and negative attitudes may prolong an episode of low back pain and may also be a factor in the progression to chronicity (Lee *et al.*, 1989; Burton *et al.*, 1995). This may also be true of the cervical spine, thus a vital component of the management process is to help address any inappropriate attitudes and beliefs. Chronic pain is a complex phenomenon involving not only tissue damage but attitudes to pain, coping strategies, previous experience of pain and alteration of central processing mechanisms. It should be a paramount aim in the management of acute patients to avoid progression to chronicity.

Classification

In order to achieve the stated aims, a variety of technical approaches may be utilized, depending on the individual needs of the patient. Three broad classes of manual procedures are used more or less universally, but there are other techniques, beyond the scope of this chapter, that are used by some osteopaths. Advice, in its various forms, should be considered a part of the therapeutic process; this is a guideline procedure of low back pain (Bigos *et al.*, 1994) and arguably should be for cervical pain.

Soft tissue

This term refers to direct-contact techniques applied to muscle and ligamentous tissue. Three types of muscle techniques are used: cross-fibre stretch, longitudinal stretch and deep pressure. Cross-fibre stretch is force applied at right angles to the muscle fibres in order to relax the muscle or increase the elasticity of the muscle fibres. The mechanism by which muscle tone is reduced is not fully understood, but it is thought that the Golgi tendon apparatus has a role to play in adjusting muscle tone. Longitudinal stretch is force applied along the length of the muscle in order to increase elasticity by breaking cross-linkages and stretching fibrous tissue. Deep pressure is applied to so-called trigger points, to specific muscles and to areas of fibrosis to increase local circulation and alter afferent input to the neuromuscular reflex. Ligamentous tissue can be also be stretched across the fibres, longitudinally or with deep pressure.

Articulation

This term refers to passive joint movement. The joints involved (zygapophysial) are moved within their normal physiological range; in practice, articulation may be combined with soft-tissue techniques. If the joint capsule or intersegmental ligaments are to be stretched then the joint can be moved beyond its resistance. Joint movement is normally carried out with the patient lying supine.

High-velocity thrust

This term refers to a specific joint manipulation. The zygapophysial joint is the focus of the thrust. The aim of HVT techniques is to separate the joint surfaces at right angles to the plane of the facets. The joint is brought to a point of tension using a combination of movements – flexion–rotation and side-bending with or without compression/traction. If a thrust is delivered to the right side of a patient's cervical spine, the neck would be flexed and side-bent to the right and rotated to the left. The intention is to focus to a single spinal level; careful palpation is used to guide the leverage and bring the joint concerned to that point of tension where the soft tissues begin to limit motion; this will always be within the normal physiological range of the joint. At this point of tension a force is applied either in rotation left or side-bending right with a high velocity but a very small amplitude, thus gapping the left zygapophysial joint and producing cavitation (Tomlinson, 1971). It is emphasized that the joint should not be moved outside its normal physiological range. The process of cavitation produces a temporary separation of the joint surfaces, allowing an increase in the range of movement available (Unsworth *et al.*, 1971). A longer-lasting effect is thought to be brought about by afferent input altering the feedback in the neuromuscular reflex arc, thus changing the efferent message to the muscle spindles, resulting in a reduction of muscle tone. This technique applies to the middle and lower zygapophysial joints. The techniques are subtly modified for different cervical regions.

Upper cervical spine

The occiput–atlas–axis form a specific function in the cervical spine: these joints combine to form a versatile complex which allows a large range of flexion–extension and rotation. Soft-tissue treatment is focused at the group of suboccipital muscles. Articulating techniques are carried out with reference to the normal values of joint mobility. The occipitoatlantal joint can be manipulated as a direct thrust through the joint, with slight side-bending and rotation, or as a combined leverage using side-bending and rotation, with slight extension (Hartman, 1985). The atlantoaxial joint is manipulated in rotation.

Mid cervical spine

The mid cervical spine consists of typical cervical vertebrae, meaning that the standard osteopathic techniques for the cervical spine can be used (Hartman, 1985).

Frequency

How often should a patient be treated? This varies quite considerably between practitioners, but the condition being treated must influence the decision. There is no reliable evidence base for the number of treatments; it depends on individual beliefs and teaching. A wide range have been reported for osteopathic practice, with an average of six treatments being typical (Burton *et al.*, 1995). In cases with acute tissue damage, treatment twice a week seems the norm, with support for the patient essential in alleviating fears and concerns. Some considerable encouragement will be needed to help the patient return to normal activities as quickly as possible. Maintenance visits, particularly in chronic or recurrent cases, are used by many osteopaths to monitor a patient over time. The interval may be 2–4 months, and the visit may consist of an assessment only or may involve some treatment; whether this helps or hinders is unknown.

Osteopathic treatment of whiplash

As with any presenting condition, a detailed structured interview must take place before any decisions are made. There is a high probability that a whiplash type of injury resulting from a road traffic accident will include litigation. With this in mind, a particularly detailed interview is necessary, followed by the physical examination and appropriate investigations; then a management plan can be formed.

As with all osteopathic management of cervical conditions, assessment of the thoracic spine is an important part of the procedure. Often with acute cervical dysfunction, initial treatment is focused on the thoracic and thoracocervical junction. Manipulation of the thoracic spine will include HVT, articulation and soft-tissue techniques. The aim behind the thoracic treatment, is to encourage full mobility within the vertebral zygapophysial and costovertebral joints. Appropriate soft-tissue treatment is needed to complement the increase in joint mobility.

Clearly any bony fractures, joint instability, brain damage or progressive neurological signs preclude osteopathic treatment. Treatment applied directly to the cervical spine is aimed at reducing dysfunction. In the clinic this would comprise stretching cervical muscles, articulating zygapophysial joints, applying HVT to zygapophysial joints and advice regarding exercises and working conditions.

Expected recovery

There have been a number of studies carried out looking at the expected course of recovery from whiplash injuries. The outcome at 3 months seems to act as a good predictor for the next 2 years (Gargan and Bannister, 1994). Over 90% of asymptomatic cases at 3 months after the road traffic accident remained asymptomatic over the next 2 years. Nearly 90% of those who were symptomatic at 3 months remained symptomatic for the next 2 years. Factors which relate to poor recovery include radicular irritation, intensity of neck pain, previous history of head trauma and initial injury-related cerebral reac-

tions (sleep disturbance, reduced speed of information processing and nervousness; Radanov *et al.*, 1994). Severe persisting neck pain with radiation in the arm is indicative of disc protrusion, and requires further investigation. There is evidence that cervical disc protrusion responds well to surgical management (Barnsley *et al.*, 1995).

Osteopathic treatment of headaches

Assuming that the headache is not of pathological origin, but due to mechanical dysfunction, then manipulation of the neck has been shown to decrease the pain and improve the range of movement of the spine (Stodolny and Chmielewski, 1989). Manipulation has also been shown to decrease the symptoms of migraine leading to a reduction in frequency and duration of induced disability (Parker *et al.*, 1978).

Treatment consists of soft-tissue techniques, i.e. longitudinal and cross-fibre stretches to the cervical muscles as well as the upper and lower fibres of trapezius; articulation of the individual zygapophysial joints as well as those gross articulations of the neck in all ranges of movement bar extension; specific joint manipulations to areas determined by palpation to be dysfunctional.

Efficacy and outcome of cervical treatment

With respect to osteopathic manipulation of the cervical spine, studies have demonstrated that results are similar to that of treatment of the lumbar spine (Howe *et al.*, 1983; Koes *et al.*, 1992). It must be said that more research has been reported with respect to low back pain. In one of the early trials investigating manipulation of the cervical spine, it was found that spinal manipulation produced a significant immediate improvement in symptoms in those patients with pain/paraesthesia in the shoulder and some improvement in those with pain/paraesthesia in the arm or hand (Howe *et al.*, 1983). Manipulation also produced a significant increase in measured rotation that was maintained for 3 weeks, together with an immediate improvement in lateral flexion; however this increase was not maintained (Howe *et al.*, 1983). Exercises are often recommended to maintain cervical spine flexibility: it has been shown that long-term benefit requires continual use (McCarthy *et al.*, 1996).

Chronic neck problems, in common with chronic low back problems, prove to follow a fluctuating course. One study found that subjects treated by manipulation showed no consistently favourable response (Sloop *et al.*, 1982), while another found that manipulation increased local paraspinal pain threshold levels (Vernon *et al.*, 1990).

Complications to manipulation

There are some inherent dangers associated with manipulating the cervical spine. Assuming that all pathological conditions have been eliminated, i.e. all contraindications have been noted, complications have still been reported following HVT.

One reported complication is Horner's syndrome. The proposed theory is that local forceful thrusts to the base of the neck led to a traction/avulsion injury to the white ramus communicans between the thoracic nerve and the sympathetic ganglion (Grayson, 1987). The author states that, although mishaps occur, manipulation should not be discouraged.

The second, more worrying complications are cerebrovascular accidents and, although uncommon, they have been reported. The general consensus of opinion is that vertebrobasilar competence should be assessed before HVTs are performed; however, recent evidence has suggested that these tests are not reliable (Thiel *et al.,* 1994). Since vertebral artery occlusion occurs in extremes of extension and rotation, it is probably safer to manipulate the neck in flexion (Danek, 1989; Thiel, 1991; Chapter 12).

It must be noted that it is not uncommon for the patient to feel slightly light-headed, dizzy or nauseous after treatment. These symptoms can occur after soft-tissue techniques, passive joint articulations or HVTs; it is proposed that stimulation of arterial reflex or altered sympathetic activity is responsible. This is usually short-lived, although if reported, care should be taken with the patient at subsequent treatment.

Summary

In osteopathic practice, neck pain is a common presenting symptom, often of mechanical origin. The osteopath will assess the individual and attempt to exclude the possibility of a serious pathology. Assuming no 'red flags' are apparent, a detailed musculoskeletal assessment will conclude with a management (treatment) plan. There is reasonable evidence to support the use of spinal manipulation with cervical conditions of mechanical origin. However, further clinical trials are absolutely necessary to investigate the effects on acute and chronic neck conditions. As clinicians, the duty of care for our patients is of paramount importance: treatment and advice should be given, based on sound biomechanical principles and all available research literature.

References

Alaranta, H., Hurri, H., Heliovaara, M., Soukka, A., Harju, R. (1994) Flexibility of the spine: normative values of goniometric and tape measurements. *Scand. J. Rehabil. Med.* **26:** 147–154.

Allen, M.E., Weir-Jones, I., Motiuk, D.R. *et al.* (1994) Acceleration perturbations of daily living: a comparison to whiplash. *Spine* **19:** 1285–1289.

Barnsley, L., Lord, S., Bogduk, N. (1993) The pathophysiology of whiplash. *Spine: State of the Art Reviews* **7:** 329–353.

Barnsley, L., Lord, S.M., Wallis, B.J., Bogduk, N. (1995) The prevalence of chronic cervical zygapophysial joint pain after whiplash. *Spine* **20:** 20–25.

Bigos, S., Bowyer, O., Breen, G. *et al.* (1994) *Acute Low-back Problems in Adults. Clinical Practice Guideline.* Quick reference guide number 14. AHCPR publication no. 95-0643. Rockville, MD: US Department of Health and Human Services, Public Health Service, Agency of Health Care Policy and Research.

Bogduk, N. (1986) The anatomy and pathophysiology of whiplash. *Clin. Biomech.* **1:** 92–101.

Burns, K. and Lyttelton, L.K. (1994) Osteopathy on the NHS: one practice's experience. *Complement. Ther. Med.* **2:** 200–203.

Burton, A.K. (1981) Back pain in osteopathic practice. *Rheumatol. Rehabil.* **20:** 239–246.

Burton, A.K. (1987) *Patterns of lumbar sagittal mobility and their predictive value in the natural history of back and sciatic pain.* Doctoral thesis: Huddersfield Polytechnic/CNAA.

Burton, A.K., Tillotson, K.M., Main, C.J., Hollis, S. (1995) Psychosocial predictors of outcome in acute and sub-chronic low back trouble. *Spine* **20:** 722–728.

Clinical Standards Advisory Group (1994) *Back Pain. Report of a CSAG committee on Back Pain.* London: HMSO.

Conlon, P.W, Isdale, I.C., Rose B.S (1966) Rheumatoid arthritis of the cervical spine. *Ann. Rheum. Dis.* **25:** 120.

Corrigan, B., Maitland G.D.(1991) *Practical Orthopaedic Medicine.* Oxford: Butterworth-Heinemann.

Danek, V. (1989) Haemodynamic disorders within the vertebrobasilar arterial system following extreme positions of the head. *Man. Med.* **4:** 127–129.

Dreyfuss, P.M.M., Fletcher D. (1994) Atlanto-occipital and lateral atlanto-axial joint pain patterns. *Spine* **19:** 1125–1131.

Ehni, G., Brenner, B. (1984) Occipital neuralgia and the C1–2 arthrosis syndrome. *J. Neurosurg.* **61:** 961–965.

Elvey, R. (1994) The investigation of arm pain: signs of adverse responses to the physical examination of the brachial plexus and related neural tissues. In: *Grieve's Modern Manual Therapy* (Boyling, J.D., Palastanga, N., eds). Edinburgh: Churchill Livingstone, pp. 577–586.

Gargan, M.F., Bannister, G.C. (1994) The rate of recovery following whiplash injury. *Eur. Spine J.* **3:** 162–164.

Grayson, M.F. (1987) Horner's syndrome after manipulation of the neck. *Br. Med. J.* **295:** 1381–1382.

Grieve, G.P. (1981a) Common patterns of clinical presentation. In: *Common Vertebral Joint Problems* (Grieve, G.P., ed.). London: Churchill Livingstone, pp. 206–208.

Grieve, G.P. (1981b) Clinical features. In: *Common Vertebral Joint Problems* (Grieve, G.P., ed.). London: Churchill Livingstone, p. 182.

Grieve, G.P. (1991) *Mobilisation of the Spine – A Primary Handbook of Clinical Medicine,* 5th edn. London: Churchill Livingstone.

Hartman, L.S. (1985) *Handbook of Osteopathic Technique,* 2nd edn. London: Chapman & Hall.

Howe, D.H., Newcombe, R.G., Wade, M.T. (1983) Manipulation of the cervical spine – a pilot study. *J. R. Coll. Gen. Pract.* **33**: 574–579.

Jackson, R. (1977) *The Cervical Syndrome*, 4th edn. Springfield, IL: Charles C Thomas.

Jerrett, W. (1979) Headaches in general practice. *Pract. Med.* **222**: 549–555.

Kahn, J.F., Monod, H. (1989) Fatigue induced by static work. *Ergonomics* **32**: 839–846.

Koes, B.W., Bouter, L.M., van Mameren, H. *et al.* (1992) The effectiveness of manual therapy and treatment by the general practitioner for non-specific back and neck complaints: a randomised clinical trial. *Spine* **17**: 28–35.

Langworthy, J., Breen, A. (1992) *The Grouping of Case History Variables for Back Pain Classification.* London: Society for Back Pain Research.

Lee, P.W.H., Chow, S.P., Lieh-Mak, F., Chan, K.C., Wong, S. (1989) Psychosocial factors influencing outcome in patients with low-back pain. *Spine* **14**: 838–843.

McCarthy, P.W., Olsen, J.P., Smelby, I. (1996) *Effects of Stretching Exercises on Active Range of Motion (ROM) in the Cervical Spine.* Bournemouth, Dorset: AECC.

McRae, R. (1990) *Clinical Orthopaedic Examination.* Edinburgh: Churchill Livingstone.

Martinez, J.L., Garcia, D.J. (1968) A model for whiplash. *J. Biomech.* **1**: 23–32.

Merskey, H., Bogduk, N. (1994a) Suboccipital and cervical musculoskeletal disorders. In: *Classification of Chronic Pain,* 2nd edn (Merskey, H., Bogduk, N., eds). Seattle: IASP Press, pp. 93–97.

Merskey, H., Bogduk, N. (1994b) Primary headache syndromes, vascular disorders, and cerebrospinal fluid syndromes. In: *Classification of Chronic Pain,* 2nd edn (Merskey, H., Bogduk, N., eds). Seattle: IASP Press, pp. 77–89.

Mounstephen, A.H., Harrison, R.K. (1995) A study of migraine and its effects in a working population. *Occup. Med.* **45**: 311–317.

Neumann, H.D. (1989) *Introduction to Manual Medicine.* Berlin: Springer Verlag.

Parker, G.B., Tupling, H. Pryor, D.S. (1978) A controlled trial of cervical manipulation for migraine. *Aust. N.Z. J. Med.* **8**: 589–593.

Radanov, B.P., Sturzenegger, M., de Stefano, G., Schnidrig, A. (1994) Relationship between early somatic, radiological, cognitive and psychosocial findings and outcome during a one-year follow-up in 117 patients suffering from common whiplash. *Br. J. Rheumatol.* **33**: 442–448.

Sharp, J., Purser, D.W. (1961) Spontaneous atlanto-axial dislocation in ankylosing spondylitis and rheumatoid arthritis. *Ann. Rheum.. Dis.* **20** 47.

Sloop, P.R., Smith, D.S., Goldenberg, E., Dore, C. (1982) Manipulation for chronic neck pain. *Spine* **7**: 532–535.

Spitzer, W.O., Skovron, M.L., Salmi, L.R. *et al.* (1995) Scientific monograph of the Quebec Task Force on whiplash-associated disorders: redefining "whiplash" and its management. *Spine* **20** (Suppl): 8S–73S.

Star, M.J, Curd, J.G., Thorne R.P. (1992) Atlantoaxial lateral mass osteoarthritis: a frequently overlooked cause of severe occipitocervical pain. *Spine* **17** (suppl): S71–S76.

Stodolny, J., Chmielewski, H. (1989) Manual therapy in the treatment of patients with cervical migraine. *J. Man. Med.* **4**: 49–51.

Thiel, H.W.T. (1991) Gross morphology and pathoanatomy of the vertebral arteries. *J. Manip. Physiol. Ther.* **14**: 133–141.

Thiel, H., Wallace, K., Donat, J., Yong-Hing, K. (1994) Effect of various head and neck positions on vertebral artery blood flow. *Clin. Biomech.* **9**: 105–110.

Tonlinson, A.M.D. (1971) Osteopathic technique – a new approach. *Br. Osteopath. J.* **5**: 20–25.

Unsworth, A., Dowson, D., Wright, V. (1971) Cracking joints: a bioengineering study of cavitation in the metacarpophalageal joint. *Ann. Rheum. Dis.* **30**: 348–358.

Vernon, H.T., Aker, P., Burns, S., Viljakatlantoaxialnen, S., Short, L. (1990) Pressure pain threshold evaluation of the effect of spinal manipulation in the treatment of chronic neck pain: a pilot study. *J. Manip. Physiol. Ther.* **13**: 13–16.

Weber, H., Burton, A.K. (1986) Rational treatment of low back trouble? *Clin. Biomech.* **1**: 160–167.

11

Physiotherapy management of neck pain of mechanical origin

G. A. Jull

Physiotherapy management of cervical spine disorders aims to care for patients by addressing their pain and pathology, which is manifested in local and regional movement dysfunctions in the articular, muscular and neural systems. The global aims of physiotherapy management are to alleviate patients' pain, reverse the dysfunction and restore optimal muscle and joint function to prevent recurrent episodes. Within this management, patients are provided with precise and relevant exercise and lifestyle strategies to assist them with effective, preventive self-management.

The nature and scope of the musculoskeletal dysfunctions in the cervical region are vast, ranging from acute minor sprains to chronic advanced degenerative pathology compromising the spinal cord. The cervical spine, through physiological and mechanical links, reflects and imposes postures on the whole spinal region. Likewise, dysfunction in cervical structures may secondarily affect or be affected by the structures of the upper limb. The neck's involvement in some shoulder pain syndromes and its possible role in various forearm and hand disorders have been described (Upton and McComas, 1973; Schneider, 1989; Hawkins *et al.*, 1990; Yaxley and Jull, 1993). Furthermore, a neck condition may directly involve the vascular system in the thoracic inlet or via the vertebral artery. The neck and shoulder region may also be the site for pain referral from non-musculoskeletal pathologies (Grieve, 1988). The variety and potential complexity of dysfunctions underlie the need for careful and specific differential diagnosis in the first instance, followed by a comprehensive yet individualized management programme.

The model of clinical practice followed by physiotherapists encompasses a problem-solving approach. The patient's presenting signs, symptoms and history are analysed to determine first of all whether or not their complaint is arising from musculoskeletal dysfunction and, if so, whether it is suitable for, and amenable to, physical treatment. The model highlights the importance of a precise physical examination to elicit the dysfunctions in the neuromuscular-articular systems which are linked to the patient's pain and disability. The treatment methods selected are precise and dysfunction-based, addressing both the unique as well as interrelated dysfunction in the three major systems. Improvement in the patient's pain and disability should parallel the changes in the physical dysfunctions. In this way, treatment outcomes are judged on improvement in both symptoms and function as well as in the physical impairments. Continued development of the understanding of the relationships between pain, physical impairment and response to a treatment method advances clinical practice.

Examination of the neck pain patient

Examination of patients with neck pain syndromes encompasses the clinical examination which includes a comprehensive history of the nature, behaviour and onset of symptoms and a physical examination. In addition, any of a variety of radiological imaging and laboratory tests can be performed as required. The clinical examination is of primary importance. It is conducted with a background knowledge steeped in the physical, behavioural and medical sciences. The methods of clinical reasoning used by the physiotherapist in decision-making during the examination involve a combination of hypothesis testing and pattern recognition (Jones *et al.*, 1995).

Subjective examination

Patients most frequently present for management with the complaint of pain. Neck pain with headache, neck pain alone or neck and arm pain are the broad clusters of patients' disorders. In taking a systematic history from the patient, the clinician seeks patterns that are characteristic of cervical disorders and notes features which are out of pattern. These latter evoke the creation of an alternative set of hypotheses to diagnose differentially the patient's complaint. While emphasis here will be placed on the physical disorder, it is necessary for the clinician to understand any psychosocial aspect of the patient's disorder.

Decision-making from the subjective examination revolves around four basic questions:

1. Is cervical spine dysfunction the origin of the patient's pain?
2. What is the likely nature and location of the structural compromise?
3. Are there factors provoking and perpetuating the condition?
4. Are there features in the patient's history or general medical condition which either caution restraint or direct particular management?

Discussion of each question will highlight aspects of clinical reasoning.

The origin of the patient's pain

The phenomenon of referred pain requires the clinician's alertness to alternative sources of pain in otherwise common cervical musculoskeletal distributions. It is well known that the neck, the upper thoracic region and the upper limbs can be the site of referred pain from, for example, the diaphragm, the heart or tumours in the apex of the lung (Grieve, 1988). A basic tenet in examination of musculoskeletal disorders is that a relationship usually exists between fluctuations in pain and specific mechanical provocation of the region. This should be lacking when, for example, heart disease is responsible for the neck and arm pain as, conversely, signs of heart disease are absent in patients with cervical angina or, as it is otherwise known, pseudoangina (Jacobs, 1990).

These are relatively overt examples of non-musculoskeletal referred pain not amenable to physical therapies. The symptom of headache is, in the main, more benign in nature yet differential diagnosis is equally important to determine a primary, partial or no role for cervical dysfunction in a patient's headache syndrome. There is considerable symptomatic overlap between the common benign headache forms of migraine without aura, tension headache and cervicogenic headache (Jull, 1994). People may suffer mixed headache forms or two concurrent headaches (Boquet *et al.*, 1989; Vernon *et al.*, 1992a; Kidd and Nelson, 1993). The history of a patient presenting with headache is a good example of clinical reasoning and pattern recognition in diagnosing cervical involvement in a patient's headache.

To predict a role for cervical dysfunction in the pathogenesis of a patient's headache, the clinician would expect to hear a pattern incorporating many of the following features. The headache described is classically a unilateral headache (Sjaastad *et al.*, 1983) but it can be bilateral (Jull, 1986a; Watson and Trott, 1993). Cervicogenic headache has side consistency and will not change sides within or between headache attacks as can occur with migraine or cluster headaches (Sjaastad *et al.*, 1989a; D'Amico *et al.*, 1994). It is associated with suboccipital or neck pain (Bogduk and Marsland, 1986; Jull, 1986a) with spread of pain to, most commonly, the frontal, retro-orbital and temporal areas. The onset of pain is most typically in the neck with subsequent spread of pain to the head. This is in contrast to the more classical migraine which has been shown to start most frequently in the head with subsequent spread to the neck (Sjaastad *et al.*, 1989b). The intensity of cervicogenic headache can be mild, moderate or severe. Its intensity can fluctuate, which is different to migraine which, if left uncontrolled, will inevitably build to a severe headache with each attack. Cervical dysfunction does not produce the excruciating pains characteristic of cluster headaches or true neuralgias (Lance, 1993). There may be other symptoms associated with the headache such as visual disturbances, nausea, dizziness, lightheadedness, but they are not a dominant feature, as in migraine with aura or cluster headache (Sjaastad and Bovim, 1991).

The temporal pattern of headache is often diagnostic of a particular headache form, as is readily evident in migraine with aura and cluster headache (Lance, 1993). A feature of cervicogenic headaches is the lack of a regular pattern (Sjaastad, 1992). They are typically precipitated mechanically by sustained neck postures or movements, but provocative factors are sometimes difficult to identify (Sjaastad *et al.*, 1983; Jull, 1986a; Pfaffenrath *et al.*, 1987). Equally, the patient may have difficulty identifying relieving factors, although the headache's lack of response to medications used for other headache forms may add to the picture of cervicogenic headache (Bovim and Sjaastad, 1993; Sjaastad *et al.*, 1993). The history of onset of cervicogenic headache commonly relates to trauma, postural strain to the neck or degenerative joint disease (Braaf and Rosner, 1975; Bogduk, 1994; Lord *et al.*, 1994) although an incident is not always identified by the patient. Age of onset is variable and there is not a familial tendency to this headache form, as is usual for migraine.

This pattern should be present to confirm the probability that cervical dysfunction is a major, if not sole, cause of the patient's headache syndrome. The clinician listens for such patterns in the differential diagnosis of all neck pain syndromes. If patterns are not clear, a number of hypotheses are proposed to continue the problem-solving process of the clinical examination.

The nature and location of the structural compromise

Over the past decade there has been an acceleration in research into the nature of the pathology causing the cervical dysfunction relating to both degenerative and traumatic causes. *In vivo* and postmortem studies in particular have revealed a host of lesions. These have ranged from ligamentous strains and contusions, to disc disruptions and zygapophysial joint fractures, to very chronic venous changes around the cervical nerves (Jónsson *et al.*, 1991, 1994; Barnsley *et al.*, 1993 (for review); Taylor and Finch, 1993). Following trauma, patients often have multiple lesions at multiple levels (Bogduk and Aprill, 1993; Jónsson *et al.*, 1994). However, it seems that imaging technology has not yet advanced to the stage where a definite pathoanatomical diagnosis can be made in all cases of patients presenting with neck pain (Jónsson *et al.*, 1991). Furthermore, the relationship between imaged structural lesions and clinical signs and symptoms can be poor (Barton *et al.*, 1993; Pettersson *et al.*, 1994). Positional observations, such as a straightened cervical spine, or a rotated C2 vertebra, also have a very tenuous association with cervical dysfunction (Boquet *et al.*, 1989; Macpherson and Campbell, 1991; Nagasawa *et al.*, 1993; Borchgrevink *et al.*, 1995). The current state indicates that the clinical examination is of primary importance, with the radiographic examination being an adjunct to diagnosis. It also means that a precise pathoanatomical diagnosis is, for many patients, a clinician's working hypothesis rather than a proven fact. What can always be gained, however, is a clinical pattern of symptoms which can incriminate certain structural compromise.

Pain is a multidimensional experience and, while the clinician must be cognizant of the psychological aspects and the central pain phenomenon, peripheral nociception still seems to be a major factor in the pain syndromes of patients presenting to general physiotherapy practices. All structures of the cervical spine are innervated and studies of experimentally induced pain in various somatic and neural structures have provided basic patterns of segmental reference which are used to provide initial directions in clinical diagnosis (Feinstein *et al.*, 1954; Cloward, 1959; Dwyer *et al.*, 1990). Broadly, structures supplied by the upper three cervical nerves cause neck pain with referral into the head. The segmental reference for pain from the mid and lower cervical regions includes the shoulder, scapular area, anterior chest and upper limb.

While structures with the same nerve supply will have similar segmental reference, other factors may qualify the source of symptoms. For example, patients may be able to pinpoint the site of their neck pain with a fingertip, localizing it to a specific zygapophysial joint. They may report an intense spot of pain on the medial border of the scapula, consistent with the areas of referred pain which Cloward (1959) recorded with cervical disc stimulation. Once pain is referred into a limb, a segmental level may become more apparent and the quality, nature and intensity of pain may suggest whether or not the pain has a neuropathic source.

Conversely, the pain may not have a clear anatomical pattern but have characteristics which might suggest a particular syndrome or structural compromise. For example, Smythe (1994) documented a predictable pattern of tender points associated with chronic C6-7 dysfunction. Physiotherapists are well-acquainted with the array of neuropathic or neurogenic pain patterns that can be associated with altered dynamics of the nervous system (Elvey, 1986; Quintner, 1989; Butler, 1991, 1994). Clues of mechanosensitivity of neural structures are gained when patients report lines of pain along the anatomical path of nerves, areas of pain at sites where nerves are vulnerable to irritation, for example, the intervertebral foramen or the path through the scalenes (Butler, 1991). A pattern where proximal and distal symptoms link up could suggest a double crush phenomenon, so well-demonstrated by the association of cervical spondylosis with carpal tunnel syndrome (Upton and McComas, 1973). Pain patterns and responses from any origin may become further heightened or widespread when there is central nervous system sensitization (Quintner and Elvey, 1993; Quintner and Cohen, 1994; Hall and Quintner, 1995) or with the phenomenon of sympathetically maintained pain (Janig, 1990).

Careful analysis of symptom responses to movements or postures can also contribute important information to clinical patterns. Based on a knowledge of cervical mechanics and kinematics, neck movements producing pain are analysed for their structural compromise of the zygapophysial joint, disc complex and intervertebral canal and nerve root complex. When patients present with neck and arm pain, differentiation is made between intrinsic cervical and other sources. Neck movements may produce all symptoms, suggesting local cervical compromise. However, upper limb movements may provoke arm symptoms. This could still reflect cervical causes, as arm movements, tension or traction of mechanosensitive nerves (Quintner, 1990). Conversely, the arm pain could be arising from the shoulder joint where dysfunction may be primary or secondary to a cervical disorder. Schneider (1989) observed that in patients with neck and arm pain, with restricted arm movement, those with disproportionately limited external rotation responded to treatment of the C5–6 segment. Those with proportional movement loss in the conventional capsular pattern required specific glenohumeral joint management.

The patterns of dysfunction and structural hypothesis proposed from the location, nature and behaviour of symptoms will be further clarified with detailed movement analysis and differential testing in the physical examination.

Factors provoking or perpetuating the condition

Recurrent chronic pain is a burden to society in terms of personal suffering, lost work productivity and health care costs. Hasvold and Johnson (1993) determined that over 50% of the female and 35% of the male population suffered headache, neck or shoulder pain on a regular basis; that is, at least monthly. Half of these people reported pain on a weekly or daily basis. The challenge to the health care worker is not in providing temporary symptomatic relief, but in successfully intervening in the chronic and recurrent pattern of neck pain and headache.

There is complexity in causal and provocative factors both in neck pain syndromes of both insidious and traumatic onset. Intrinsic, environmental and psychosocial factors variously have their roles and the physiotherapist seeks a clear and complete picture of patients and their environment in understanding what provokes and aggravates their pain syndrome.

Intrinsically, contributing factors may arise in the nervous, muscular or articular systems. A fixed cervicothoracic spine can overstrain adjacent cervical segments. A patient's acquired deficit in neural tissue elasticity may cause otherwise normal movements and postures to provoke pain (Butler, 1991). It is believed that a major factor contributing to the perpetuation of pain syndromes is poor neuromotor control (Janda, 1994; Jull, 1994; Richardson and Jull, 1994; White and Sahrmann, 1994; Hodges and Richardson, 1996). Evidence is accumulating that lack of stability function of the deep spinal and postural muscles is a key deficit in chronic back and neck pain (Beeton and Jull, 1994; Richardson and Jull, 1995a,b; Hides et al., 1996; Hodges and Richardson, 1996) and a precise physical examination can reveal these problems. Furthermore, evidence is growing to suggest that precise rehabilitation of the muscle dysfunction can successfully intervene in the chronic pain state.

Work sites and practices can also place provocative cyclic or fatigue loading, or overload, on cervicobrachial neuromuscular–articular structures (La Ban and Meerschaert, 1989). The introduction of ergonomically designed work stations and changes in work practices has contributed to reducing these stressors (Grandjean, 1988). However, they have not eliminated the problem and the physiotherapist carefully

analyses the movement and motor patterns the patient uses in performing tasks. Here often lies the key to particular structural overload.

The nature of injury may also have a significant influence on the likelihood of progression to a chronic condition. Sturzenegger and colleagues (Radanov et al., 1993; Sturzenegger et al., 1994, 1995) studied 117 consecutive patients presenting with a whiplash injury to identify which factors may be associated with long term and chronic problems. At the 1-year follow-up, 24% of subjects had persistent symptoms. The initial symptomatic and accident mechanisms which predicted longer-term problems included a higher intensity of neck pain, the presence of headache, not being prepared for the accident, an inclined or rotated head position, and a stationary car at impact. Such information helps identify patients at risk for more severe problems. For such patients, a treatment programme directed towards enhancing muscle control and support to substitute for the possible loss of osseoligamentous integrity is essential (Derrick and Chesworth, 1992).

Features indicating caution, restraint or a particular direction in treatment

There can be features presenting in patients' symptomatology, in the history of their neck disorders, or in their medical history, which alert the physiotherapist to pathologies which may give definitive directions in management.

Care is always warranted when patients present with signs and symptoms of physical compromise of the nervous system. Such syndromes can range from irritation or compression of the spinal nerve or nerve root through to compromise of the spinal cord. While the former are amenable to carefully applied physical therapy techniques, the presence of cord signs dictates thorough medical investigation and possible surgical management.

There are a host of symptoms which can accompany cervical musculoskeletal disorders. These include dizziness, lightheadedness, nausea, visual, auditory, sensory and balance disturbances and poor concentration (Hinoki and Niki, 1975; Barnsley et al., 1993). The basis of these symptoms is not always certain, although many are likely to relate to convergence in the central nervous system of neck afferents with, for example, the trigeminal nucleus and vestibular nuclei (Dieterich et al., 1993; Bogduk, 1994; Karlberg et al., 1995). Cervical proprioceptive input has considerable influence on posture through the tonic neck reflex and eye movement and accommodation through the cervico-ocular and iliospinal reflexes.

When the origin of symptoms such as lightheadedness, or visual disturbances, lies in cervical musculoskeletal dysfunction, they can be alleviated by treatment of the neck. However, such symptoms can have other causes and the crucial factor in examination is to differentiate a cervical cause of these symptoms from other causes. For example, dizziness is a symptom of which all practitioners using manipulative therapy to treat neck dysfunction are highly mindful. Differentiation between cervical vertigo and dizziness of vertebrobasilar, or vestibular, origin is necessary. As head and neck movements can invoke symptoms from any system, cervical vertigo is often provisionally diagnosed through exclusion of neurological and labyrinthine signs (Coman, 1986; Dieterich *et al.*, 1993; Bogduk, 1994).

Conclusion of subjective examination

The information gained from all aspects of the subjective examination provides an evolving clinical pattern. The clinical reasoning process continues in the physical examination to gain a working physical diagnosis on which to base selection of physiotherapy treatment techniques.

Physical examination

The physiotherapist tests the function of the articular, neural and muscular systems and performs tests of other systems as appropriate to the patient's condition. The aims are to diagnose differentially both the immediate source of pain and factors contributing to and perpetuating the cervical syndrome. The dysfunctions linked to the condition are identified and these guide the selection of specific and precise treatment procedures.

The physical examination encompasses several procedures. The assessments of posture and active movements can reflect dysfunction in any or all of the neuromuscular–articular systems. The articular system receives more specific attention via a manual examination of the spinal segments. Two functions of the nervous systems are tested, namely tests of normal conduction and tests of free movement and extensibility (neuromechanics). The muscle system is examined through a variety of tests, including tests specific to particular muscles through to patterns of muscle activity and kinesthetic awareness.

A checklist of physical examination procedures belies the potential complexity of musculoskeletal dysfunction and the level of problem-solving required to reach an accurate physical diagnosis. There are several factors which should be considered concurrently in decision-making both for diagnosis and treatment.

1. Cervical pain syndromes represent multisystem dysfunction. Joint pain and dysfunction cannot occur in isolation and will induce reactions in the neuromuscular system (Stokes and Young, 1984; Watson and Trott, 1993; Hides *et al.*, 1994).

Similarly, mechanosensitivity of neural structures will induce protective muscle activity (Hall *et al.*, 1993). If muscle control is poor, joint strain and pain may result (Panjabi, 1992a). In consequence, examination or treatment which focuses on one system, to the exclusion of others, is misdirected.

2. There is considerable variability in cervical structure and function within the asymptomatic normal population. Ranges of movement are highly variable and hypomobility, segmentally and regionally, will increase with age (Jull, 1986b; Hole *et al.*, 1995). Neural tissues have variable flexiblity (Yaxley and Jull, 1991; Edgar *et al.*, 1994). Slight tightness in cervical axioscapular muscles is probably as common in asymptomatic as in symptomatic subjects (Treleaven *et al.*, 1994). Neck muscle strength varies across subjects with and without symptoms (Vernon *et al.*, 1992b; Watson and Trott, 1993). Therefore the implications of any variation from an ideal must be questioned. Variations become relevant when they have a direct link to the pain state.

3. The sensitivity and specificity of any physical test to discriminate relevant dysfunction must be appreciated to make meaningful decisions.

4. Any movement of the head and neck will stress each and every structure of the neuromuscular-articular system. Any structure can be involved in a painfully limited movement. Careful differential examination is required to identify the compromised structure accurately.

5. Any physical examination of the cervical region should consider the musculoskeletal system as a whole. There is an interdependence in cervical, thoracic and lumbar postural form, as well as an interdependence between upper limb and spinal movement (Crawford and Jull, 1993; Stewart *et al.*, 1995). The nervous system is a continuous tissue track and movement distal to the cervical region can affect local neural tissue structures (Brieg, 1978). Local muscle dysfunctions may reflect more widespread problems (Janda, 1994).

To highlight the integrated nature of the dysfunction, the description of the physical examination in this text will highlight some examples of differential testing rather than repeat physical examination proformas which can be found in standard physiotherapy texts (Maitland, 1986; Grieve, 1988; Boyling and Palastanga, 1994; Grant, 1994a). An emphasis is deliberately given to assessment of the neuromuscular system as it is believed that this is an area of considerable change in current therapeutics.

Postural assessment

Postural form provides information in both the acute and chronic pain states. Acute pain from joints, neural tissues or muscles can be reflected in familiar antalgic postures such as the acute wry neck, or the raised shoulder, which relieves tension from the neurovascular bundle.

In patients able to assume their normal standing and sitting positions, posture is analysed for basic structural form, the interrelationship of spinal curves and muscle form (Kendall *et al.*, 1993; Janda, 1994; White and Sahrmann, 1994). There is an assumption that a deviation from an ideal or neutral posture, in which there is minimal stress or strain, is capable of causing adverse strain and subsequently pain in spinal structures (Kendall *et al.*, 1993). There have been numerous studies revealing a wide variation in human postural shape, indicating that there is a certain painfree tolerance when postural form alone is considered. Other variables may have to be considered along with postural form. The specific links between postural factors and pain need to be identified to depict the aspects of posture, position and control that require rehabilitation. These links are also necessary to justify any emphasis on postural re-education in management and preventive programmes.

On a regional level the forward head posture, associated with an increased kyphosis in the upper thoracic or thoracic region, is regarded as the most common poor postural form in neck pain syndromes (Sweeney *et al.*, 1990; Kendall *et al.*, 1993; Janda, 1994; Raine and Twomey, 1994; White and Sahrmann, 1994). Nevertheless, Dalton and Coutts (1994) found that it was also a factor of age, indicating some painfree adaptation. This would be consistent with the findings of Griegel-Morris *et al.* (1992) that it was those of their population with a more exaggerated forward head posture that had the greater incidence of headache and cervicothoracic pain.

An important link between the forward head posture and muscle dysfunction was reported by Watson and Trott (1993) in their study of cervicogenic headache patients. They found that a lack of endurance capacity of the upper cervical and deep neck flexors was correlated with a forward head posture. Longus colli has been shown to have an important supporting and postural function on the cervical curve, working with the cervical extensors to stabilize the cervical segments in all positions of the head (Mayoux-Benhamou *et al.*, 1994). This link between a pain state, poor postural form and dysfunction in a muscle with a primary supporting role of the cervical segments guides a specific rehabilitation direction. The direction is to improve the supporting capacity of this deep muscle in the quest for improvement in postural form and active joint support for alleviation of joint strain and pain (Jull, 1994; Richardson and Jull, 1995a).

The well-coordinated activity of the muscles of the upper thoracic and scapular region is vital for well-supported cervicothoracic posture, as well as for upper limb function and proper transfer of loads from the upper limb to the trunk (Johnson *et al.*, 1994). Clinically, imbalances in levels of activity of the axioscapular muscles are not uncommonly observed (Janda, 1994; White and Sahrmann, 1994). Most particularly, muscles such as levator scapulae can become overactive, the overactivity creating poor scapular mechanics as well as resolving into unnecessary compressive loads through the upper cervical joints (Behrsin and Maguire, 1986). Such overactivity can be recognized by viewing hypertrophy of the levator scapulae in its bulk towards its insertion into the superomedial border of the scapula (Janda, 1994). A lack of supporting function of important shoulder girdle muscles, such as serratus anterior and the mid and lower portions of the trapezius, can be in evidence during observation of postural form. An abducted and winged position of the scapula may be observed, accompanied by a lack of muscle bulk in the interscapular region (Janda, 1994).

The shape of the shoulder region is also of interest. Some unevenness in shoulder height may reflect the very common occurrence of a slight scoliosis, thereby having little, if any, dysfunctional significance (Vercauteren *et al.*, 1982). An acutely sloping shoulder may indicate poor upper trapezius activity in concert with an overactive levator scapulae. Conversely, the upper trapezius may appear hypertonic. This may be part of a problem of poor neuromotor control and a poor pattern of muscle activity (Janda, 1994). Alternatively, the hypertonicity of the upper trapezius accompanied by a subtle elevation of the shoulder girdle could be protective of mechanosensitive cervical nerve trunks. This warrants an inspection of the scalenes which may also be reactive.

Considerable information can be gained from analysing postural relationships and muscle form. There are multiple factors influencing posture and the clinician seeks those which have a link to the patient's pain syndrome.

Tests of neuromotor control

There are a variety of tests which can be used in a clinical setting to gain an insight into a patient's kinesthetic awareness and pattern of muscle use and control. These can include head and neck repositioning sense (Revel *et al.*, 1991), patterns of muscle recruitment (Janda, 1994) and postural and movement control. Examination of movement patterns can reveal inappropriate use of some muscles substituting for others, which usually reflects a lack of control by muscles with a prime stability function. Conversely, patients may adopt inappropriate regional movement strategies, again reflecting poor muscle stability capacity and control. Such poor muscle and movement environments are conducive to perpetuating strains and recurrent and chronic pain.

One set of tests assesses the efficiency of the axioscapular muscles to control proximal girdle stability. The pattern of glenohumeral abduction, for example (Janda, 1994), can reveal inappropriate overuse of scapular elevators, creating an environment for local muscle pain as well as exposing the cervical spine to unnecessary and repetitive compressive and tensile loads (Behrsin and Maguire, 1986). Forwards arm elevation can reveal not only poor axioscapular control, but also a loss of deep cervical flexor control as the patient shows subtle to marked signs of forward head and neck displacement during the full arm movement.

The pattern of control of the muscles intrinsic to the spine can be assessed through movement and postural patterns. The interaction between the cervical flexor synergists, for example, is gauged from the pattern of control during neck flexion from extension to neutral. Insufficiency of the upper cervical and deep neck flexors, so important to cervical segmental control (Mayoux-Benhamou *et al.*, 1994), is readily in evidence when the head remains in extension and as the neck is brought into neutral (Fig. 11.1). This indicates dominant activity in the sternocleidomastoid (which is a neck flexor, but upper cervical extensor), rather than a balanced activity in the neck flexor synergy. Testing the patient's ability to assume a neutral spinal postural position in either a sitting, or four-point kneeling, position can alert the clinician to a patient's inadequate deep and postural muscle control and joint position sense. The patient will be observed to use inappropriate muscle and movement strategies in attempting to assume a balanced postural position (Fig. 11.2). The postural analysis and these preliminary tests of neuromotor control begin to point to the dysfunction in the patient's muscle system and direct the clinician to more precise and exacting tests of muscle function.

Examination of active cervical movements

An appreciation of the patient's basic flexibility is gained before specific examination of the cervical region.

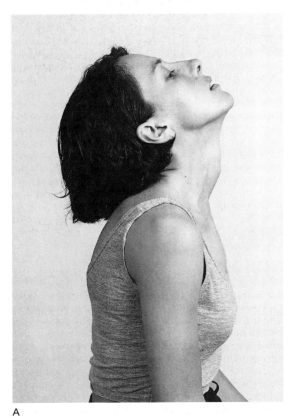
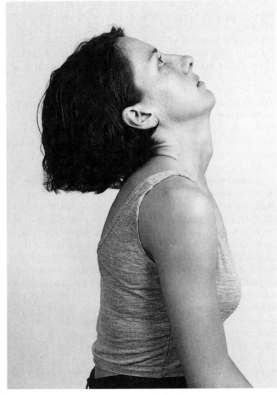

A   B

Fig. 11.1 Return from extension to the upright position. (A) The movement is dominated by sternocleidomastoid and the upper cervical region remains in extension. (B) A good pattern of movement is demonstrated, in which the upper cervical and deep neck flexors initiate the return from extension and control and protect the craniocervical region.

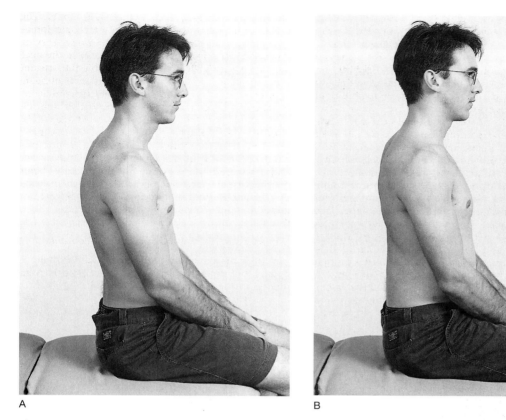

A   B

Fig. 11.2 An assessment of the patient's ability to assume a neutral spine posture. (A) A well-balanced posture. (B) Note the lumbar pelvic region is flexed, with the patient extending in the lower thoracic area to achieve an upright posture. This is indicative of poor neuromotor control.

Active movements of the cervical region stress articular, muscle and neural tissues of the region as well as giving indications of muscle control. Interpretation of examination findings is built on an ever-increasing understanding of the anatomy, mechanics and kinematics of the region. New knowledge continues to mould and develop clinical concepts leading clinicians towards better pathoanatomical hypotheses (Mercer and Jull, 1996). Using such knowledge, the physiotherapist examines movements in single and combined planes, continuing to focus on gaining a pattern of dysfunction which is linked to the patient's symptomatic complaints and functional impairment.

The functional cervical spine incorporates the region from the atlanto-occipital articulations to the upper thoracic region. Movement is examined in each of the three primary planes of motion. There is both interdependence and independence in the segmental movement of the cervical regions. Total movement, as well as movement focused to the upper cervical and cervicothoracic regions, is examined. Several principles and practices are followed in examination of active movement which apply to each direction of movement and which are in line with the global principles of examination.

Observation and measurement of movement

In examination of cervical movement, the clinician assesses the pattern and distribution of movement, the gross range of motion and its relationship to the patient's symptoms. A symptomatic segmental block to movement may be recognized via a distortion of an otherwise smooth curve of the neck. Excessive movement may be observed in the C4–6 region during sagittal plane motion as the patient pivots the head and neck over a hypomobile and fixed cervicothoracic region. Restoration of some mobility in this region would be part of a treatment programme designed to relieve stress from the C4–6 segments. Likewise, observation of this poor pattern and control of motion would signal poor supporting capacity of neck musculature (Fig. 11.1).

There are now clinically applicable and affordable measurement tools to provide repeatable, although gross, measures of cervical motion (Hole *et al.*, 1995). Although there is undoubted merit in aims to have quantification of physical factors, measures of gross movement often provide very poor links between dysfunction and functional outcome. Clinicians have not embraced these tools widely and often continue to rely more on visual analysis. Indeed, Hindle *et al.* (1990) endorsed the clinicians' sentiments when they found that it was not absolute range of motion which distinguished back pain from non-back pain subjects, but rather the aberrant patterns of movement through range.

Regionalization of active movement examination

Reactions of pain and abnormal or limited motion contribute more to a clinical pattern when they can be localized to a segment or region of the spine. Sagittal plane motion is focused to the cranioverterbral region by testing flexion and extension of the head rather than the head–neck complex. A subtle neck retraction action will better induce extension in the cervicothoracic area. The regional location of a limitation of axial rotation can be gauged by the patient performing head rotation with a fully flexed cervical spine (C1–2), with the upper cervical spine in flexion (C2–3), as compared with rotation performed in a neutral sagittal position (Fig. 11.3).

Examination of movements in combination

Normal function involves complex loading, rather than movements in a pure plane, suggesting that a pattern or position of combined movement may be more compromised in a dysfunctional segment. The joints of the cervical region are therefore also examined with a combination of movements. The combination of added movements is derived from the joint's movement and pain as well as kinematic relationships (Edwards, 1992). For example, there is related zygapophysial joint and uncovertebral joint motion in lateral flexion and ipsilateral axial rotation of the mid and lower cervical spine (Penning and Wilmink, 1987). Added extension will take the

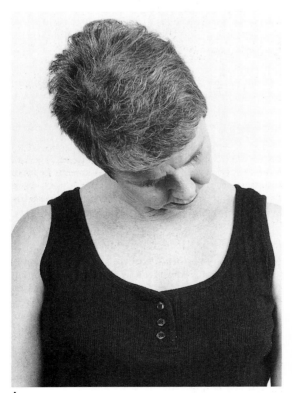
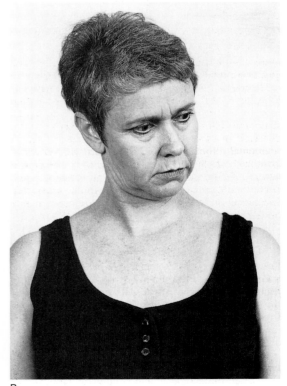

A   B

Fig. 11.3 Examination of cervical axial rotation (A) focused to the C1–2 segment; (B) focused to the C2–3 segment.

zygapophysial joint towards its close-packed position. The concept of combined movement examination is guided by knowledge of kinematics derived principally from *in vitro* research (White and Panjabi, 1990). Nevertheless, clinical presentation must always override the theoretical state. This was well-illustrated in recent *in vivo* studies where, for example, lateral flexion and axial rotation displayed a contralateral couple in some subjects at both C2–3 and in the upper thoracic region, rather than the expected ipsilateral couple (Penning and Wilmink, 1987; Mimura *et al.*, 1989; Willems *et al.*, 1996).

The application of overpressure

There is a difference in magnitude between ranges of active and passive motion. Physiotherapists have long applied gentle passive pressure to guide the patient's movement to the end of range so that a clear estimation of range and any pain response can be gained (Maitland, 1986). The merit of this practice was well-illustrated by Dvorak *et al.* (1993). They found quite marked differences in the frequency of segments judged hypomobile, normal and hypermobile in their X-ray analysis of subjects performing voluntary full range of cervical motion versus motion taken passively to the limit of range.

Differentiation of structural restraint to motions

Differential analysis of the structure limiting motion increases the accuracy of the physical findings, which guides optimal treatment selection. Restricted cervical lateral flexion, for example, could be the result of joint restriction, muscle tightness or lack of painfree movement or extensibility of neural tissues. Initial structural differentiation is made by observing if the decrease in lateral flexion is associated with a segmental block, or the whole motion is more symmetrically limited (muscle or neural tissues). The latter is further differentiated by pretensioning the nervous system by supporting the arm in abduction and external rotation and investigating its influence on the range of lateral flexion (Elvey, 1986).

Manual examination of segmental motion

Examination of active range of movement provides information about the region's impairment and gives preliminary directives towards the nature and site of the physical dysfunction. Manual examination of segmental motion and tissue compliance provides more detailed information on the location and nature of the physical dysfunction in the spinal segment.

The techniques of manual spinal segmental examination are well-described in physiotherapy texts (Maitland, 1986; Grieve, 1988; Edwards, 1992; Boyling and Palastanga, 1994; Grant, 1994a). In summary, motion at the segment is tested and palpated in each

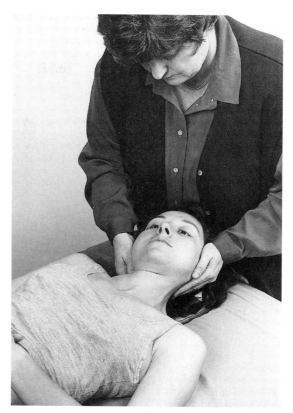

Fig. 11.4 The downward and medial excursion of the C2 and C3 facet is tested in lateral flexion to detect end-of-range motion loss.

of the three planes of primary motion. In addition, the segment is directly stressed with gentle manual forces applied in anteroposterior, posteroanterior and lateral directions in the zygapophysial joint facet planes. The joints are also examined in positions of combined movements as directed by the findings of the active movement examination (Fig. 11.4). The tissue resistance to motion, its nature and any pain response to testing are assessed to make decisions about the location and problems of the segments which are linked to the patient's symptoms. As well, any excess motion or hypomobility which could be contributing to the problem is sought in adjacent segments or regions. In this way, the articular component of the patient's symptoms, movement impairment and functional disability are identified and recorded. Specific directives for treatment are gained, as well as impairments documented which can be expected to change with improvement in the patient's symptoms.

Manual examination has shown good sensitivity and specificity to detect the symptomatic level in spinal pain patients when compared to other medical diagnostic techniques such as nerve or joint blocks and even mobility X-rays (Jull *et al.*, 1988; Jensen *et al.*, 1990; Janos and Ray, 1992; Phillips and Twomey, 1996). It has also proved sensitive in the detection of cervical joint dysfunction in some patients suffering post concussional headaches (Treleaven *et al.*, 1994). While manual examination may be able accurately to detect the presence of a painful zygapophysial joint, or central intervertebral joint, it is not pathology-specific. Rather, it provides the essential physical parameters upon which physical treatment can be selected and evaluated.

Examination of the nervous system

The effect of any pathology or trauma on the nervous system is assessed by testing two functions. A clinical neurological examination is performed as a basic test for normal conduction of the central and peripheral nervous systems. Any signs of central nervous system compromise, as may occur with spinal canal stenosis from any cause, require immediate medical consultation, if not already diagnosed. Signs of spinal nerve, or nerve root, irritation or compression likewise require careful monitoring by the treating clinician. Its presence provides direction to physical management.

The second function of the nervous system which is tested is that of its free movement and extensibility. The role of adverse neuromechanics or mechano-sensitivity of the nervous system in upper quadrant pain syndromes has received considerable attention over the past decade (Elvey, 1986; Butler, 1991). As a clinical phenomenon, it is not uncommon, especially in patients with neck and arm pain. It has also been attributed a role in some chronic upper limb disorders (Upton and McComas, 1973; Elvey, 1986; Quintner, 1990; Yaxley and Jull, 1993). The nerves themselves may become sensitized from the pathology in neighbouring articular or muscular structures (Butler, 1991) or, in some cases, the nerves themselves may have suffered some direct strain through, for example, a traction element in injury (Quintner, 1990). What is being revealed clinically, as well as in the laboratory, is that in these situations the nerves are sensitive to movement, evoking considerable protective muscle response (Hall *et al.*, 1993; Hall and Quintner, 1995).

The role of mechanosensitivity of the upper quadrant nervous system is elicited through the application of the brachial plexus tension test (Elvey, 1986). The test involves an ordered sequence of movement of the shoulder and girdle, the forearm, wrist and hand (Fig. 11.5). The test stresses the trunks of the brachial plexus and the cervical nerve roots, with most effect on C5 and C6. It is applied gently, and when positive, the clinician perceives the onset of muscle guarding, which attempts to elevate the

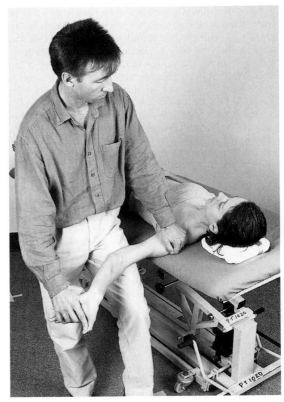

Fig. 11.5 The brachial plexus tension test involves the ordered application of gentle shoulder girdle depression, shoulder abduction (90°) and external rotation, wrist and hand extension followed by elbow extension. The sequence can be varied.

girdle and prevent arm extension, and notes any reproduction of the patient's symptoms. The test potentially stresses many other muscular, fascial and ligamentous structures of the cervicobrachial region and upper limb (Moses and Carman, 1996). Therefore, a stress more selective to the nervous system is added via contralateral cervical lateral flexion. Its influence on patients' arm symptoms, as well as the limitation to lateral flexion, is assessed. Selvaratnam *et al.* (1994) proved the discriminate validity of this sensitizing manoeuvre and the brachial tension test to detect mechanosensitivity in the upper quadrant nervous system. They conducted an experiment where the test was used successfully to differentiate between normal control subjects and subjects with shoulder and arm pain where mechanosensitivity of the nervous system could (patients after open heart surgery) and could not (patients with supraspinatus tendinitis) be expected to be part of the cause of the pain syndrome.

There are several variations to the original brachial plexus tension test which have been developed with the aim of placing more selective tension on the peripheral nerve trunks (Butler, 1991). In addition, neuromeningeal structures in the spinal canal can be tested in a cephalocaudad direction to assess their contribution to a pain syndrome (Maitland, 1986; Troup, 1986; Butler, 1991). Careful differentiation of a restriction of upper cervical flexion is often required, particularly in patients with cervicogenic headache. The articular, muscular and neuromeningeal structures of the upper cervical area are all stressed with a passive upper cervical flexion test which often reproduces head pain. Connective tissue attachments have also recently been identified between the rectus capitus posterior minor and dura mater (Hack *et al.*, 1995), thereby increasing the intimacy of the relationship. Some differentiation between restriction of motion due to muscle or neural tissues can be made by repeating the upper cervical flexion test with the nervous system pretensioned caudally through a straight leg raise. An increase in resistance to the movement suggests a greater involvement of neural tissues in the dysfunction.

Examination of the muscle system

Control of head and neck postures in normal function is a complex neuromotor task (Keshener *et al.*, 1989). As with every other region in the body, muscles will react to pain, trauma and pathology. In patients with cervical pain disorders, the challenge is to identify dysfunctions in the muscle system which are linked to the patient's pain, pathology and functional disability. Identifying such links directs which functions of these muscles are critical to test.

There has been a far greater volume of research into back and abdominal muscle function in low back pain patients than there has been into muscle function of the neck and shoulder girdle complex. It has been the interest in the role of instability in back pain, particularly the hypothesis of lack of control of the segment's neutral zone motion (Panjabi, 1992a,b), that has prompted new directions in clinical research. In trying to solve the muscle dysfunction associated with low back pain and, therefore, devise the most efficacious rehabilitation, both clinicians and researchers have recently focused on muscle control and active stabilization (Saal and Saal, 1989; Robison, 1992; Richardson and Jull, 1994; Wilke *et al.*, 1995).

In normal function, all muscles have a role in producing movement and in postural and spinal control, although some functional divisions between muscles have been suggested (Bergmark, 1989; Richardson and Jull, 1994). Bergmark (1989) grouped the trunk muscles into a global and local system. The global system incorporated the more superficial muscles which have a primary role in torque production and control of the whole trunk. The local system includes the deep muscles which have direct attachments to the vertebrae and which have the ability to support and control or actively stabilize the spine both as a whole and at the segmental level.

There has been a significant clinical breakthrough with the recent discovery of a dysfunction in the stabilizing capacity of some deep muscles of the trunk, the lumbar multifidus and the deep transversus abdominis (Hides *et al.*, 1994, 1996; Hodges and Richardson, 1996). The problem in the segmental multifidus in the acute, first-episode low back pain patients was thought to relate to reflex inhibition while that in transversus abdominis was identified as a deficit in motor control. A manifestation of these dysfunctions, which can be elicited in the clinical setting, is the inability of the patient to hold a setting or low-load isometric contraction of the muscle. It has been argued that this reflects a loss of tonic or postural supporting function of the muscles, related to lessening of type I muscle fibre action (Richardson and Jull, 1994, 1995b).

In the neck, there are likewise many muscles connecting the head to the vertebral column and evidence is emerging to support the model of a broad grouping into global and local muscles based on their anatomical location and some of their more important functions. Conley *et al.* (1995) studied the function of individual neck muscles through exercise-induced contrast shifts in T2-weighted magnetic resonance images. They showed that the more superficial muscles (global system) such as sternocleidomastoid (ventrally) and semispinalis capitus and splenius capitus (dorsally) made a greater contribution to torque production than their deeper synergists (local system) longus capitus and longus colli and semispinatus cervicus and multifidus respectively. Conley *et al.* (1995) found that, while these muscles did not contribute as much to torque production, they were the ones which demonstrated resting activity. The authors attributed this to their postural, supporting role. Mayoux-Benhamou *et al.* (1994) have also supported the importance of the longus colli for postural control of the cervical curve. These deep muscles, including those of the craniocervical region, are well-placed to offer spinal segmental control and stabilization.

The critical question to ask is: what is the muscle dysfunction associated with neck pain? There has been comparatively little research into the cervical musculature in patients with neck pain syndromes. However, in line with clinical theory (Janda, 1983), a dysfunction which has emerged is a lack of endurance of the neck flexor group (Silverman *et al.*, 1991; Watson and Trott, 1993; Treleaven *et al.*, 1994). In an assessment of gross muscle function, Vernon *et al.* (1992b) found that patients with neck pain demonstrated generally less torque production in all planes, but there was a greater loss in strength of the cervical flexors as opposed to the cervical extensors. From our clinical and research findings of the nature of the dysfunction in the deep muscles in the lumbar spine, we developed a clinical test for the cervical region to focus more specifically on the deep craniocervical and cervical flexors, namely, rectus capitus anterior and lateralis and longus capitus and colli (Jull, 1994). In line with their normal function of tonic or postural support, the test examines these muscles' ability to maintain a low-level tonic contraction by maintaining a precise upper cervical flexion position (see p. 181 for a full description of the test). Preliminary studies of deep neck flexor holding capacity in asymptomatic subjects and subjects with neck pain indicated marked differences in performance (unpublished data). Furthermore, initial indications are that restoration of their tonic (supporting) capacity parallels a reduction in neck pain and headache (Beeton and Jull, 1994).

Laboratory-based evidence is emerging to support the clinical evidence of a more intricate muscle dysfunction in neck pain patients rather than merely a gross uniform reaction in all muscles. Uhlig *et al.* (1995) studied muscle fibre composition and muscle fibre transformation in biopsy studies of selected neck muscles of patients with persistent cervical pain of various pathologies. They found that there was an increased relative amount of type IIC fibres in all muscles studied, indicating that muscle fibre transformation occurred with neck pain. Fibre transformation always proceeded in the direction from type I (slow oxidative fibre) to type IIB (fast glycolytic fibre), which functionally suggests a loss of the tonic or postural supporting capacity of the neck muscles as a dysfunction in neck pain patients, a dysfunction akin to that found clinically in back pain patients. Notably, there was a much higher prevalence of transitional fibres (type II C) in the neck flexors than the extensors and changes in the flexors were present and most evident in the early stages of the neck disorder (<2 years' duration). Within the neck flexors, there was more evidence of transformation in the longus colli, a muscle of the deep local system, than in the sternocleidomastoid (global system). Fibre transformation in the extensors was far less than in the flexors and occurred consistently over many years. Of the neck extensors examined (rectus capitus posterior minor, obliquus capitus inferior, splenus capitus, trapezius), fibre transformations were most evident in obliquus capitus inferior but, in contrast to the flexors, this occurred at later stages of the disorder (symptoms >2 years). The higher percentage of fast-type IIB fibres persisted as a permanent feature in these patients' muscles, even though transformation activity ceased with time. Notably, neck pain also persisted.

This laboratory evidence supports the clinical observations and preliminary data which suggest that a primary dysfunction in the neck muscles is a loss of tonic supporting capacity, that the dysfunction is relatively greater in the neck flexors and within the neck flexors: it is the deep muscles, which have the important segmental supporting function, that display the greatest dysfunction. Importantly, Uhlig *et al.* (1995) found that the muscle dysfunction was not pathology-specific and suggested that pain was probably the stimulus for this pattern of muscle reaction. This work supports the current new directions in therapeutic exercise for spinal patients which target these supporting muscles (Richardson and Jull, 1995a).

There are other dysfunctions in the muscles of the neck and shoulder girdle complex which can occur in neck pain patients. Loss of tonic postural function in the lower scapular stabilizers (e.g. the mid, lower trapezius, serratus anterior muscles), so important for upper quadrant postural form and control, is a frequent finding clinically (Beeton and Jull, 1994; Janda, 1994; Jull, 1994; White and Sahrmann, 1994). It is considered that this is another key muscle group for rehabilitation of the neck pain patient.

Other muscles can become overactive and tight, themselves becoming a source of pain as well as imposing unnecessary additional stresses on articular or neural structures. These include many of the axioscapular muscles such as the levator scapulae, scalenes, upper trapezius and various girdle muscles such as the pectorals and latissimus dorsi. The upper cervical extensors may also become shortened. Any of these muscles may become overactive as a guarding response to joint pain or neural mechanosensitivity. Alternatively, their increase in activity may reflect abnormal neuromotor control which may have a central programming origin or arise from a not-ideal peripheral environment (Hall *et al.*, 1993; Edgar *et al.*, 1994; Janda, 1994; White and Sahrmann, 1994). While clinical theories of dysfunctional imbalances in activity levels of the axioscapular muscles are well-developed, there is little research into their prevalence. This probably reflects, in part, the difficulty in obtaining quantifiable measures of this muscle characteristic. However, it does seem that, while the loss of tonic supporting function of the neck muscles, particularly the deep neck flexors, is a universal reaction to neck pain and pathology, the presence of tightness in particular muscles is not (Treleaven *et al.*, 1994). Rather, other additional influences (e.g. problems of motor patterning, neural tissue mechanosensitivity or extensibility) are likely to be at play when these muscle dysfunctions are present and contributing to the problems. Such a situation highlights the need for dysfunction-based prescription of exercises for successful outcomes and underscores the shortcomings of providing patients with general exercise sheets.

Tests of muscle function

Dysfunction in the muscle system is sought clinically through a series of testing procedures. Those relevant to the rehabilitation of active stabilization and neuromotor control will be emphasized.

Tests of holding capacity of the deep segmental and postural supporting muscles

While all muscles have a postural supporting role, the deep neck flexors of the craniocervical and cervical region and the lower stabilizers of the scapula are those which exhibit the early and often quite marked dysfunction. The muscles' tonic holding capacity is examined by testing their ability to hold a low load, isometric contraction which replicates their function. Testing must be precise and accurate to isolate the target muscles as much as possible from non-dysfunctioned synergists which might attempt to substitute for and mimic the correct action.

The deep neck flexors of the craniocervical and cervical regions are tested through the patient's ability to hold a precise inner-range upper cervical flexion action. For clinical testing, the patient is positioned supine, crook lying to eliminate load (head weight). This ensures the muscles are tested in as much isolation as possible from synergists (e.g. sternocleidomastoid) which are necessarily recruited when resistance is added. The patient's head is supported on a folded towel placed under the occiput only, of a height such that there is a neutral head–neck starting position. The muscles to be tested are deep and are unable to be seen or uniquely palpated to determine if a correct contraction is occurring. Therefore, an indirect method to assess their performance was devised which monitored the subtle movement produced by the muscle action. The upper cervical flexion action causes a very slight flexion or flattening of the cervical curve. This subtle displacement is monitored with an inflatable pressure sensor (Stabilizer, Chattanooga, South Pacific) which is positioned suboccipitally behind the neck (Fig. 11.6). For the baseline starting position, the sensor is inflated to fill the space between the plinth and neck without pushing the neck forwards (20 mmHg).

The testing action is a pure head nod which the clinician must carefully teach to the patient. The gentleness and precision of the action need to be reinforced. When the patients have poor activation capabilities of their deep neck flexors, they will try to use substitution strategies to mimic the correct holding contraction. These must be identified and corrected. The common substitutions to mask poor deep neck flexors include recruiting the superficial flexors, sternocleidomastoid and scalenes and even the hyoids and platysma. Alternatively, the patient may perform an incorrect chin retraction action or may try to compensate for poor tonic function by performing the action too quickly.

Subjects are required to attempt 10 10-s holds of the upper cervical flexion action. A performance score is calculated by multiplying the pressure increase (from the baseline of 20 mmHg) by the number of successfully completed 10-s holds. An ideal performance would constitute a 10 mmHg increase of pressure with the patient able to perform the 10 sets of holds, giving a performance score of 100. As mentioned, our preliminary data suggest that neck pain patients are well below this level.

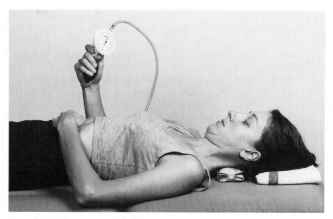

Fig. 11.6 The test of holding capacity of deep neck flexors is performed by maintaining a precise upper cervical flexion position. Performance is quantified indirectly by monitoring the patient's ability to hold the neck position via a pressure sensor placed behind the neck.

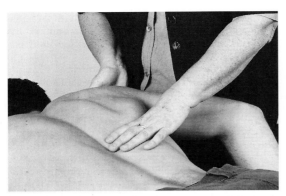

Fig. 11.7 The test of tonic holding capacity of the lower scapular stabilizers. Note that the arm is in slight abduction with the elbow flexed to discourage substitution with latissimus dorsi.

The tonic holding capacity of the lower scapular stabilizers (mid, lower trapezius, serratus anterior) is tested with a modified classic grade 3 muscle test (Kendall *et al.*, 1993). The major modification is that the arm load is eliminated by resting the arm by the side. The patient is required to hold the scapula against the chest wall in a position of retraction and depression (Fig. 11.7). The patient's ability to perform 10 10-s holds of the scapular position is tested. The patient's performance is inadequate when he or she loses control of scapular position or substitutes the correct performance with other muscle action, i.e. the latissimus dorsi, upper trapezius or rhomboids.

Tests of muscle length

The axioscapular, girdle and neck muscles prone to hypertonicity and tightness are tested and these procedures are well-described in clinical texts (Janda, 1983; Travell and Simons, 1983). Careful differential testing is required of those muscles which have a close relationship to major neural structures, notably the upper trapezius, scalenes and deep suboccipital extensors. Edgar *et al.* (1994) revealed that people with normally less flexibility in their upper-quadrant neural systems had less apparent extensibility in their upper trapezii. This was reasoned to be a normal protective phenomenon and the authors caution both clinicians and patients against routine stretching without knowing precisely the underlying cause for the muscle response.

Special investigations

There are factors in the patient's symptoms and history which direct the inclusion of other specific tests which are either structure- or systems-related.

Clinical and radiological tests of craniovertebral

ligaments can be indicated for a patient following acute trauma, such as from a motor vehicle accident. The upper cervical area is not uncommonly injured in whiplash injury and the injury mechanism exposes the alar ligaments to injury (Dvorak *et al.*, 1987; Jónsson *et al.*, 1991). The clinical and radiological stress tests involve lateral flexion or axial rotation (Reich and Dvorak, 1986; Dvorak *et al.*, 1987; Aspinall, 1989). The sensitivity and specificity of these tests have not been established and both present problems *in vivo*, resulting from pain and patient guarding.

The symptom of dizziness and any other signs of vertebrobasilar insufficiency are foremost in the mind of any practitioner using manipulative therapy procedures for the cervical spine. Injury to the vertebral artery is a very real, albeit rare risk which can have disastrous consequences. Testing protocols exist to attempt to identify the at-risk patient (Lewit, 1985; Australian Physiotherapy Association Protocol, 1988; Grant, 1994b), although their sensitivity and specificity are unknown. The validity of some tests is in doubt (Thiel *et al.*, 1994). The ethical issue is whether the benefits of high-velocity manipulative thrust procedures outweigh the risks (Powell *et al.*, 1993) and data are lacking to debate this issue rationally.

The presence of arm pain, hypoaesthesia and other vascular symptoms can direct the inclusion of a number of tests. These may aim to compromise the intervertebral foramen and structures in the thoracic inlet or reveal dysfunction in the sympathetic nervous system. Other medical and radiological examinations can be undertaken as relevant to differential diagnosis in support of the clinical examination.

Conclusion of examination

The problem-solving process of the clinical examination culminates with the physiotherapist gaining an understanding of patients themselves, their neck problem and their expectations of treatment outcome. Both a provisional pathoanatomical and a physical diagnosis are made. The latter depicts and defines the dysfunctions in the articular, muscular and nervous systems which are linked to patients' pain and functional limitations. The presence and nature of the dysfunctions guide the treatment strategies selected in management.

It is essential that the clinician has indicators to guide the progress of treatment and to evaluate the efficacy of the management programme. To the patient, the most important outcome is permanent relief of the pain and disability for which they sought treatment. The specific functional disabilities reported by the patient are used as primary outcome measures of treatment effectiveness. The physiotherapist seeks the same outcomes but is also interested in the changes in physical impairments which are as a result of their treatment. The links between changes in impairments (or dysfunction) and changes in symptoms guide intelligent treatment selection and application. Physical impairments need to be quantitatively or at least qualitatively documented so that changes can be monitored.

Physiotherapy management

Physiotherapy management aims to reverse the dysfunction causing the patient's neck pain and disability as well as prevent recurrent episodes of pain. All systems may require active management and physiotherapy management is inclusive of the following therapies: manipulative therapy, specialized therapeutic exercise and muscle function strategies, re-education of posture and neuromotor control, ergonomic and lifestyle advice, the application of electrophysical agents and other physical aids as required.

Management is dysfunction-based, precise and comprehensive, to cope with the often complex dysfunctions which may present in the integrated cervical neuromuscular–articular system. There is now unequivocal evidence that intervention in one system alone does not guarantee resolution of dysfunction in other systems (Hides *et al.*, 1996) and all systems require exacting management.

The talent in management of neck pain syndromes is to recognize where it is most effective to intervene into the cycle of interrelated dysfunction (Fig. 11.8). The model used in physiotherapy practice to guide treatment selection, application and progression is the process of repeated assessment of effect of an intervention on the dysfunction in each system (Maitland, 1986). More specifically, the effect of manipulating a dysfunctional cervical joint or inhibiting a hypertonic muscle, as examples, is evaluated by assessing any change in joint pain and movement. In turn, the effect that this pain relief or increased joint

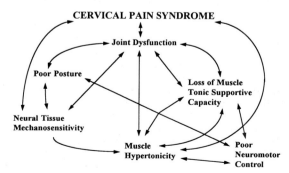

Fig. 11.8 The cycle of interrelated dysfunction in the articular, muscular and nervous systems which is manifest in the cervical pain syndrome.

movement has on impairments in the other systems is assessed. In this way, the dysfunction in each system is monitored and precise treatment added as appropriate.

Treatment of articular dysfunction

A combination of manipulative therapy, active mobilizing exercises and exercise to improve muscle support and control for the cervical segments are the principal therapies physiotherapists use to manage joint dysfunction and its resultant symptoms.

Manipulative therapy incorporates the techniques of passive segmental joint mobilization (rhythmical, low-velocity procedures), and high-velocity, low-force, small-amplitude joint manipulation techniques. The aims of manipulative therapy are to relieve joint pain, restore motion and alleviate the effect that the painful joint dysfunction may have on other structures in the neural and muscular systems. Selection of a particular technique is guided by the nature of the articular dysfunction elicited in the examination, which manifests physically as abnormal motion in specific planes and abnormal tissue resistance to induced motion. This could be caused by muscle reactivity or spasm, or increased or decreased collagenous tissue stiffness (Thabe, 1986; Jull *et al.*, 1988; Shirley and Lee, 1993) and will usually be accompanied by pain. Technique selection is also directed by the location of the segmental dysfunction, whether the dysfunction originates in the upper cervical joints, the cervical zygapophysial joints or the disc complex. Other influences are the history, the acuteness or chronicity of the problem, the proposed pathoanatomical lesion and the presence of any conditions which might contraindicate certain manipulative procedures.

Precise descriptions of techniques can be found in manipulative physiotherapy texts and will not be described in detail (Maitland, 1986; Grieve, 1988; Edwards, 1992; Kaltenborn, 1993). Manipulative therapy techniques are applied specifically to the assessed dysfunction and, in the main, they relate specifically to the direction of motion loss or its related movement. For instance, restoring the downward and medial glide of the superior facet of a zygapophysial joint to restore lateral flexion should also aid in the return of the segment's axial rotation range.

Manipulative therapy techniques are chosen to utilize both the proposed manipulation-induced analgesic and biomechanical effects of passive movement to ease joint pain and restore its motion (Vernon, 1989; Zusman *et al.*, 1989; Herzog *et al.*, 1993; Lee *et al.*, 1993; Petersen *et al.*, 1993; Vicenzino *et al.*, 1994; Wright, 1995). The nature of the technique will reflect the intention of its effect. In situations of acute pain and joint tissue damage, for

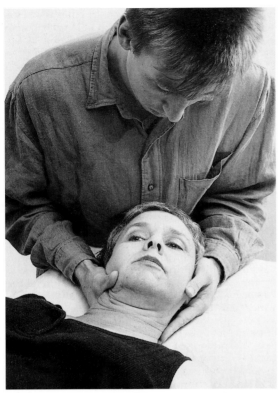

Fig. 11.9 A high-velocity, low-amplitude manipulative thrust technique to restore right lateral flexion to the (right) C2–3 zygapophysial joint.

example, movement is applied very gently and rhythmically in a painfree manner to utilize analgesic effects of movement and encourage movement for its mechanical effects. Conversely, acute pain with joint locking, purportedly from a meniscus entrapment or extrapment (Mercer and Bogduk, 1993), may direct use of a gentle high-velocity manipulative thrust technique to gap the joint, to inhibit the muscle activity and permit the joint and meniscus to move fully again. In other dysfunction, techniques may need to be applied at the end of a joint's abnormal hypomobile range to restore normal physiological ranges of motion. Such techniques may be in the form of either specific low-velocity or high-velocity procedures (Fig. 11.9).

It is imperative that movement gained by a manipulative therapy technique is reinforced by both the mechanical and neurophysical benefits of active movement. It has been shown that movement gained by a specific manipulative technique performed in isolation will be lost within 48 h (Nansel *et al.*, 1990). The patient must perform active movements directed as locally and precisely as possible to the affected segment to maintain movement gains. Either the neck can be positioned to focus movement at a particular level (Fig. 11.3) or patients can be taught to use their own fingers as a proprioceptive cue for a particular joint.

There is commonly a need for a number of segments to be treated concomitantly, using different techniques for different rationales. A simple example is where gentle passive mobilization techniques are being used to treat the pain arising from a segment with subtle translational instability. Simultaneously, neighbouring segments are mobilized to reduce hypomobility so that movement will be distributed more normally between segments, alleviating strain from the symptomatic segment. However, local manipulative therapy treatment to joints will be in vain if the segmental instability problem is not addressed through correct muscle stabilization training. Muscle retraining is an integral component of treatment of joint dysfunction.

Treatment of neural tissue dysfunction

There have been considerable advances in therapeutics within physiotherapy for the recognition, diagnosis and manual therapy treatment of pain syndromes particularly related to pathomechanics of the nervous system (Elvey, 1981; Butler, 1991; Quintner and Elvey, 1993; Hall and Quintner, 1995). A text has been devoted to the subject (Butler, 1991). For the purposes of discussion here, a simplified treatment paradigm will be used. This will serve to provide an insight into the type of management which might be used to address this form of neural tissue dysfunction – that related to adverse mechanics with resulting pain and mechanosensitivity of neural tissues. For detailed reading on nerve injury, neuromechanics and pathomechanics, the reader is referred to landmark texts such as Brieg (1978), Sunderland (1978) and Lundborg (1988).

Neural tissues of the upper forequarter can be injured directly in association with joint and muscle injury. As more commonly occurs, neural tissues can be compromised by the sequelae of joint pathology, injury and the repair process. The broad options for management therefore include treating the related joint dysfunction, directly mobilizing the neural tissues or using a combination of both methods (Elvey, 1986; Butler, 1991). The model of immediate assessment of effect of an intervention on a positive neural tissue test as well as other joint and muscle signs again guides treatment selection and progression. Adverse neural mechanics and mechanosensitivity can contribute to both acute and chronic pain states.

Manipulative therapy treatment of the joint dysfunction may successfully resolve the sensitivity in

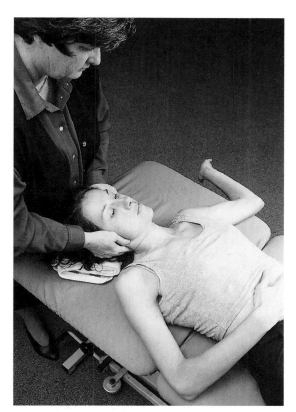

Fig. 11.10 A combined articular and neural tissue technique. The C5–6 segment is mobilized into contralateral lateral flexion. To maximize effects on neural tissues, they are pretensioned with the arm positioned in a submaximal test position.

neural structures, allowing free painless movement to return. Often techniques need to be devised which aim simultaneously to move the joint and neural structures to resolve the dysfunction. For example, anteroposterior glides (Fig. 11.4) to a mid to lower dysfunctioned cervical segment may be performed while the trunks and roots of the brachial plexus are moved by the patient performing active elbow flexion and extension in the brachial plexus tension test position (Fig. 11.5). Conversely, a joint may be moved to deliberately move neural tissue simultaneously, such as will occur with a cervical, segmental contralateral lateral flexion technique. The effect on neural tissues could be enhanced during the mobilization by pretensioning them, by positioning the patient's painful arm in a calculated proportion of a full-tension test position (Fig. 11.10). The sensitivity in the neural tissues may also be addressed by devising sequences of upper limb movements directly to move neural structures (Butler, 1991). The

most potent single movement for the cervical nerves and brachial plexus is scapular depression.

Any technique chosen which directly addresses neural structures is always performed gently and in an exploratory manner. Any treatment progression is carefully guided by the re-evaluation of the response in the neural tissue tension test. Overenthusiastic application of technique can provoke, rather than relieve, the pain associated with the neural tissue dysfunction. The advent of direct movement therapy to the nervous system together with a greater understanding of the scope of neural tissue dysfunction has broadened and furthered the management of musculoskeletal disorders. Research documenting the nature of the syndromes and the nature and validity of the clinical neural tissue tests is increasing. However, the mechanism of action of successful neural tissue therapeutics is an important area of future research which is only beginning (Slater *et al.*, 1994; Vicenzino *et al.*, 1994).

Treatment of the muscle system and neuromotor control

Proper functioning of the muscle system is essential to offer the joints support and control and to prevent adverse strain, reinjury and further pain. Achievement of muscle control is frequently commensurate with pain control (Derrick and Chesworth, 1992; Beeton and Jull, 1994; Richardson and Jull, 1995a) and is a fundamental component of joint treatment.

Specific muscle and movement dysfunctions have been identified in patients with cervical dysfunction, as previously described. Based on our clinical and research work, therapeutic exercise strategies have been devised specifically to address those muscles which are dysfunctioned in neck pain and to exercise them according to their functional demands (Jull, 1994; Richardson and Jull, 1995a,b). This places an emphasis on stabilization training and movement control directly to address the major muscle dysfunctions linked with neck pain and pathology. Additionally, active stability is a predominant functional requirement in this proximal spine and girdle region so that the forces from the actions of the head and upper extremities are accepted here without undue strains. The exercise programme includes progressive components which are added as the muscles respond to the retraining. Some details of the newer aspects of training will be given.

Retraining the tonic holding capacity of the deep stability and postural muscles

The dysfunction of loss of tonic holding capacity of the deep neck flexors and lower scapular stabilizers is addressed in the first instance to restore their postural and joint-supporting function. Optimally, training is commenced in the first treatment, the only factor mitigating against this is if pain is created by the upper cervical flexion action or by scapular depression and retraction. This could occur if neural structures are quite mechanosensitive or if the upper cervical joints are acutely painful. In these cases pain must be settled as a first priority, as it will be inhibitory to muscle action.

The functional demands of these muscles is restored by training their tonic holding capacity with an isometric contraction without load (Richardson and Jull, 1995a). In one of the first components of rehabilitation, the muscles are exercised for their precise function but in a non-functional position. This trains them in as much isolation as possible from their synergists to ensure that they specifically are exercised and that their dysfunction is unequivocally reversed.

The deep neck flexors are trained in the formal test position of supine crook lying, utilizing feedback from the pressure sensor (Fig. 11.6). Patients should commence by training at a level they can achieve, for if the task is too difficult they will substitute with unwanted actions or muscles, as previously described. For example, patients may be able initially to increase the pressure by 4 mmHg and perform three 10-s holds before fatigue. They should initially train at this level, performing the formal exercise in supine lying at least once, preferably twice, per day. The exercise should be carefully monitored and performance quantified at each treatment session. Progression is by increasing the time the contraction can be held. Achievement of 10 10-s holds is the first aim and this is followed by improving the strength of contraction, which will increase the pressure recorded. This is to a maximum of 10 mmHg, as pressures above this level are indicative of a substitution strategy, usually that of an incorrect head retraction action.

The lower scapular stabilizer function is trained utilizing the same principles. If patients cannot control the scapula flat against the chest wall in depression and retraction in prone test position (Fig. 11.7), their training may need to begin in side lying. The therapist often needs to use various facilitation strategies to activate the muscle and inhibit its synergists, such as latissimus dorsi and even, in some patients, the scapular elevators. Performance is improved by increasing the holding time (10 10-s holds) and progressing position from no added load in the prone test position to adding gradual increments of arm load. Progression is until the patient can control scapular position and support arm load in 140° abduction – the classic grade 3 muscle test position for lower trapezius (Kendall *et al.*, 1993).

The essence of testing and training the deep and postural supporting muscles is precision, accuracy and control. If patients are permitted to change to a substitution strategy to hold the neck or scapular position, bad patterns are reinforced and the training becomes ineffectual and counterproductive. The clinical skill required accurately to facilitate and activate the deep muscle parallels that required for a delicate high-velocity manipulation of a cervical segment. The precision of training needs to be thoroughly comprehended by both clinician and patient.

Integration of holding capacity training into postural control and functional activities

It is necessary for patients to train the holding capacity of the deep neck flexors and lower scapular stabilizers several times per day to improve their tonic function and to improve patterns of neuromotor control. Postural retraining requires patients to assume a correct upright, neutral spine position to which is added, in training, a conscious activation and hold of the supporting muscles, the lower scapular stabilizers and the deep abdominal, transversus abdominis (Richardson and Jull, 1995a). Assumption of the correct neutral spine, postural position with the low-level activation of these muscles corrects the head position and seems automatically to subtly activate the deep neck flexors and indeed the deep lumbar extensors, such as multifidus.

Retraining a correct, neutral spinal posture can be difficult in patients with poor proprioception and motor control. Re-education usually begins in the lumbopelvic region and the patient trains to assume an upright neutral position of the pelvis with a normal, discrete low lumbar lordosis. Too often patients use the chest-out, shoulders-back postural correction. This is a poor method as it usually results in an incorrect thoracolumbar or thoracic lordosis (Fig. 11.2b) rather than the correct lumbopelvic position which will encourage balanced, thoracic and cervical curves. The postural muscle activation is added to the correct spinal position. The patient is taught the correct muscle activation and scapular position. A common fault is that patients will try too hard, overactivate the muscles and substitute the correct muscle action with thoracic extension or even with scapular retraction and elevation. The correct muscle action needs to be facilitated with an emphasis that only a muscle contraction of 10–15% of maximum is required to retrain the postural tonic supporting role of the muscles. Again the subtlety and precision of control need to be well-understood by the patient.

Frequent repetition is necessary to retrain a new postural and muscle skill and improve holding capacity of the supporting muscles. To maximize compliance, practice must not be too intrusive into the patient's usually busy lifestyle. Patients need to incorporate practice into their everyday activities and the clinician should help them identify cues and times to practise, for example, whenever they answer the telephone, when stationary in the car at traffic lights, etc. Patients must incorporate training and ultimately the postural habit into their lifestyle.

Exercise and postural training are usually not a problem when patients realize that it relieves their neck pain. This is easily and potently shown by simply demonstrating the effects of muscle reciprocal relaxation. The painful and tight levator scapulae muscles, for example, are palpated near the superomedial border of the scapula. Allow the patient to feel the pain relief and relaxation in the muscles on repalpation following assumption of a correct postural position with gentle activation of the lower scapular stabilizers.

Muscle-lengthening procedures

The technical aspects of muscle-lengthening procedures are well-addressed by Travell and Simons (1983). More importantly, the possible cause of the muscle overactivity needs to be identified. Addressing this issue will influence the treatment approach and help to achieve a more permanent effect than is ever achieved by instituting a routine stretching programme alone. Factors which might underlie the presence of a tight or hypertonic muscle which require primary attention include adaptive length changes to poor postural form, protective hypertonicity of mechanosensitive or shortened neural tissues (note especially upper trapezius, scalenes, suboccipital extensors), lack of stability function of synergistic muscles, and poor patterns of muscle activity (Hall *et al.*, 1993; Edgar *et al.*, 1994; Janda, 1994; Jull, 1994; White and Sahrmann, 1994).

Re-education of patterns of muscle activity and movement control

Poor patterns of muscle and movement control are considered to be problems of the central nervous system programming (Janda, 1994) as well as the result of pain and the inhibitory and excitatory effects of injuries on the muscle system. The muscle system will also be affected by disuse post-injury (Richardson and Jull, 1994). These poor patterns are usually linked to inadequate stability capacity of the deep and postural supporting muscles of the spine and girdles. Once these muscles have been activated and trained, both in isolation and in static postural control, the stabilization programme is continued to ensure their appropriate timing and function during movement with and without load. There are three basic patterns which may require re-education or which are used to train the interaction between local and global muscles. These are:

1. Re-education of the synergistic action between the deep and superficial neck flexors in the through range control of cervical flexion.

2. Re-education of the pattern of axioscapular muscle sequencing and activity during arm movements (Janda, 1994). This is usually begun with short-lever arm action into abduction and progressed to long levers in all planes with or without added load.
3. Re-education of core neck and trunk control with superimposed gravitational and upper-limb load. These tasks replicate patients' working, sporting or recreational activities.

Co-contraction exercises

Muscle co-contraction of agonist and antagonist is a strategy for active joint stabilization (Keshner *et al.*, 1989; Andersson and Winters, 1990). It is linked to increasing joint stiffness and support independent of the torque-producing role of the muscles (Carter *et al.*, 1993). There are many facilitation strategies used by physiotherapists to encourage co-contraction (Sullivan and Markos, 1987). Exercises can be performed in a variety of positions, for example, sitting, four-point kneeling and prone, propped on elbows. For any exercise, the spine should be positioned in its correct neutral position. Some gentle presetting of the deep and postural muscles seems to enhance the effect of exercise. An effective exercise for home use is a self-applied gentle, sustained rotatory resistance applied rhythmically to alternate sides of the head to co-activate the neck flexor and extensor muscles.

Throughout the entire exercise programme, the holding capacity of the deep neck flexors and lower scapular stabilizers continues to be tested with their specific tests (Figs 11.6 and 11.7) as it is difficult with any other method to check if they have maintained this important function. Patients continue to train and maintain this function of these muscles groups specifically throughout the whole treatment and indeed as part of their continuing preventive programme after discharge from active treatment. It is the deep muscles whose function is so vital for segmental support and control and ironically it is these muscles whose function is most compromised by joint pain and pathology.

Ergonomic advice

Ergonomic and lifestyle advice should be offered to all persons and it should cover their working, domestic and recreational environments. However excellent the work site and equipment may be, it will not compensate for poor postural and movement control and poor joint support. Patients must understand that they hold in their muscle systems the key to effective joint support and protection from recurrent pain.

Conclusion

The key issue in the physiotherapy management of patients with cervical pain syndromes is recognition of a complex dysfunction in the neural, muscular and articular systems. Examination is a problem-solving exercise which aims to provide a provisional patho-anatomical diagnosis. Most importantly, it depicts the exact dysfunctions in the three systems which are linked to the patient's pain and disability. The major symptoms, functional disabilities and impairments are documented so that the efficacy and outcome of treatment can be evaluated objectively.

Treatment is precise and dysfunction-based. Selection and progression of techniques are guided by an assessment of effects model. The initial aim of physiotherapy management is to relieve the patient's current neck pain and disability. The long-term aim is to prevent recurrent and chronic pain. All patients are provided with knowledge of key issues in the prevention of recurrent neck pain together with an exercise programme that focuses, at discharge, on maintenance of joint protection and control. They are encouraged to continue simple exercises which activate their deep and postural muscles in everyday postures as a lifelong preventive habit, just as they have trained themselves to clean their teeth as a lifelong preventive measure against tooth decay.

References

Andersson, G.B.J., Winters, J.M. (1990) Role of muscle in postural tasks: spinal loading and postural stability. In: *Multiple Muscle Systems* (Winters, J.M., Woo, S.L.-Y., eds). New York: Springer-Verlag pp. 375–395.

Aspinall, W. (1989) Clinical testing for cervical mechanical disorders which produce ischemic vertigo. *J. Orthop. Sports Phys. Ther.* **11:** 176–182.

Australian Physiotherapy Association (1988) Protocol for pre-manipulative testing of the cervical spine. *Aust. J. Physiother.* **34:** 97–100.

Barnsley, L., Lord, S., Bogduk, N. (1993) The pathophysiology of whiplash. In: *Spine*: State of the Art Reviews 7, pp. 329–353 Philadelphia: Hanley and Belfus.

Barton, D., Allen, M., Finlay, D. *et al.* (1993) Evaluation of whiplash injuries by technetium 99m isotope scanning. *Arch. Emerg. Med.* **10:** 197–202.

Beeton, K., Jull, G.A. (1994) The effectiveness of manipulative physiotherapy in the management of cervicogenic headache: a single case study. *Physiotherapy* **80:** 417–423.

Behrsin, J.F., Maguire, K. (1986) Levator scapulae action during shoulder movement: a possible mechanism for shoulder pain of cervical origin. *Aust. J. Physiother.* **32:** 101–106.

Bergmark, A. (1989) Stability of the lumbar spine. *Acta Orthop. Scand.* **60:** 1–54.

Bogduk, N. (1994) Cervical causes of headache and dizziness. In: *Grieve's Modern Manual Therapy of the*

Vertebral Column (Boyling, J.D. and Palastanga, N., eds). Edinburgh: Churchill Livingstone, pp. 317–332.

Bogduk, N., Aprill, C. (1993) On the nature of neck pain, discography and cervical zygapophysial joint blocks. *Pain* **54:** 213–217.

Bogduk, N., Marsland, A. (1986) On the concept of third occipital headache. *J. Neurol. Neurosurg. Psychiatry* **49:** 775–780.

Boquet, J., Boismare, F., Payenneville, G. *et al.* (1989) Lateralisation of headache: possible role of an upper cervical trigger point. *Cephalalgia* **9:** 15–24.

Borchgrevink, G., Smevik, O., Nordby, A. *et al.* (1995) MR Imaging and radiography of patients with cervical hyperextension – flexion injuries after car accidents. *Acta Radiol.* **36:** 425–428.

Bovim, G., Sjaastad, O. (1993) Cervicogenic headache: responses to nitroglycerin, oxygen, ergotamine and morphine. *Headache* **33:** 249–252.

Boyling, J.D., Palastanga, N. (eds) (1994) *Grieve's Modern Manual Therapy*, 2nd edn. Edinburgh: Churchill Livingstone.

Braaf, M.M., Rosner, S. (1975) Trauma of the cervical spine as a cause of chronic headache. *J. Trauma* **15:** 441–446.

Brieg, A. (1978) *Adverse Mechanical Tension in the Central Nervous System*. Stockholm: Almqvist and Wiksell.

Butler, D.S. (1991) *Mobilisation of the Nervous System*. Melbourne: Churchill Livingstone.

Butler, D.S. (1994) The upper limb tension test revisited. In: *Physical Therapy of the Cervical and Thoracic Spine* (Grant, R., ed.). New York: Churchill Livingstone pp. 217–244.

Carter, R.R., Crago, P.E., Gorman, P.H. (1993) Non linear stretch reflex interaction during a contraction. *J. Neurophysiol.* **69:** 943–952.

Cloward, R.B. (1959) Cervical discography. A contribution to the etiology and mechanism of neck, shoulder and arm pain. *Ann. Surg.* **150:** 1052–1064.

Coman, W.B. (1986) Dizziness related to ENT conditions. In: *Modern Manual Therapy of the Vertebral Column* (Grieve, G.P., ed.). Edinburgh: Churchill Livingstone, pp. 303–314.

Conley, M.S., Meyer, R.A., Bloomberg, J.J. *et al.* (1995) Noninvasive analysis of human neck muscle function. *Spine* **20:** 2505–2512.

Crawford, H.J., Jull, G.A. (1993) The influence of thoracic posture and movement on range of arm elevation. *Physiother. Theory Pract.* **9:** 143–148.

D'Amico, D., Leone, M., Bussone, G. (1994) Side-locked unilaterality and pain localization in long-lasting headaches: migraine, tension-type headache, and cervicogenic headache. *Headache* **34:** 526–530.

Dalton, M., Coutts, A. (1994) The effect of age on cervical posture in a normal population. In: *Grieve's Modern Manual Therapy*, 2nd edn (Boyling, J.D., Palastanga, N., eds.). Edinburgh: Churchill Livingstone, pp. 361–370.

Derrick, L., Chesworth, B. (1992) Post-motor vehicle accident alar ligament instability. *J. Orthop. Sports Phys. Ther.* **16:** 6–10.

Dieterich, M., Pöllmann, W., Pfaffenrath, V. (1993) Cervicogenic headache: electronystagmography, perception of verticality and posturography in patients before and after C2-blockade. *Cephalalgia* **13:** 285–288.

Dvorak, J., Panjabi, M., Gerber, M. *et al.* (1987) CT – Functional diagnostics of rotary instability of the upper cervical spine. *Spine* **12:** 198–205.

Dvorak, J., Panjabi, M.M., Grob, D. *et al.* (1993) Clinical validation of functional flexion/extension radiographs of the cervical spine. *Spine* **18**: 120–127.

Dwyer, A., Aprill, C., Bogduk, N. (1990) Cervical zygapophyseal joint pain patterns I: a study in normal volunteers. *Spine* **15**: 453–457.

Edgar, D., Jull, G., Sutton, S. (1994) The relationship between upper trapezius muscle length and upper quadrant neural tissue extensibility. *Aust. J. Physiother.* **40**: 99–103.

Edwards, B.C. (1992) *Manual of Combined Movements.* Edinburgh: Churchill Livingstone.

Elvey, R.L. (1981) Brachial plexus tension tests and the pathoanatomical origin of arm pain. *Proceedings of Aspects of Manipulative Therap.* (Idczack, R.M., ed.). Australia: Lincoln Institute of Health Sciences, pp. 105–110.

Elvey, R.L. (1986) Treatment of arm pain associated with abnormal brachial plexus tension. *Aust. J. Physiother.* **32**: 225–230.

Feinstein, B., Langton, J.N.K., Jameson, R.M. *et al.* (1954) Experiments on referred pain from deep somatic tissues. *J. Bone. Joint Surg.* **36A**: 981–987.

Grandjean, E. (1988) *Fitting the Task to the Man.* Taylor and Francis.

Grant, R. (ed.) (1994a) *Physical Therapy of the Cervical and Thoracic Spine,* 2nd edn. New York: Churchill Livingstone.

Grant, R. (1994b) Vertebral artery concerns: premanipulative testing of the cervical spine. In: *Physical Therapy of the Cervical and Thoracic Spine* (Grant, R., ed.). Churchill Livingstone, pp. 145–165.

Griegel-Morris, P., Larson, K., Mueller-Klaus, K. *et al.* (1992) Incidence of common postural abnormalities in the cervical, shoulder and thoracic region and the association with pain in two age groups of healthy subjects. *Phys. Ther.* **72**: 425–431.

Grieve, G.P. (1988) *Common Vertebral Joint Problems,* 2nd edn. Edinburgh: Churchill Livingstone.

Hack, G.D., Koritzer, R.T., Robinson, W.L. *et al.* (1995) Anatomic relation between the rectus capitis posterior minor muscle and the dura mater. *Spine* **20**: 2484–2486.

Hall, T., Quintner, J.L. (1995) Mechanically evoked EMG responses in peripheral neuropathic pain: a single case study. In: *Proceedings of the Ninth Biennial Conference of the Manipulative Physiotherapists Association of Australia* (Jull, G., ed.). Gold Coast, Queensland, pp. 42–47.

Hall, T.M., Pyne, E.A., Hamer, P. (1993) Limiting factors of the straight leg raise test. *Proceedings of the 8th Biennial Conference, Manipulative Physiotherapists Association of Australia.* (Singer, K., ed.). Perth, Australia, pp. 32–39.

Hasvold, T., Johnson, R. (1993) Headache and neck or shoulder pain – frequent and disabling complaints in the general population. *Scand. J. Prim. Health Care* **11**: 219–224.

Hawkins, R.J., Bilco, T., Bonutti, P. (1990) Cervical spine and shoulder pain. *Clin. Orthop.* **258**: 142–146.

Herzog, W., Zhang, Y.T., Conway, P.J. *et al.* (1993) Cavitation sounds during spinal manipulative treatments. *J. Manipul. Physiol. Ther.* **16**: 523–526.

Hides, J.A., Stokes, M.J., Saide, M. *et al.* (1994) Evidence of lumbar multifidus wasting ipsilateral to symptoms in patients with acute/subacute low back pain. *Spine* **19**: 165–172.

Hides, J.A., Richardson, C.A., Jull, G.A. (1996) Multifidus muscle recovery is not automatic following resolution of acute first episode low back pain. *Spine* **21**: 2763–2769.

Hindle, R.J., Pearcy, M.J., Gross, A.T. *et al.* (1990) Three-dimensional kinematics of the human back. *Clin. Biomech.* **5**: 218–228.

Hinoki, M., Niki, H. (1975) Neurological studies on the role of the sympathetic nervous system in the formation of traumatic vertigo of cervical origin. *Acta Otolaryngol. Suppl. (Stockh.)* **330**: 185–196.

Hodges, P.W., Richardson, C.A. (1996) Inefficient muscular stabilization of the lumbar spine associated with chronic low back pain: a motor control evaluation of transversus abdominis. *Spine* **21**: 2640–2650.

Hole, D.E., Cook, J.M., Bolton, J.E. (1995) Reliability and concurrent validity of two instruments for measuring cervical range of motion: effects of age and gender. *Manual Ther.* **1**: 36–42.

Jacobs, B. (1990) Cervical angina. *N.Y. State J. Med.* **90**: 8–11.

Janda, V. (1983) *Muscle Function Testing.* London: Butterworths.

Janda, V. (1994) Muscles and motor control in cervicogenic disorders: assessment and management. In: *Physical Therapy of the Cervical and Thoracic Spine* (Grant, R., ed.). New York: Churchill Livingstone, pp. 195–216.

Janig, W. (1990) The sympathetic nervous system in pain: physiology and pathophysiology. In: *Pain and the Sympathetic Nervous System* (Stanton-Hicks, M., ed.). Kluwers, pp 17–91.

Janos, S.C., Ray, C.D. (1992) Mechanical examination of the lumbar spine and mechanical discography/mechanical facet joint injection. *Proceedings International Conference, IFOMT.* Vail, Colorado, p. A92.

Jensen, O.K., Justesen, T., Nielsen, E.F. *et al.* (1990) Functional radiographic examination of the cervical spine in patients with post-traumatic headache. *Cephalalgia* **109**: 275–303.

Johnson, G., Bogduk, N., Nowitzke, A. *et al.* (1994) Anatomy and actions of the trapezius muscle. *Clin. Biomech.* **9**: 44–50.

Jones, M., Jensen, G., Rothstein, J. (1995) Clinical reasoning in physiotherapy. In: *Clinical Reasoning in the Health Professionals* (Higgs J., Jones M., eds). Oxford: Butterworth-Heinemann, pp.72–87.

Jónsson, H., Bring, G., Rauschning, W. *et al.* (1991) Hidden cervical spine injuries in traffic accident victims with skull fractures. *J. Spinal Disord.* **4**: 251–263.

Jónsson, H., Cesarini, K., Sahlstedt, B. *et al.* (1994) Findings and outcome in whiplash-type neck distortions. *Spine* **19**: 2733–2743.

Jull, G.A. (1986a) Headaches associated with the cervical spine – a clinical review. In: *Modern Manual Therapy of the Vertebral Column* (Grieve, G.P., ed.). Edinburgh: Churchill Livingstone, pp. 322–329.

Jull, G.A. (1986b) Clinical observations of upper cervical mobility. In: *Modern Manual Therapy of the Vertebral Column* (Grieve, G.P., ed.). Edinburgh: Churchill Livingstone, pp. 315–321.

Jull, G.A. (1994) Headache of cervical origin. In: *Physical Therapy of the Cervical and Thoracic Spine,* 2nd edn. New York: Churchill Livingstone, pp. 261–286.

Jull, G.A., Bogduk, N., Marsland, A. (1988) The accuracy of manual diagnosis for cervical zygapophysial joint pain syndromes. *Med. J. Aust.* **148**: 233–236.

Jull, G.A., Treleaven, J., Versace, G. (1994) Manual examination: is pain a major cue to spinal dysfunction. *Aust. J. Physiother.* **40**: 159-165.

Kaltenborn, F.M. (1993) *The Spine. Basic Evaluation and Mobilization Techniques.* Olaf Norlis Bokhandel.

Karlberg, M., Persson, L., Magnusson, M. (1995) Reduced postural control in patients with chronic cervicobrachial pain syndrome. *Gait Posture* **3**: 241-249.

Kendall, F.P., McCreary, E.K., Provance, P.G. (1993) *Muscles Testing and Function,* 4th edn. Baltimore: Williams & Wilkins.

Keshner, E.A., Campbell, D., Katz, R.T. *et al.* (1989) Neck muscle activation patterns in humans during isometric head stabilization. *Exp. Brain Res.* **75**:335-344.

Kidd, R.F., Nelson, C.M. (1993) Musculoskeletal dysfunction of the neck in migraine and tension headache. *Headache* **33**: 566-569.

La Ban, M.M., Meerschaert, J.R. (1989) Computer generated headache. Brachiocephalgia at first byte. *Am. J. Phys. Med. Rehabil.* **68**: 183-185.

Lance, J.W. (1993) *Mechanisms and Management of Headache,* 5th edn. Oxford: Butterworth-Heinemann.

Lee, M., Latimer, J., Maher, C. (1993) Manipulation: investigation of a proposed mechanism. *Clin. Biomech.* **8**: 302-306.

Lewit, K. (1985) *Manipulative Therapy in Rehabilitation of the Motor System.* London: Butterworths.

Lord, S.M., Barnsley, L., Wallis, B.J. *et al.* (1994) Third occipital headache; a prevalence study. *J. Neurol. Neurosurg. Psychiatry* **57**: 1187-1190.

Lundborg, G. (1988) *Nerve Injuries and Repair.* Edinburgh: Churchill Livingstone.

Macpherson, B.C., Campbell, C. (1991) C2 rotation and spinous process deviation in migraine: cause or effect or coincidence? *Neuroradiology* **33**: 475-477.

Maitland, G.D. (1986) *Vertebral Manipulation,* 5th edn. London: Butterworth.

Mayoux-Benhamou, M.A., Revel, M., Vallé C. *et al.* (1994) Longus colli has a postural function on cervical curvature. *Surg. Radiol. Anat.* **16**: 367-371.

Mercer, S., Bogduk, N. (1993) Intra-articular inclusions of the cervical synovial joints. *Br. J. Rheumatol.* **32**: 705-710.

Mercer, S.R., Jull, G.A. (1996) Morphology of the cervical intervertebral disc: implications for McKenzie's model of the disc derangement syndrome. *Manual Ther.* **1**: 76-81.

Mimura, M., Moriya, H., Watanabe, T. *et al.* (1989) Three-dimensional motion analysis of the cervical spine and special reference to the axial rotation. *Spine* **14**: 1135-1139.

Moses, A., Carman, J. (1996) Anatomy of the cervical spine: implications for the upper limb tension test. *Aust. J. Physiother.* **42**: 31-36.

Nagasawa, A., Sakakibara, T., Takahashi, A. (1993) Roentgenographic findings of the cervical spine in tension-type headache. *Headache* **33**: 90-95.

Nansel, D., Peneff, A., Cremata, E. *et al.* (1990) Time course considerations for the effects of unilateral lower cervical adjustments with respect to the amelioration of cervical lateral-flexion passive end-range asymmetry. *J. Manipul. Physiol. Ther.* **13**: 297-304.

Panjabi, M. (1992a) The stabilizing system of the spine. Part 1. Function, dysfunction, adaptation and enhancement. *J. Spinal Disord.* **5**: 383-389.

Panjabi, M. (1992b) The stabilizing system of the spine. Part II. Neutral zone and instability hypothesis. *J. Spinal Disord.* **5**: 390-397.

Penning, L., Wilmink, J.T. (1987) Rotation of the cervical spine. A CT study in normal subjects. *Spine* **12**: 732-738.

Petersen, N., Vicenzino, B., Wright A. (1993) The effects of a cervical mobilisation technique on sympathetic outflow to the upper limb in normal subjects. *Physiother. Theory Pract.* **9**: 149-156.

Pettersson, K., Hildingsson, C., Toolanen, G. *et al.* (1994) MRI and neurology in acute whiplash trauma. *Acta. Orthop. Scand.* **65**: 525-528.

Pfaffenrath, V., Dandekar, R., Pollmann, W. (1987) Cervicogenic headache – the clinical picture, radiological findings and hypothesis on its pathophysiology. *Headache* **27**: 495-499.

Phillips, D.R., Twomey, L.T. (1996) A comparison of manual diagnosis with a diagnosis established by a uni-level lumbar spinal block procedure. *Manual Ther.* **1**: 82-87.

Powell, F.C., Hanigan, W.C., Olivero, W.C. (1993) A risk/benefit analysis of spinal manipulation therapy for relief of lumbar or cervical pain. *Neurosurgery* **33**: 73-78.

Quintner, J.L. (1989) A study of upper limb pain and parasthesia following neck injury in motor vehicle accidents: assessment of the brachial plexus tension test of Elvey. *Br. J. Rheumatol.* **28**: 528-533.

Quintner, J. (1990) Stretch-induced cervicobrachial pain syndrome. *Aust. J. Physiother.* **36**: 99-104.

Quintner, J.L., Cohen, M.L. (1994) Referred pain of peripheral nerve origin: an alternative to the 'myofascial pain' construct. *Clin. J. Pain* **10**: 243-251.

Quintner, J.L., Elvey, R.L. (1993) Understanding 'RSI'. A review of the role of peripheral neural pain and hyperalgesia. *J. Manual Manipul. Ther.* **1**: 99-105.

Radanov, B.P., Sturzenegger, M., Di Stefano, G. *et al.* (1993) Factors influencing recovery from headache after common whiplash. *Br. Med. J.* **307**: 652-655.

Raine, S., Twomey, L. (1994) Posture of the head, shoulders and thoracic spine in comfortable erect standing. *Aust. J. Physiother.* **40**: 25-32.

Reich, C., Dvorak, J. (1986) The functional evaluation of craniocervical ligaments in side flexion using X-rays. *J. Manual Med.* **2**: 108-113.

Revel, M., Andre-Deshays, C., Minguet, M. (1991) Cervicocephalic kinesthesic sensibility in patients with cervical pain. *Arch. Phys. Med. Rehabil.* **72**: 288-291.

Richardson, C.A., Jull, G.A. (1994) Concepts of assessment and rehabilitation for active lumbar stability. In: *Grieve's Modern Manual Therapy* (Boyling, J.D., Palastanga, N., eds). Edinburgh: Churchill Livingstone, pp. 705-720.

Richardson, C.A., Jull, G.A. (1995a) Muscle control- pain control. What exercises would you prescribe? *Manual Ther.* **1**: 2-10.

Richardson, C.A., Jull, G.A. (1995b) *An historical perspective on the development of clinical techniques to evaluate and treat the active stabilising system of the lumbar spine. Monograph no. 1. The lumbar spine.* Melbourne: Australian Physiotherapy Society, pp. 5-13.

Robison, R. (1992) The new back school prescription: stabilization training. Part 1. *Occup. Med.* **7**: 17-31.

Saal, J.A., Saal, J.S. (1989) Nonoperative treatment of herniated lumbar intervertebral disc with radiculopathy. An outcome study. *Spine* **14**: 431-437.

Schneider, G. (1989) Restricted shoulder movement: capsular contracture or cervical referral – a clinical study. *Aust. J. Physiother.* **35**: 97–100.

Selvaratnam, P.J., Matyas, T.A., Glasgow, E.F. (1994) Non-invasive discrimination of brachial plexus involvement in upper limb pain. *Spine* **19**: 26–33.

Shirley, D., Lee, M. (1993) A preliminary investigation of the relationship between lumbar postero-anterior mobility and low back pain. *J. Manual Manipul. Ther.* **1**: 22–25.

Silverman, J.L., Rodriquez, A.A., Agre, J.C. (1991) Qualitative cervical flexor strength in healthy subjects and in subjects with mechanical neck pain. *Arch. Phys. Med. Rehabil.* **72**: 679–681.

Sjaastad, O. (1992) Laterality of pain and other migraine criteria in common migraine. A comparison with cervicogenic headache. *Funct. Neurol.* **7**: 289–294.

Sjaastad, O., Bovim, G. (1991) Cervicogenic headache. The differentiation from common migraine. An overview. *Funct. Neurol.* **6**: 93–100.

Sjaastad, O., Saunte, C., Hovdahl, H. *et al.* (1983) Cervicogenic headache. An hypothesis. *Cephalalgia* **3**: 249–256.

Sjaastad, O., Fredriksen, T.A., Sand, T. *et al.* (1989a) Unilaterality of headache in classic migraine. *Cephalalgia* **9**: 71–77.

Sjaastad, O., Fredriksen, T.A., Sand, T. (1989b) The localisation of the initial pain of attack: a comparison between classic migraine and cervicogenic headache. *Funct. Neurol.* **4**: 73–78.

Sjaastad, O., Joubert, J., Elsas, T. *et al.* (1993) Hemicrania continua and cervicogenic headache. Separate headaches or two faces of the same headache? *Funct. Neurol.* **8**: 79–83.

Slater, H., Vicenzino, B., Wright, A. (1994) 'Sympathetic slump': the effects of a novel manual therapy technique on peripheral sympathetic nervous system function. *J. Manual Manipul. Ther.* **2**: 156–162.

Smythe, H. (1994). The C6-7 syndrome – clinical features and treatment response. *J. Rheumatol.* **21**: 1520–1526.

Stewart, S.G., Jull, G.A., Ng, J.K.-F. *et al.* (1995) An initial analysis of thoracic spine movement during unilateral arm elevation. *J. Manual Manipul. Ther.* **3**: 15–20.

Stokes, M., Young, A. (1984) The contribution of reflex inhibition to arthrogenous muscle weakness. *Clin. Sci.* **67**: 7–14.

Sturzenegger, M., Di Stefano, G., Radanov, B.P. *et al.* (1994) Presenting symptoms and signs after whiplash injury: the influence of accident mechanisms. *Neurology* **44**, 688–693.

Sturzenegger, M., Radanov, B.P., Di Stefano, G. (1995) The effect of accident mechanisms and initial findings on the long-term course of whiplash injury. *J. Neurol.* **242**: 443–449.

Sullivan, P.E., Markos, P.D. (1987) *An Integrated Approach to Therapeutic Exercise.* Virginia: Reston.

Sunderland, S. (1978) *Nerves and Nerve Injuries,* 2nd edn. Edinburgh: Churchill Livingstone.

Sweeney, T., Prentice, C. Saal, J.A. *et al.* (1990) Cervico-thoracic muscular stabilization techniques. *Phys. Med. Rehabil., State Art. Rev.* **4**: 335–359.

Taylor, J.R., Finch, P. (1993) Acute injury of the neck: anatomical and pathological basis of pain. *Ann. Acad. Med. Singapore* **22**: 187–192.

Thabe, H. (1986) Electromyography as tool to document diagnostic findings and therapeutic results associated with somatic dysfunctions in the upper cervical spinal joints and sacroiliac joints. *J. Manual Med.* **2**: 53–58.

Thiel, H., Wallace, K., Donat, J. *et al.* (1994) Effect of various head and neck positions on vertebral artery flow. *Clin. Biomech.* **9**: 105–110.

Travell J.G., Simons, D.G. (1983) *Myofascial Pain and Dysfunction. The Trigger Point Manual.* Williams & Wilkins.

Treleaven, J., Jull, G., Atkinson, L. (1994) Cervical musculoskeletal dysfunction in post-concussional headache. *Cephalalgia* **14**: 273–279.

Troup, J.D.G. (1986) Biomechanics of the lumbar spinal canal. *Clin. Biomech.* **1**: 31–43.

Uhlig, Y., Weber, B.R., Grob, D. *et al.* (1995) Fiber composition and fiber transformations in neck muscles of patients with dysfunction of the cervical spine. *J. Orthop. Res.* **13**: 240–249.

Upton, A.R.M., McComas, A.J. (1973) The double crush in nerve entrapment syndromes. *Lancet* **2**: 359–362.

Vercauteren, M., Van Beneden, M., Verplaetse, R. *et al.* (1982) Trunk asymmetries in a Belgian school population. *Spine* **7**: 555–562.

Vernon, H. (1989) Exploring the effect of a spinal manipulation on plasma beta-endorphin levels in normal men. *Spine* **14**: 1272–1273.

Vernon, H., Steiman, I., Hagino, C. (1992a) Cervicogenic dysfunction in muscle contraction headache and migraine: a descriptive study. *J. Manipul. Physiol. Ther.* **15**: 418–429.

Vernon, H.T., Aker, P., Aramenko, M. *et al.* (1992b) Evaluation of neck muscle strength with a modified sphygmomanometer dynamometer: reliability and validity. *J. Manipul. Physiol. Ther.* **15**: 343–349.

Vicenzino, B., Collins, D., Wright, A. (1994) Sudomotor changes induced by neural mobilisation techniques in asymptomatic subjects. *J. Manual Manipul. Ther.* **2**: 66–74.

Watson, D., Trott, P. (1993) Cervical headache: an investigation of natural head posture and upper cervical flexor muscle performance. *Cephalalgia* **13**: 272–284.

White, A.A., Panjabi, M.M. (1990) *Clinical Biomechanics of the Spine.* Philadelphia: J.B. Lippincott.

White, S.G., Sahrmann, S.A. (1994) A movement system balance approach to management of musculoskeletal pain. In: *Physical Therapy of the Cervical and Thoracic Spine* (Grant, R., ed.). New York: Churchill Livingstone, pp. 339–357.

Wilke, H.J., Wolf, S., Claes, L.E. *et al.* (1995) Stability increase of the lumbar spine with different muscle groups: a biomechanical *in vitro* study. *Spine* **20**: 192–198.

Willems, J.M., Jull, G.A., Ng, J. K-F. (1996) An *in vivo* study of the primary and coupled rotations of the thoracic spine. *Clin. Biomech.* **11**: 311–316.

Wright, A. (1995) Hypoalgesia post-manipulative therapy: a review of a potential neurophysiological mechanism. *Manual Ther.* **1**: 11–16.

Yaxley, G.A., Jull, G.A. (1991) A modified upper limb tension test: an investigation of responses in normal subjects. *Aust. J. Physiother.* **37**: 143–152.

Yaxley, G.A., Jull, G.A. (1993) Adverse tension in the neural system. A preliminary study of tennis elbow. *Aust. J. Physiother.* **39**: 15–22.

Zusman, M., Edwards, B., Donaghy, A. (1989) Investigation of a proposed mechanism for the relief of spinal pain with passive joint movement. *Manual Med.* **4**: 58–61.

12

Contraindications to cervical spine manipulation

A. G. J. Terrett

Introduction

Head-neck pain and dizziness are symptoms which spinal manipulation therapy (SMT) practitioners usually accept as possibly indicating spinal joint and/or muscle lesions, and therefore they may be indications for SMT. While this is true in many cases, these same symptoms can indicate pathologies which contraindicate SMT. This chapter discusses vertebral artery dissection (VAD), where the initial symptoms may be head-neck pain and/or dizziness, which may prompt the patient to consult a practitioner.

A rationale for the prevention of complications from SMT may be based on an understanding of:

1. The causes of reported complications from SMT.
2. The contraindications to SMT.
3. Diagnostic assessment of patients prior to SMT.
4. Avoiding certain therapies in patients thought to be at risk.
5. Avoiding those techniques which are thought to carry the greatest risk.
6. Emergency care procedures, should an injury occur.

This study is based upon 185 cases collected from the English, French, German, Scandinavian and Asian literature, which were reported from 1934 to 1995.

Incidence of vertebrobasilar stoke following SMT

The actual incidence of post-SMT vertebrobasilar stroke (VBS) is not known, but can be expected to be higher than the reported incidence.

Figures commonly quoted for serious injury following SMT have been: 1 in several tens of millions of manipulations (Maigne, 1972); 1 in 10 000 000 (Cyriax, 1978); 1 in 1 000 000 (Hosek *et al.*, 1981); and 2-3 per million (Gutmann, 1983; Dvorak and Orelli, 1985). It is to be noted that, as the subject is being better investigated, the estimated incidence is increasing.

Case analysis

Examination of cases reveals the following age and gender distribution, practitioner involved and sequelae.

Age distribution of patients who suffered VBS

It has been suggested that 'most risks of this nature are expected to be found in the elderly' because of spondylitic and arteriosclerotic changes (Taylor, 1981). Table 12.1 summarizes the age and gender of the cases reviewed. The age distribution graph of patients who suffered VBS following SMT (Fig. 12.1) easily dispels the idea that these injuries are more likely to affect the elderly. At first glance, there does appear to be a predilection for SMT accidents in the 30-45-year age group (Ladermann, 1981). Closer analysis does not reveal any greater risk in any age range (Terrett and Kleynhans, 1992; Terrett, 1996). The superimposed curve in Figure 12.1 is an age analysis of 6187 consecutive patient visits to an SMT practitioner's office (many patients are therefore recorded more than once); the horizontal line = 10%.

Table 12.1 *Age and sex distribution of people suffering vertebrobasilar stroke after spinal manipulation therapy*

Age (years)	Male		Female		Sex unknown		Total	
	Cases	Deaths	Cases	Deaths	Cases	Deaths	Cases	Deaths
6–10	1						1	
11–15								
16–20	1		1				2	
21–25	4	2	3				7	2
26–30	6		18	2			24	2
31–35	18	3	28	6	1		47	9
36–40	15	3	18	4	2		35	7
41–45	12	1	9	2	3		24	3
46–50	2		6		1		9	
51–55	7	3	4	2			11	5
56–60	1		4	1			5	1
61–65	2						2	
66–70			2				2	
Unknown	5	1	6	2	5	2	16	5
Total	74	13	99	19	12	2	185	34

The increased number of accidents reported in the 30–45-year age group appears simply to be a reflection of the age group most likely to seek the services of a practitioner of SMT.

Therefore, factors such as a patient's age and the presence or absence of degenerative osseous or vascular changes do not appear to be important in assessing a patient's risk of manipulative iatrogenesis (Terrett, 1987c, 1996; Terrett and Kleynhans, 1992).

Age of patients who suffered post-SMT VBS

Age and gender are known for 162 of the 185 patients. The age range for the patients was:

- Males (*n* = 69): 7–63, with an average of 37.8 years.
- Females (*n* = 93): 20–68, with an average of 37.1 years.

The age distribution for mortality when age and gender were known was:

- Males (*n* = 12): 23–51, with an average age of 38.0 years.
- Females (*n* = 17): 33–60, with an average age of 38.7 years.

The 5 cases of death where age was unknown were one male, two females, and in two cases the gender was not stated.

Gender distribution of patients who suffered post-SMT VBS

It has been stated that the group most at risk of VBS following SMT are young females. Of the 185 cases reviewed here, the gender was known in 180 cases, which revealed:

- 103 females (57.2%), of whom 17 died (16.5%).
- 77 males (42.8%), of whom 13 died (16.9%).

The initial impression is that there seems to be a greater risk for females. Closer examination reveals that this does not indicate a female sex predilection, but simply reflects the greater number of female patients seeking SMT. Studies have revealed the following male–female patient percentages: 40.7–59.3%; and 44.8–55.2% (Christiensen, 1993, 1994).

Practitioner involved and sequelae

Table 12.2 lists the practitioner involved and the sequelae. As is to be expected, the greater number of cases have involved chiropractors, because they perform most of this type of treatment. In the USA 94% of SMT is performed by chiropractors, 4% by osteopaths and 2% by medical practitioners (Shekelle and Brook, 1991; Shekelle *et al.,* 1991).

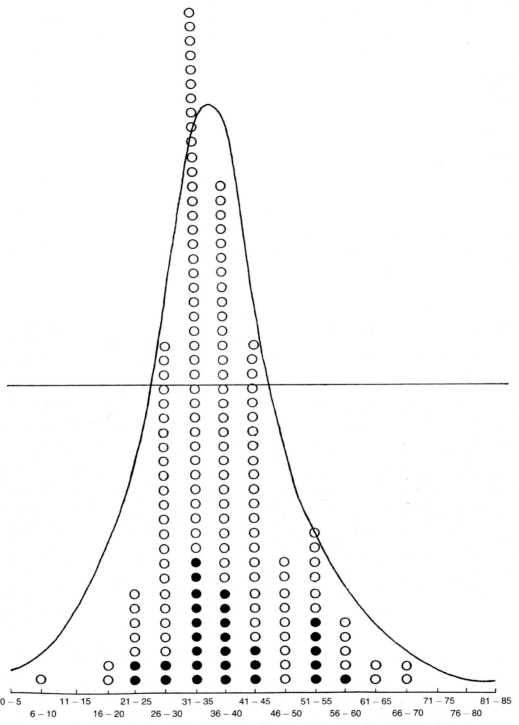

Fig. 12.1 Age distribution of post spinal manipulative therapy (SMT) vertebrobasilar stroke (VBS) cases compared to age distribution of patients attending practitioners for SMT. Open circles = post-SMT VBS case who did not die; filled circles = post-SMT VBS case who died.

Table 12.2 *Practitioner and sequelae of 185 cases of vertebrobasilar stroke (1934–1995)*

Practitioner	CR	ACR	U-K	RND	LIS-R	LIS	Death	Total
Chiropractor	6	8	9	36		5	13	77
Chiropractic	4	6	1	13	1		5	30
Medical practitioner	5		5	7			8	25
Osteopath	2		1	5	1	1	3	13
Physiotherapist	2			5				7
Self	1	1	1	2				5
Naturopath			1	1			1	3
Wife							1	1
Barber				1				1
Kung-fu practitioner			1					1
Unknown	7		1	10			3	22
Total	27	15	21	80	2	6	34	185

CR = Complete recovery; ACR = almost complete recovery; U-K = unknown; RND = residual neurological deficit; LIS-R = locked-in syndrome with recovery; LIS = locked-in syndrome/tetraplegia.
Note: One case in the death column had been a case of tetraplegia.

Mechanisms of cerebrovascular injury

Clinical anatomy

The vertebral artery (VA) courses upwards, encased within the transverse foramina of the cervical vertebrae. On exiting the foramen in the axis vertebra, the VA abandons its almost vertical course to pass upwards and laterally to reach the foramen of the atlas transverse process. The VAs are not freely movable at the C1 and C2 transverse foramina, but are relatively fixed by fibrous tissue. The VA then proceeds around the lateral mass of the atlas, enters the foramen magnum and, at the lower border of the pons, unites with the VA of the opposite side to form the basilar artery. The posterior inferior cerebellar arteries (PICAs) leave the VAs just before they join each other to form the basilar artery. The basilar artery passes up the anterior surface of the brainstem, and divides to become the posterior cerebral arteries.

Clinical biomechanics

Rotation of the cervical spine to the extent of 45–50° occurs chiefly at the atlantoaxial joint. This is about half of total cervical spine rotation (Selecki, 1969). During head rotation, because the VA is fixed at the C1 and C2 transverse foramina, it is stretched/tensioned, compressed and torqued. Research indi-cates that rotation is the single most effective movement producing decrease in blood flow – it applies the greatest stress to the VA (deKleyn and Nieuwenhuyse, 1927; deKleyn and Versteegh, 1933; Tatlow and Bammer, 1957; Toole and Tucker, 1960; Brown and Tatlow, 1963; Andersson *et al.,* 1970; Barton and Margolis, 1975; Grossman and Davies, 1982; Yang *et al.,* 1985). While cadaver studies (deKleyn and Nieuwenhuyse, 1927; deKleyn and Versteegh, 1933; Tatlow and Bammer, 1957; Toole and Tucker, 1960; Brown and Tatlow, 1963) are important, early VA compromise is not reproducible in live subjects (Refshauge, 1994; Thiel *et al.,* 1994; Haynes, 1996). In a study of 280 VAs, Haynes (1996) found that 5% lost the Doppler sounds during rotation to the end range; but none of these developed any signs or symptoms of brainstem ischaemia. It is important to note that in no case of lateral flexion was there any loss of the Doppler signals (Haynes, 1996); and the cadaver study of Toole and Tucker (1960) also indicated that lateral flexion placed less stress on the VAs. This should be considered when a rationale for the application of SMT to the upper cervical spine is developed (Terrett and Kleynhans, 1992; Terrett, 1996).

During normal daily activities the blood flow in the VAs fluctuates (Bakay and Sweet, 1953), but symptoms do not occur in healthy individuals. Therefore, occlusion of one VA does not necessarily reduce the arterial supply to the posterior fossa via the basilar or posterior cerebellar arteries. Compression or spasm of a VA from C1–2 rotation will induce symptoms only if flow in the contralateral VA is already compromised.

Table 12.3 *Non-spinal manupulative therapy vascular accidents associated with head rotation and/or extension*

Childbirth (Yates, 1959)
By surgeon or anaesthetist during surgery (Brain, 1963; Fisher, 1993; Nosan *et al.*, 1993; Tettenborn *et al.*, 1993)
Callisthenics (Nagler, 1973)
Yoga (Nagler, 1973; Hanus *et al.*, 1977)
Overhead work (Okawara and Nibblelink, 1974)
Neck extension during radiography (Fogelholm and Karli, 1975)
Neck extension for a bleeding nose (Fogelholm and Karli, 1975)
Turning the head while driving a vehicle (Easton and Sherman, 1977; Sherman *et al.*, 1981; Yang *et al.*, 1985)
Archery (Sorenson, 1978)
Wrestling (Rogers and Sweeney, 1979)
Emergency resuscitation (Saternus and Fuchs, 1982)
Star gazing (Barty, 1983)
Sleeping position (Hope *et al.*, 1983)
Swimming (Tramo *et al.*, 1985)
Rap dancing (Dorey and Mayne, 1986)
Fitness exercise (Pryse-Phillips, 1989)
Beauty parlour stroke (Weintraub, 1992, 1993)
Tai chi (Oh, 1993)

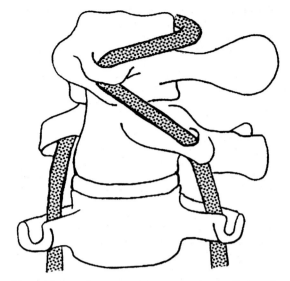

Fig. 12.2 Stretch, torque and compression applied to the vertebral artery between the atlas and axis vertebrae with contralateral rotation.

Normally, during daily head movements, occlusion due to compression does not produce a sufficient decrease in flow to produce ischaemic signs and symptoms, or the development of infarction. In most cases the development of infarction indicates an underlying arteriopathic process, other than brief occlusion.

There have been a number of cases where sustained or repetitive head position during normal activities has produced brainstem ischaemic accidents in the absence of SMT (Table 12.3). Functional tests may have screened out some, but could have precipitated VBS in others. These cases would no doubt have been high-risk had they been treated by SMT, and even though the outcome may have been identical, the practitioner most likely would have been held responsible.

Injury sites

Injury to the VAs can occur anywhere along their path, by stretching, shearing or crushing. Various authors postulate that there are seven potential sites in the cervical spine at which the VA can be compressed or injured by spinal movement (Terrett and Kleynhans, 1992; Terrett, 1996). Rotation applies the greatest stress to the arterial structures in the upper cervical spine. The most reported site of post-SMT VA damage is between C1 and C2 transverse processes, where the VAs are relatively fixed at the C1 and C2 transverse foramina (Fig. 12.2).

Injury to the internal carotid artery by the C1 transverse process has also been reported. Only 5 cases of internal carotid artery injury associated with SMT have been reported (Lyness and Wagman, 1974; Beatty, 1977; Murthy and Naidu, 1988; Braune *et al.*, 1991; Peters *et al.*, 1995).

Arterial wall trauma

The mechanism of injury to the nervous system from a vertebrobasilar accident is brainstem ischaemia, which may be due to:

1. Trauma to the arterial wall producing transient vasospasm.
2. Trauma to the arterial wall producing damage to the arterial wall.

There have been cases of VBS following SMT which were subsequently examined by angiograms, and Doppler sonography in which no evidence of vascular injury could be found (Terrett, 1996). In these cases it is believed that transient arterial spasm may have been the mechanism for the neurological sequelae. Even in cases where arterial damage is found, the onset of symptoms is often immediate – too quick for clotting to have occurred, and this most likely indicates spasm. Spasm would be particularly deleterious in the presence of hypoplasia or arteriopathy of the contralateral VA, or if the contralateral VA terminates in the PICA.

Fortunately, in most cases this spasm is transient and, if not accompanied by severe arterial damage, or retraumatized, the patient soon recovers without any deficit. This appears to be a much more common happening than has been reported.

In most cases of VBS following SMT where angiography or autopsy findings are available, there is found to be damage to the artery wall. One of the following mechanisms may occur:

1. Compression and/or stretching of the VA wall may apply enough force to disrupt the vasa vasorum, resulting in subintimal haematoma. This may decrease VA blood flow by occlusion of the lumen (Fig. 12.3a). Intramural haematoma may also result in vasospasm.
2. Intimal tear. The intima is the least elastic layer of the vessel wall, and the most likely to tear when the vessel is stretched and/or compressed. Exposure of the subendothelial tissue leads to the cascade mechanism, resulting in clot formation (thrombosis). The clot frequently remains adherent to the tear with propagation distally and/or proximally, and may lead to vessel occlusion (Fig. 12.3b). Following the intimal tear, the vessel (if not further traumatized) may undergo repair with no further symptoms, or it may go into spasm. Spasm may be induced following blood coagulation due to the release of thrombin, which is a potent constrictor of cerebral vessels (White *et al.,* 1980). Such spasm may then produce thrombosis (Blaumanis *et al.,* 1976).
3. Intimal tear with embolic formation. The propagating clot extends into the lumen. The blood flow may 'break off' part and form an embolus (Fig. 12.3c), which can then cause arterial occlusion distally, leading to infarction of the area supplied.
4. Vessel wall dissection with subintimal haematoma. When the intima and the internal elastica are disrupted, allowing blood to dissect between them and the muscularis, a dissecting aneurysm is formed. The intramedial blood frequently compresses the true lumen, which accounts for the narrowed appearance angiographically. This also exposes the subendothelial tissue, which may result in thrombosis and occlusion of the vessel (Fig. 12.3d). Dissecting haemorrhage can rupture through the intima, establishing communication with the true lumen (Fig. 12.3e). Recanalization may occur, enlarging the true and/or false lumen.
5. Vessel wall dissection with pseudoaneurysm formation. When the muscularis as well as the intima and internal elastica are disrupted, a pseudoaneurysm may form, as the remaining adventitia distends. As well as producing the changes above, this disruption may propagate distally to occlude the PICA (Fig. 12.3f).

6. Perivascular bleeding (false saccular aneurysm). Disruption in the continuity of the arterial wall allows blood to leak into the surrounding soft tissue and produce a periarterial haemorrhage, which is contained in the fascia. These changes may produce external compression of the vessel, resulting in either occlusion of the lumen or turbulence, which may initiate thrombus and embolus formation (Fig. 12.3g).

Onset of signs and symptoms

The time between the application of SMT and the onset of signs and symptoms can vary from immediately to many days. The interval is probably related to the differing mechanisms of injury. When brainstem ischaemia is due to vasoconstriction, symptoms would be expected immediately, whereas those (other than the pain of dissection) due to thrombus and/or embolus formation resulting from a vessel wall dissection would only become symptomatic after some time.

A review of the 185 cases reveals that the time between SMT and the onset of symptoms was given in 138 cases, and indicates:

- 69% during SMT.
- 3% within moments or minutes of SMT.
- 8.5% within 1 h of SMT.
- 8.5% 1–6 h after SMT.
- 5% 7–24 h after SMT.
- 6% 24 h or more after SMT.

Signs and symptoms of vertebrobasilar ischaemia (VBI) produced by SMT usually occur in the practitioner's office (72%), and should be immediately recognized by the practitioner.

The major signs and symptoms of VBI are the five *D*s *A*nd 3 *N*s:

1. *D*izziness/vertigo/giddiness/light-headedness.
2. *D*rop attacks/loss of consciousness.
3. *D*iplopia (or other visual symptoms).
4. *D*ysarthria (speech difficulties).
5. *D*ysphagia.
6. *A*taxia of gait (walking difficulties/incoordination of the extremities/ataxia/falling to one side).
7. *N*ausea (with possible vomiting).
8. *N*umbness on one side of the face and/or body.
9. *N*ystagmus.

Dizziness is the most common symptom of VBI and may be unaccompanied by any other signs or symptoms.

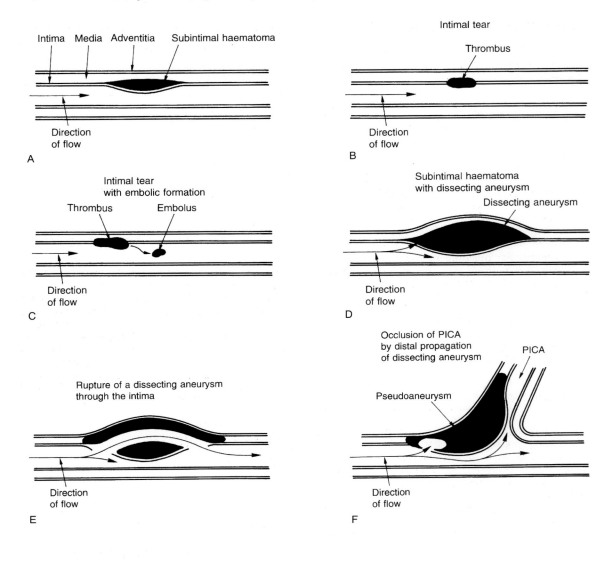

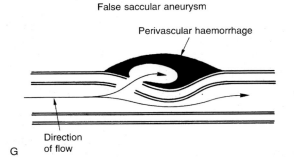

Fig. 12.3 (A) Subintimal haematoma; (B) intimal tear; (C) intimal tear with embolic formation; (D) subintimal haematoma with dissecting aneurysm; (E) rupture of a dissecting aneurysm through the intima; (F) occlusion of posterior inferior cerebellar artery (PICA) by distal propagation of dissecting aneurysm; (G) false saccular aneurysm. From Terrett (1997) with permission.

Post-SMT stroke syndromes

Post-SMT central nervous system injury (stroke) usually conforms to one of the following syndromes:

1. Wallenberg (dorsolateral medullary or retro-olivary) syndrome (occlusion of the PICA). The acute signs and symptoms usually disappear within several weeks. Most patients have a significant degree of recovery, but often experience residual neurological deficits.
2. Locked-in syndrome (cerebromedullospinal disconnection, occlusion of the basilar artery). Most patients with locked-in syndrome die early in the course of the disease. The survivors usually remain in a chronic locked-in state, as the medullary vital centres automatically maintain respiratory and cardiovascular function, although a few cases of substantial recovery have been reported (Khurana *et al.*, 1980; McCusker *et al.*, 1982; Carmody *et al.*, 1987; Povlsen *et al.*, 1987; Bell *v.* Griffiths, 1994).
3. Other brainstem syndromes.
4. Occipital lobe injury.
5. Cerebellar injury.
6. Thalamus injury.

Patient history

Tables have been produced which attempt to identify pre-existing pathological and/or altered physiological risk factors of VBS if SMT is proceeded with (George *et al.*, 1981; Terrett, 1983; Kleynhans and Terrett, 1985; Henderson and Cassidy, 1988). It is now apparent that very few of the factors, either alone or in combination, specifically increase the susceptibility to post-SMT VBS.

Different facets of the history will be reviewed.

Presenting complaint

The presenting complaint of patients who suffered VBS after SMT was given in 137 (74%) cases (Table 12.4). It can be seen that there is little that could alert the astute practitioner of an impending VBS, as most patients were young healthy individuals, suffering from musculoskeletal complaints such as head and/or neck and/or shoulder pain, without any predisposing VBS risk factors.

Transient ischaemic attacks (TIAs)

When a review of systems reveals transient ischaemic symptoms, it strongly suggests the necessity for medical referral and for the exclusion of SMT.

Table 12.4 *Major presenting complaint of patients who subsequently had a spinal manipulative therapy-induced vertebrobasilar stroke (n = 137)*

Presenting complaint	Percentage
Neck pain and/or stiffness	47.4
Neck pain/stiffness and headache	19.7
Headache	16.8
Torticollis	5.8
Low back pain	2.2
Abdominal complaint	2.2
Scoliosis/kyphoscoliosis	1.5
Head cold/cold in the head	1.5
Upper thoracic pain	1.5
Upper-limb numbness	0.7
Hayfever	0.7

Patients with vertebrobasilar TIAs may have many attacks before they suffer a VBS (Weiner, 1981). Symptoms due to VA compromise (five *D*s *A*nd 3 *N*s) should alert the practitioner not to manipulate the neck, and that the patient may require immediate medical referral (Weiner, 1981). If the patient suffers from carotid TIAs, medical referral is imperative as patients may suffer a complete stroke after only a few episodes – 10% in the first 6 months, then 6% in 1 year (Weiner, 1981). Signs and symptoms of carotid artery ischaemia include:

1. Hemianaesthesia.
2. Hemiparesis or monoparesis.
3. Headache.
4. Dysphasia.
5. Visual field disturbance.
6. Confusion.

Bruits

If, during review of symptoms, a patient states that an audible bruit has recently developed (which may be associated with symptoms such as headache and neck pain), the patient should not be manipulated, as this may indicate signs of an impending spontaneous dissecting aneurysm (Mas *et al.*, 1985, 1987).

Contraceptives

Several authors have listed oral contraceptives as a potential risk factor. VBS following SMT in women taking oral contraceptives has been reported in only 4 cases (Mueller and Sahs, 1976; Ladermann, 1981; Brownson *et al.*, 1986; Peters *et al.*, 1995), indicating most likely no causal relationship. Also noted is that only one of these women was reported as a smoker.

Women taking oral contraceptives are at a greater risk of vertebrobasilar thrombosis than those not taking contraceptives (Bickerstaff, 1975). However, as the source of emboli in these cases is not from the VAs (Ask-Upmark and Bickerstaff, 1976), taking the contraceptive pill would not appear to predispose such patients to any greater risk of post-SMT VBS.

Cigarette smoking and atherosclerosis

In patients with other stroke risk factors, such as hypertension, hyperlipidaemia, heart disease and/or diabetes mellitus, chronic smoking enhances the decrease in cerebral blood flow (Rogers *et al.*, 1983).

A review of the 185 cases reveals that 11 patients were recorded as smokers:

● Females – seven cases (29–41 years), average age 37 years.
● Males – four cases (33–55 years), average age 42 years.

Only one patient smoked over the age of 45 years. Although chronic smoking appears to increase the risk of cerebral stroke, it does not appear to increase the risk of VBS after SMT; otherwise such injuries would be expected to be more common in older age groups.

Osteoarthritis

Osteoarthritis does not appear to increase the risk of VBS after SMT. If it did, it would be expected that:

1. The older age group would be at a significantly greater risk, which they are not (Terrett and Kleynhans, 1992; Terrett, 1996).
2. Osteoarthritic compromise of the vertebral artery would be most likely to occur at the C4–6 spinal levels.

Radiographs of elderly patients with a diagnosis of VBI secondary to cervical spondylosis, when compared to age- and gender-matched controls (Adams *et al.*, 1986), failed to demonstrate any difference in the severity of radiographic changes. It was concluded that radiographs of the cervical spine were of little value, only confirming the high incidence of cervical spondylosis in the elderly.

Postpartum

Only four of the 103 females were reported as being postpartum (Masson and Cambier, 1962; Parkin *et al.*, 1978; Modde, 1985; Mas *et al.*, 1987). Considering the number of women who present to SMT practitioners offices after childbirth complaining of neck pain, this would not appear to indicate any causal relationship.

Migraine headaches

Strokes in migraine patients are rare, but can occur, and are usually in the posterior cerebral artery (distal branches of the VAs; Broderick and Swanson, 1987; Gilroy, 1990). Several authors have mentioned that a history of migraine may be an important precipitating factor in some cases of post-SMT VBS (Zimmermann *et al.*, 1978; Anonymous, 1980; Krueger and Okazaki, 1980; Solomon and Spaccavento, 1982; Carmody *et al.*, 1987; Mas *et al.*, 1987; Cashley, 1993). Migraines are a stroke risk factor in young adults (Spaccavento *et al.*, 1981; Solomon and Spaccavento, 1982), vascular spasm in migraine patients may exacerbate injuries (Zimmermann *et al.*, 1978), and migraneurs have been shown to be hypercoagulable (Dalessio, 1978). While no definite predisposition can be demonstrated in migraneurs, it would appear to be unwise to stress or irritate the VAs during a migraine attack, when arteries are in an irritable state.

Important risk factors

The most important VBS risk factors to identify in the history are:

1. Sudden severe pain in the side of the head and or neck, which is different from any pain the patient has had before.
2. Dizziness, unsteadiness, giddiness, vertigo.

Sudden severe head and/or neck pain

Many SMT practitioners are not aware that the earliest symptom of VAD (with or without SMT) is usually severe head and/or neck pain, usually described as different from any previously experienced, which can occur minutes, hours, days or even weeks prior to the onset of neurological dysfunction. Mokri *et al.* (1988) found the initial manifestation of VAD (not associated with SMT) was head pain in 60% of cases, vertigo and oscillopsia in 20%, and focal neurological deficits in 20%. Sturzenegger (1994) found headache was the prominent symptom in 86% of patients. Nicholls *et al.* (1993) indicated that irritation of the VA can produce pain from the forehead/cheek to the occiput/neck, and to the upper trapezius region. Report of this distinct type of pain, although non-specific as an isolated symptom, should raise suspicion of the possibility of an underlying VAD. As long as symptoms of brainstem ischaemia are absent, head and/or neck pain due to VAD will rarely be correctly diagnosed.

While the majority of cases of head and/or neck pains are major indications for SMT, in some circumstances the same symptom which prompts the patient to seek care may be due to VAD, which is a major *contraindication* to SMT. The problem for the practitioner is that often the head and/or neck pain due to VAD cannot be differentiated from a musculoskeletal region. This is a dilemma for the practitioner, as severe head and/or neck pain of a musculoskeletal origin (without signs of brainstem ischaemia) which will respond to SMT is very common, whereas VAD is uncommon. The incidence of VAD has been reported to be only about 1–6 patients per year in a large hospital (Hart and Easton, 1985; Biller *et al.*, 1986; Mas *et al.*, 1987; Mokri *et al.*, 1988; Sturzenegger, 1994,).

To complicate the problem further, VAD may be totally asymptomatic. One study found three patients with asymptomatic VAD while investigating other suspected lesions (Mokri *et al.*, 1988). These silent VADs appear to occur predominantly in cases of multiple dissections of cervical arteries (Hart and Easton, 1983; Chiras *et al.*, 1985; Mas *et al.*, 1987). This finding raises the possibility of an as yet unknown underlying arteriopathy which predisposes to vessel dissection. Evidence of fibromuscular dysplasia has been found in 23% and 33% of patients in two studies (Hart and Easton, 1983; Mas *et al.*, 1987).

A review of 27 cases of non-SMT VAD (where central nervous system dysfunction was not one of the earliest signs) revealed that the delay in the onset of central nervous system dysfunction after the onset of headache or neck pain was:

● 30% after less than 1 day.
● 15% 1, 2 or 3 days later.
● 30% 1–2 weeks later,
● 25% 3 weeks or more.

These findings suggest that many cases of VAD attributed to SMT practitioners may have existed prior to treatment, and may have been the cause of the symptoms which prompted the patient to seek care (or they may have been silent). Therefore, the practitioner who was blamed for the arterial and neurological damage may not have had any effect on the course of the disease process, or at worst may have hastened the inevitable. Because these scenarios are possible, it is suggested that techniques which excessively stress the VAs should not be used on any patient.

Dizziness, unsteadiness, vertigo, giddiness

The signs of VBI (five *D*s *A*nd three *N*s) should be known to all SMT practitioners.

Observant SMT practitioners would be aware that patients suffering from dizziness often respond dramatically following upper cervical SMT (Davis, 1953;

Jepson, 1963; Wing and Hargrave-Wilson, 1974; Cote *et al.*, 1991; Fitz-Ritson, 1991) but other possible causes of dizziness have to be kept in mind, and a differential diagnosis should be made (Giles, 1977). The problem for the practitioner is:

1. Dizziness is usually the prominent symptom of VBI, and often unaccompanied by any of the other signs and/or symptoms.
2. There is no simple method available to the SMT practitioner to determine whether the dizziness is due to VBI (contraindication to SMT) or whether it is due to a disturbance of articular and/or muscle proprioceptive input (an indication for SMT).

Many cases have been reported where SMT was proceeded with in a dizzy patient, with disastrous results (Terrett, 1990a, 1996; Terrett and Kleynhans, 1992). In these cases, the practitioner may have had no effect, or may have aggravated existing VA pathology, resulting in VA damage, but is blamed as having caused the VBS. Because available assessment methods do not enable SMT practitioners to be absolutely sure whether or not the symptom of dizziness/giddiness/unsteadiness/vertigo (or even head/neck pain) that the patient is suffering from is due to arterial wall pathology or not, in such patients it is recommended that treatment methods which excessively stress the VA walls not be used. It is suggested that SMT should be modified, or other forms of therapy used (soft-tissue therapy, accessory joint play movements, heat, ice, physiological therapeutics, etc.). If, after one or two treatment sessions, the dizziness decreases, then this most likely indicates that VBI was not the cause, and that normal SMT methods can then be used. One case is presented here to illustrate a not uncommon scenario, where dizziness in the history should alert the practitioner to modify or alter treatment.

> A 31-year-old female consulted a medical practitioner, suffering signs of a TIA (nausea, headache, vertigo, slurred speech, ataxia of gait). The practitioner recognized the nature of the TIA attack and referred the patient to a neurologist for a lumbar puncture. However, the practitioner did not recognize the TIA as a contraindication to cervical SMT and manipulated the cervical spine. Immediately following cervical SMT the patient had a VBS, due to dissection of both VAs (right artery 100% blocked, left artery 80% blocked). After 2 weeks in intensive care, the patient then improved, but was left with a permanent neurological deficit, and impairment to higher-level thinking (previously a gifted screenwriter, now a file clerk; Saltzberg *v.* Hawkins 1991).

This scenario, of brainstem signs and/or symptoms which should have alerted the practitioner, may be much more common than the literature suggests, but because the reports are written by authors more interested in the neurology, post-mortem, angiographic, computed tomographic or magnetic resonance imaging scan findings, most likely this important point for SMT practitioners was not commented upon.

Patient examination

Three major tests have been described as being able to detect those patients at risk of VBS following SMT. They are:

1. Blood pressure measurement.
2. Neck auscultation.
3. Functional vascular tests.

Blood pressure measurement

Review of cases reveals that the victims are usually young, and there is no consistently found hyper- or hypotension. Therefore, the taking of blood pressure does not appear to be particularly useful in determining any increased risk of VBS following SMT.

Neck auscultation

Review of cases of post-SMT VBS reveals that the neck was auscultated for bruits in 18 cases (Terrett, 1996). In *none* of these was a VA bruit heard. Seventeen cases involved VA damage, of which 10 were confirmed by angiography and one was confirmed at postmortem. One case involved carotid artery damage (Murthy and Naidu, 1988) with positive arteriography and surgical findings, and yet no carotid bruit was heard on neck auscultation.

As there were no arterial bruits detected after the arterial damage, it would be highly unlikely that a bruit would have been detected prior to SMT. Therefore, it is the author's opinion that the taking of blood pressure, and listening for bruits, leads practitioners into a false sense of security that they are doing a relevant vertebrobasilar screening examination.

Functional vascular tests

There are at least four variations of the VA patency tests (Houle, 1972; Kleynhans, 1980; George *et al.*, 1981; Terrett and Webb, 1982; Terrett, 1983; Grant, 1988; Henderson and Cassidy, 1988). In all, the patient's head is held for 30 s in the premanipulative position (e.g. rotation, rotation with extension) before SMT, and the patient is observed for any signs, such as nystagmus, and asked to report any symptoms

of VBI. Dizziness is the most common symptom of VBI, and may be unaccompanied by any other symptoms or signs; therefore the absence of other brainstem signs and/or symptoms does not always exclude the possibility of a vascular cause.

When positive, these tests only indicate that rotation has possibly produced brainstem ischaemia, possibly due to compression of one VA, and inadequate patency of the opposite artery. However, when signs and symptoms are present, there is a risk to the patient, so further evaluation is indicated and manipulation should not be performed.

There are four major problems with these procedures as a predictor of VBS after SMT:

1. Even if you have a negative test result, VBS may still occur because these tests reproduce some of the stresses of SMT on the osseous–articular–musculo–ligamentous–vascular structures, but cannot predict the effect of thrust, which may further stretch the VA, and damage the vessel wall (Fig. 12.3).

   Bolton *et al.* (1989) demonstrated the limited diagnostic value of these tests. In a patient in whom the pre-SMT tests failed to identify any VA problem, subsequent digital subtraction angiography revealed occlusion of one VA.

   Haynes (1996) in a study of 280 VAs found that in 14 (5%) the Doppler sound stopped during neck rotation, but none of these patients developed any signs or symptoms of brainstem ischaemia.

   A negative test result cannot be interpreted to mean that there is no arteriopathic process in the VAs. Therefore, these tests appear to be inadequate in all but the most grossly pathological or highly susceptible cases. There have been at least two cases where patients suffered VA trauma after negative test results (Parkin *et al.*, 1978; Lindy, 1984).
2. There is a problem of false-positive tests (Terrett, 1983), as vertigo and nystagmus of cervical origin (joint and/or muscle) are well-documented, with theories being related to the stimulation of cervical sympathetics or to cervical muscle and joint receptors (Gayral *et al.*, 1954; Gray, 1956; de Jong, 1977; Liedgren and Odkvist, 1979; Maeda, 1979; Hulse, 1983; Thiel *et al.*, 1994). This type of dizziness can be expected to respond well to SMT.

   The author has often experienced cases where testing before SMT produced dizziness, but the dizziness could not be reproduced after soft-tissue therapy and gentle SMT, indicating vertebrogenic dizziness.

   Thiel *et al.* (1994) had an experimental group of 12 subjects who had positive functional vertebrobasilar tests and a history of dizziness and/or related symptoms during certain positions of the head and neck. Using duplex Doppler ultrasound, no decrease in VA blood flow was detected in these patients (or in the 30 subjects in the control group) during the functional vascular test position.

3. There is no evidence to suggest that these tests, when positive, indicate any underlying arterio-pathy or altered anatomy which would predispose to arterial wall damage and VBS if SMT were proceeded with.

4. There have been cases where merely placing the head into the rotated position has induced a stroke (Roche *et al.,* 1963; Gatterman, 1982; Danesh-mend *et al.,* 1984; see Table 12.2).

While we have to admit these inadequacies, it is still considered that when a positive result is found, caution is prudent.

Risk reduction

There appear to be two major problems occurring with SMT associated with VBS, which are:

1. Rotational SMT.
2. Continuing to treat a person with SMT after signs and/or symptoms of arterial damage have become evident.

Changes in SMT technique can easily be made so as to minimize the the risks of SMT.

Rotational SMT

Of the 185 cases, the method of SMT was described in 76 cases (41%), which reveals that rotation was used in 65.8% of cases, rotation with extension, flexion and/or traction was used in 29%, and toggle recoil repeated three times was used in 1.3%. Traction was used in 3.9%. In 94.8% of cases rotation, with or without other movements, was used in the treatment.

That rotation is the cervical movement most likely to damage the VA wall is supported by review of five sources:

1. Haemodynamic studies in cadavers.
2. Haemodynamic studies in live subjects.
3. The mechanism involved in non-SMT VA damage is usually neck rotation, or rotation with extension.
4. Post-SMT angiography consistently reveals the VA damage to be between C1 and C2 because rotation compresses and stretches the VA most at this level.
5. Post-SMT VBS autopsy investigations consistently reveal the VA damage to be between C1–2.

Regarding traction, some have considered that this makes rotation SMT safer. This belief is not supported by one study of 41 cadavers (82 VAs), where extension and rotation occluded five (6%) VAs; when traction was then added, another 27 complete occlusions occurred (*n* = 32 or 39%); all occurred above C2 level (Brown and Tatlow, 1963).

Continued treatment of a patient after signs of arterial damage have become evident

It has been documented (Terrett, 1987b, 1990b, 1996; Terrett and Kleynhans, 1992) that many cases of VBS after SMT could have been avoided had the practitioner understood that the symptoms post-SMT were due to arterial trauma, and that further trauma to an artery already undergoing pathological change can only be expected to aggravate the condition.

The signs of VA damage can present in one of three ways:

1. Sudden onset of severe head and/or neck pain.
2. Vertebrobasilar ischaemia (the five *D*s *A*nd three *N*s).
3. Both the above occurring together.

As already described, the earliest sign of damage to the VA wall is often head and/or neck pain. If head and/or neck pain occurs following upper cervical SMT, the practitioner should not remanipulate the neck in the mistaken belief that the first treatment was not done correctly. Those patients in whom head pain (usually occipital) and/or neck pain began during SMT usually describe the pain as:

1. Immediate, sudden, during SMT.
2. Distinctly different from pains previously suffered.
3. Sharp discomfort, excruciating, intense, violent, severe.

If pain occurs without the signs of ischaemia, it is difficult for the practitioner to know whether it is a joint and/or muscle pain reaction to the SMT, but the author suggests that SMT should not be repeated in case the pain is due to VAD.

Symptoms after cervical SMT, such as fainting and nausea, have been called by Maigne (1972) sympathetic storms. Several authors have postulated that irritation of the cervical sympathetic nerves may cause spasm of the vertebrobasilar arteries and their branches (Neuwirth, 1955; Stewart, 1962; Maigne, 1972; Jackson, 1977). Although this is an attractive theory for various head, chest and arm symptoms, it needs to be supported by research. A study of the neural control of VA blood flow found no evidence to support the contention that cervical lesions could affect hind-brain blood flow (Bogduk *et al.,* 1981). VA blood flow was found to be profoundly unresponsive to stimulation of any component of the cervical sympathetic system and it was concluded that the theory that irritation of cervical sympathetic nerves can alter VA blood flow is untenable. Therefore, practitioners should be careful before ascribing post-SMT reactions to sympathetic storms, and be aware that they most likely indicate either alteration of upper cervical proprioceptive input or, more dangerously, brainstem ischaemia induced by VA trauma (Terrett, 1990a, 1996; Terrett and Kleynhans, 1992).

The problem for the practitioner is that dizziness is usually the prominent symptom in both cases and, in the absence of other signs of ischaemia, it is not possible to determine the cause. These patients may subsequently respond well to SMT and suffer no ill effect, as dizziness usually responds well to SMT (Davis, 1953; Jepson, 1963; Wing and Hargrave-Wilson, 1974; Cote *et al.,* 1991; FitzRitson, 1991). However, it is suggested that in such cases, because of the possibility of serious damage, it would be irresponsible to proceed with rotation thrust SMT techniques, which are the most likely to stress the VA wall. It seems to be courting possible disaster, as there are no diagnostic methods available to determine whether the symptoms of post-SMT pain or dizziness are due to cervical proprioceptive or sympathetic system stimulation or to VAD. In these patients other forms of therapy to the upper cervical spine should be used.

To illustrate that to continue manipulation of the neck after the onset of signs of brainstem ischaemia is irresponsible, the following case is presented as a not uncommon scenario. (For other cases, see Terrett, 1990a,b, 1996; Terrett and Kleynhans, 1992.)

> A previously healthy 31-year-old male underwent a cervical manipulation from a medical practitioner for a headache and stiff neck, which he had developed after playing tennis. Two hours after the first manipulation he returned to the practitioner who injected him intravenously with Valium and manipulated his neck again. He became disoriented and did not regain full consciousness. The practitioner again manipulated his neck about $2\frac{1}{2}$ h later, when the patient gave a large groan and developed pins and needles in the arms and legs. His arms and legs went stiff, he went into spasm, and the right side of his face and shoulder dropped. He later vomited. An ambulance was called, and he was admitted to hospital 4 h after the second cervical manipulation. His condition deteriorated and he suffered brain death. Respiratory support was removed 3 days later (Terrett, 1987a, 1996).

If any adverse signs and/or symptoms occur during treatment – *stop*. There is nothing to be gained from continuing to retraumatize an artery already undergoing pathological change. Left alone, the patient may recover. Continuing to treat the patient may result in death, tetraplegia or permanent neurological deficit.

Emergency care

A practitioner may still be unfortunate enough to have a patient develop signs of brainstem ischaemia even after all precautions have been taken.

If post-SMT VBI signs occur (Terrett, 1987b, 1990a, 1996; Terrett and Kleynhans, 1992):

1. *Do not remanipulate the patient's neck.* There is nothing to gain from retraumatizing an artery undergoing pathological change, and it may in fact result in further arterial damage and disaster.
2. *Observe the patient.* The symptoms may resolve within a short time, indicating either transient VBI, possibly due to spasm, or proprioceptive dizziness.
3. *Refer the patient.* If the symptoms do not subside, do not panic and remanipulate the patient's neck.

    If the patient's symptoms progress and do not abate, he or she needs to be hospitalized.

    The practitioner's assistance in describing what happened may be helpful in instituting the correct therapy quickly.

Conclusion

Several authors have mentioned that patients with signs and/or symptoms of VBI can respond beneficially following SMT. The author agrees that many cerebral and cranial nerve-type signs and/or symptoms can respond to SMT (Terrett, 1984, 1988, 1989, 1993, 1994, 1995), but readers should appreciate that a patient whose symptoms are due to VAD, and thrombus formation, is not likely to respond beneficially to SMT.

This issue has been confused by some writing about transient rotational occlusion producing transient brainstem symptoms. What is trying to be prevented here is trauma to arterial structures resulting in intramural haemorrhages, lacerations, dissections, aneurysms, thrombus and embolus formation with resultant central nervous system damage – not episodes of transient ischaemia.

As practitioners better understand the pathology, warning signs in the review of systems and history, warning signs during and after treatment which indicate that treatment should be altered or ceased, and the need in some cases for the patient to be hospitalized, the incidence of these injuries should decrease.

It has been stated that all thrust techniques are ruled out as dangerous, and that 'we should stay our hand until indications for thrust techniques are quite unequivocal' (Grieve, 1986). It is the author's opinion that it is not thrust that is the most dangerous component of the manipulation, but that it is extreme rotation. Techniques can be modified to abandon that component which appears to carry greatest risk for our patients.

Regarding post-SMT VBS, the following conclusions are offered:

1. VBS following SMT is very rare (nobody knows what the true incidence is), but many cases could have been avoided.
2. There does not appear to be any age group or gender that is predisposed to post-SMT VBS.
3. Cadaver and *in vivo* studies on haemodynamic changes with neck movement indicate that rotation applies greater stress on the VAs than lateral flexion. While cadaver and *in vivo* studies both come to this conclusion, it is apparent that cadaver studies do not accurately reflect changes *in vivo*.
4. Current knowledge is limited, and prediction of patients at risk by currently used patient assessment methods requires much further research, and possibly the adoption in practice of new diagnostic methods (e.g. Doppler ultrasound).
5. In many cases, the patient may have presented with an existing VAD, which may have caused the symptoms (head and/or neck pains) which prompted the patient to consult the practitioner. The practitioner, who is then held responsible for causing the injury, may have had no effect on the final outcome, or merely hastened the inevitable. It is possible, though, that without the artery being traumatized, its wall may have healed with no occurrence of stroke.
6. Many of the cases of patient injury could have been prevented had the practitioner been aware of VBI signs and symptoms, which should have been elicited during the review of systems, or case history, and which should have indicated that SMT should not be proceeded with. This may have occurred more commonly than the literature suggests.
7. Many of the cases of patient injury may have been prevented had the practitioner performed a physical examination, including holding the head in the premanipulative position while observing for signs and/or symptoms of VBI.
8. The most severe injuries following SMT are not cases of transient ischaemia due to compression or vasospasm, but of vessel wall laceration, dissection, etc., possibly predisposed by an as yet unknown arteriopathy.

9. Post-SMT dizziness may have many causes. The patient who develops post-SMT dizziness should not be remanipulated, but transported to hospital for observation.
10. Many cases of patient injury were caused or made worse because the practitioner did not stop treatment, which had the effect of further traumatizing an artery undergoing pathological change.
11. It is not possible to predict all patients who may be presenting to our offices with pre-existing vertebral artery dissections (or other arteriopathic processes which may predispose to arterial dissection), as they may be silent, or may in fact be causing the head and/or neck pains (without other warning signs) prompting the patient to seek help. The absence of reported contraindications does not mean that the patient will not suffer post-SMT VBS and, in fact, most of the reported cases did not document the supposed contraindications. Therefore, we cannot absolutely protect these patients by pretreatment screening.
12. Many of the cases which occurred in predisposed patients (pre-existing VA dissection, with or without examination findings) may not have occurred had the practitioners used a method of SMT which did not stress the VA walls.

References

Adams, K.H.R., Yung, M.W., Lye, M., Whitehouse, G.H. (1986) Are cervical spine radiographs of value in elderly patients with vertebrobasilar insufficiency? *Age Aging* **15:** 57–59.

Andersson, R., Carleson, R., Nylen, O. (1970) Vertebral artery insufficiency and rotational obstruction. *Acta Med. Scand.* **188:** 475–477.

Anonymous (1980) Chiropractors urged to consider stroke risk. *Med. World News* (March 17): 23.

Ask-Upmark, E., Bickerstaff, E.R. (1976) Vertebral artery occlusion and oral contraceptives. *Br. Med. J.* **1:** 487–488.

Bakay, L., Sweet, W.H. (1953) Intra-arterial pressures in the neck and brain. *J. Neurosurg.* **10:** 353–359.

Barton, J.W., Margolis, M.T. (1975) Rotational obstruction of the vertebral artery at the atlantoaxial joint. *Neuroradiology* **9:** 117–120.

Barty, G.M. (1983) Expert testimony. Klippel *v.* Alchin. Wagga Wagga, Australia. 12 Aug 1983, 33.

Beatty, R.A. (1977) Dissecting hematoma of the internal carotid artery following chiropractic cervical manipulation. *J. Trauma* **17:** 248–249.

Bell *v.* Griffiths (1994) Hunter J (Judgement). Supreme Court, Common Law Division, Sydney: 14 Sep 1994. Case also reported in: Anonymous. John Bell: "Buried alive." *New Idea* (Magazine) 1987 (Aug 29), 21.

Bickerstaff, E.R. (1975) *Neurological Complications of Oral Contraceptives*. Oxford: Clarendon Press, pp. 57–58.

Biller, J., Hingtgen, W.L., Adams, H.P. *et al.* (1986) Cervicocephalic arterial dissections. *Arch. Neurol.* **43:** 1234–1238.

Blaumanis, O.R., Gertz, S.D., Grady, P.A., Nelson, E.R. (1976) Thrombosis in acute experimental cerebral vasospasm. *Stroke* **7:** 9–10.

Bogduk, N., Lambert, G., Duckworth, J.W. (1981) The anatomy and physiology of the vertebral nerve in relation to cervical migraine. *Cephalalgia* **1:** 1–14.

Bolton, P.S., Stick, P.E., Lord, R.S.A. (1989) Failure of clinical tests to predict ischemia before neck manipulation. *J. Manipul. Physiol. Ther.* **12:** 304–307.

Brain, L. (1963) Some unsolved problems of cervical spondylosis. *Br. Med. J.* **1:** 771–777.

Braune, H.J., Munk, M.H., Huffmann, G. (1991) Hirninfarkt im stromgebiet der arteria cerebri media nach chirotherapie der Halswirbelsaule. *Dtsch. Med. Wochenschr.* **116:** 1047–1050.

Broderick, J.P., Swanson, J.W. (1987) Migraine related strokes: clinical profile and prognosis in 20 patients. *Arch. Neurol.* **44:** 868–871.

Brown, B.S.J., Tatlow, W.F.T. (1963) Radiographic studies of the vertebral arteries in cadavers. *Radiology* **81:** 80–88.

Brownson, R.J., Zollinger, W.K., Madiera, T., Fell, D. (1986) Sudden sensorineural hearing loss following manipulation of the cervical spine. *Laryngoscope* **96:** 166–170.

Carmody, E., Buckley, P., Hutchinson, M. (1987) Basilar artery occlusion following chiropractic cervical manipulation. *Irish Med. J.* **80:** 259–260.

Cashley, M.A.P. (1993) Basilar artery migraine or cerebral vascular accident? *J. Manipul. Physiol. Ther.* **16:** 112–114.

Chiras, J., Marciano, S., VegaMolina, J. *et al.* (1985) Spontaneous dissecting aneurysm of the extracranial vertebral artery (20 cases). *Neuroradiology* **27:** 327–333.

Christiensen, M.G. (ed.) (1993) *Job Analysis of Chiropractic: A Project Report, Survey Analysis and Summary of the Practice of Chiropractic within the United States.* 901 54th Ave, Greeley, Colorado. National Board of Chiropractic Examiners, p. 58.

Christiensen, M.G. (ed.) (1994) *Job Analysis of Chiropractic in Australia and New Zealand: A Project Report, Survey Analysis and Summary of the Practice of Chiropractic within Australia and New Zealand.* 901 54th Ave, Greeley, Colorado, National Board of Chiropractic Examiners, p. 72.

Cote, P., Mior, S.A., Fitz-Ritson, D. (1991) Cervicogenic vertigo: a report of three cases. *J. Can. Chiro. Assoc.* **35:** 89–94.

Cyriax, J. (1978) *Textbook of Orthopaedic Medicine,* vol. 1. *Diagnosis of Soft Tissue Lesions,* 7th edn. London: Baillière Tindall, p. 165.

Dalessio, D. (1978) Migraine, platelets, and headache prophylaxis. *J.A.M.A.* **239:** 52–53.

Daneshmend, T.K., Hewer, R.L., Bradshaw, J.R. (1984) Acute brain stem stroke during neck manipulation. *Br. Med. J.* **288:** 189.

Davis, D. (1953) A common type of vertigo relieved by traction of the cervical spine. *Ann. Intern. Med.* **38:** 778–786.

de Jong, P.T.V.M. (1977) Ataxia and nystagmus induced by injection of local anaesthetic in the neck. *Ann. Neurol.* **1:** 240–246.

deKleyn, A., Nieuwenhuyse, P. (1927) Schwindelanfaelle und nystagmus bei einer bestimmten stellung des kopfes. *Acta Otolaryngol.* **11:** 155.

deKleyn, A., Versteegh, C. (1933) Ueber verschiedene formen von Menieres syndrom. *Dtsche Ztschr.* **132:** 157.

Dorey, R.S.A., Mayne, V. (1986) Break dancing injuries. *Med. J. Aust.* **144:** 610–611.

Dvorak, J., Orelli, F. (1985) How dangerous is manipulation of the cervical spine? *Manual Med.* **2:** 1–4.

Easton, J.D., Sherman, D.G. (1977) Cervical manipulation and stroke. *Stroke* **8:** 594–597.

Fisher, M. (1993) Basilar artery embolism after surgery under general anesthesia: a case report. *Neurology* **43:** 1856.

Fitz-Ritson, D. (1991) Assessment of cervicogenic vertigo. *J. Manipul. Physiol. Ther.* **14:** 193–198.

Fogelholm, R., Karli, P. (1975) Iatrogenic brainstem infarction. *Eur. Neurol.* **13:** 6–12.

Gatterman, M.I. (1982) Extreme caution advised. *J Chiropract.* **19:** 14.

Gayral, L., France, T., Nuewirth, E. (1954) Oto-neuro ophthalmologic manifestations of cervical origin. Posterior cervical sympathetic syndrome of Barre Lieou. *N.Y. State J. Med.* **54:** 1920–1926.

George, P.E., Silverstein, H.T., Wallace, H., Marshall, M. (1981) Identification of the high risk pre-stroke patient. *J. Chiropract.* **15:** S26–S28.

Giles, L.G.F. (1977) Vertebral-basilar artery insufficiency. *J. Can. Chiropractic Assoc.* **21:** 112–117.

Gilroy, J. (1990) *Basic Neurology,* 2nd edn. New York: Pergamon Press, p. 157.

Grant, R. (1988) Dizziness testing and manipulation of the cervical spine. In: *Physical Therapy of the Cervical and Thoracic Spine* (Grant, R., ed.). New York: Churchill Livingstone, pp. 111–124.

Gray, L.P. (1956) Extralabyrinthine vertigo due to cervical muscle lesions. *J. Laryngol.* **70:** 352–360.

Grieve, G.P. (1986) Incidents and accidents of manipulation. In: *ModernManual Therapy of the Vertebral Column* (Grieve, G.P., ed.). London: Churchill Livingstone, pp. 873–884.

Grossman, R.I., Davies, K.R. (1982) Positional occlusion of the vertebral artery: a rare cause of embolic stroke. *Neuroradiology* **23:** 227–230.

Gutmann, G. (1983) Verletzungen der arteria vertebralis durch manuelle therapie. *Manuelle Med.* **21:** 2–14.

Hanus, S.H., Homer, T.D., Harter, D.H. (1977) Vertebral artery occlusion complicating yoga exercises. *Arch. Neurol.* **34:** 574–575.

Hart, R.G., Easton, J.D. (1983) Dissection of the cervical and cerebral arteries. *Neurol. Clin.* **1:** 155–182.

Hart, R.G., Easton, J.D. (1985) Dissections. *Stroke* **16:** 925–927.

Haynes, M.J. (1996) Doppler studies comparing the effects of cervical rotation and lateral flexion on vertebral artery flow. *J. Manipul. Physiol. Ther.* (in press).

Henderson, D.J., Cassidy, J.D. (1988) Vertebral artery syndrome. In: *Upper Cervical Syndrome: Chiropractic Diagnosis and Treatment* (Vernon, H., ed.). Baltimore: Williams & Wilkins, pp. 194–206.

Hope, E.E., Bodensteiner, J.B, Barnes, P. (1983) Cerebral infarction related to neck position in an adolescent. *Pediatrics* **72:** 335–337.

Hosek, R.S., Schram, S.B., Silverman, H., Meyers, J.B. (1981) Cervical manipulation. *J.A.M.A.* **245:** 922.

Houle, J.O.E. (1972) Assessing hemodynamics of the vertebrobasilar complex through angiothlipsis. *Digest Chiropractic Economics* **15:** 14–15.

Hulse, M. (1983) Disequilibrium caused by a functional disturbance of the upper cervical spine. Clinical aspects and differential diagnosis. *Man. Med..* **1:** 18–23.

Jackson, R. (1977) *The Cervical Syndrome*. Springfield, IL: Thomas, pp. 245–246.

Jepson, O. (1963) Dizziness originating in the columna cervicalis. *Nordisk Med.* **6**: 675–676. Translated in: *J. Can. Chiro. Assoc.* **11**: 7–8, 25.

Khurana, R.K., Genut, A.A., Yannakakis, G.D. (1980) Locked-in syndrome with recovery. *Ann. Neurol.* **8**: 439–441.

Kleynhans, A.M. (1980) The prevention of complications from spinal manipulative therapy. In: *Aspects of Manipulative therapy* (Idczak, R.M., ed.). Melbourne: Lincoln Institute of Health Sciences, pp. 133–141.

Kleynhans, A.M., Terrett, A.G.J. (1985) The prevention of complications from spinal manipulative therapy. In: *Aspects of Manipulative Therapy*, 2nd edn (Glasgow, E.F. *et al.*, eds). London: Churchill Livingstone, pp. 161–175.

Krueger, B.R., Okazaki, H. (1980) Vertebral-basilar distribution infarction following chiropractic cervical manipulation. *Mayo Clin. Proc.* **55**: 3220–3232.

Ladermann, J.P. (1981) Accidents of spinal manipulation. *Ann. Swiss Chiropractors Assoc.* **7**: 161–208.

Liedgren, C., Odkvist, L. (1980) The morphological and physiological basis for vertigo of cervical origin. In: *Differential Diagnosis of Vertigo* (Claussen, C., ed.). Proceedings of the 6th scientific meeting of the NES, Finland 1979. New York: Walter de Gruyter, pp. 567–587.

Lindy, D.R. (1984) Patient collapse following cervical manipulation: a case report. *Br. Osteopathic J.* **16**: 84–85.

Lyness, S.S., Wagman, A.D. (1974) Neurological deficit following cervical manipulation. *Surg. Neurol.* **2**: 121–124.

McCusker, E.A., Rudick, R.A., Honch, G.W., Griggs, R.C. (1982) Recovery from the "locked-in" syndrome. *Arch. Neurol.* **39**: 145–147.

Maeda, M. (1979) Neck influences on the vestibulo-ocular reflex arc and the vestibulocerebellum. *Prog. Brain Res.* **50**: 551–559.

Maigne, R. (1972) *Orthopedic Medicine: A New Approach to Vertebral Manipulations*. Springfield, IL: Thomas, pp. 155, 169.

Mas, J.L., Goeau, C., Bousser, M.G. *et al.* (1985) Spontaneous dissecting aneurysms of the internal carotid and vertebral arteries: two case reports. *Stroke* **16**: 125–129.

Mas, J.L., Bousser, M.G., Hasboun, D., Laplane, D. (1987) Extracranial vertebral artery dissections: a review of 13 cases. *Stroke* **18**: 1037–1047.

Masson, M., Cambier, J. (1962) Insuffisance circulatoire vertebro basilaire. *Presse Med.* **70**: 1990–1993.

Modde, P.J. (1985) *Chiropractic Malpractice*. Columbia, MD: Hanrow Press, pp. 269–270, 273–275, 311–318, 322–323, 329–331, 334–337.

Mokri, B., Houser, O.W., Sandok, B.A., Piepgras, G. (1988) Spontaneous dissections of the vertebral arteries. *Neurology* **38**: 880–885.

Mueller, S., Sahs, A.L. (1976) Brain stem dysfunction related to cervical manipulation. *Neurology* (Minneap). **26**: 547–560.

Murthy, J.M.K., Naidu, K.V. (1988) Aneurysm of the cervical internal carotid artery following chiropractic manipulation. *J. Neurol. Neurosurg. Psychiatry* **51**: 1237–1238.

Nagler, W. (1973) Vertebral artery obstruction by hyperextension of the neck; report of three cases. *Arch. Phys. Med. Rehabil.* **54**: 237–240.

Nakamura, C.T., Lau, J.M., Polk, N.O., Popper, J.S. (1991) Vertebral artery dissection caused by chiropractic manipulation. *J. Vasc. Surg.* **14**: 122–124.

Neuwirth, E. (1955) The vertebral nerve in the posterior cervical syndrome. *N.Y. State J. Med.* **55**: 1380.

Nicholls, F.T., Mawad, M., Mohr, J.P. *et al.* (1993) Focal headache during balloon inflation in the vertebral and basilar arteries. *Headache* **33**: 87–89.

Nosan, D.K., Gomez, C.R., Maves, M.D. (1993) Perioperative stroke in patients undergoing head and neck surgery. *Ann. Otol. Rhinol. Laryngol.* **102**: 717–23.

Oh, V.M.S. (1993) Brain infarction and neck callisthenics. *Lancet* **342**: 739.

Okawara, S., Nibblelink, D. (1974) Vertebral artery occlusion following hyperextension and rotation of the head. *Stroke* **5**: 640–642.

Parkin, P.J., Wallis, W.E., Wilson, J.L. (1978) Vertebral artery occlusion following manipulation of the neck. *N.Z. Med. J.* **88**: 441–443.

Peters, M., Bohl, J., Thomke, F. *et al.* (1995) Dissection of the internal carotid artery after chiropractic manipulation of the neck. *Neurology* **45**: 2284–2286.

Povlsen, U.J., Kjaer, L., Arlien-Soborg, P. (1987) Locked-in syndrome following cervical manipulation. *Acta Neurol. Scand.* **76**: 486–488.

Pryse-Phillips, W. (1989) Infarction of the medulla and cervical cord after fitness exercises. *Stroke* **20**: 292–294.

Refshauge, K.M. (1994) Rotation: a valid premanipulative dizziness test? Does it predict safe manipulation? *J. Manipul. Physiol. Ther.* **17**: 15–19.

Roche, L., Colin, M., DeRougemont, J. *et al.* (1963) Lesions traumatiques de la colonne cervicale et attaintes de l'artère vertébrale. Responsabilité d'un examen medical. *Ann. Med. Leg.* **43**: 232–235. (This case is also reported in Vedrine and Spay (1968), and Jung *et al.* (1976).)

Rogers, L., Sweeney, P.J. (1979) Stroke: a neurologic complication of wrestling. *Am. J Sports Med.* **7**: 352–354.

Rogers, R.L., Meyer, J.S., Shaw, T.G. *et al.* (1983) Cigarette smoking decreases cerebral blood flow suggesting increased risk for stroke. *J.A.M.A.* **250**: 2796–2800.

Saltzberg v. Hawkins (1991) Los Angeles County Superior Court case no. 697925. Kakita J and Jury. Judgement 13 Nov 1991. (Note: case also reported in Chapman-Smith (1992) Who should manipulate? – $1.3 million award against MD. *Chiropractic Rep.* **6**: 6 and in Anonymous (1991) MD's cervical manipulation causes woman's stroke. *MPI's Dynamic Chiropractic* (Dec 20), 33.

Saternus, K.S., Fuchs, V. (1982) Ist die arteria vertebralis bei der Reanimation gefahrdet? *Man. Med.* **20**: 101–104.

Schmitt, H.P. (1978) Manuelle therapie der halswirbelsaule. *Z. Allgemeinmed.* **54**: 467–474.

Selecki, B.R. (1969) The effects of rotation of the atlas on the axis: experimental work. *Med. J. Aust.* **56**: 1012–1015.

Sherman, D.G., Hart, R.G., Easton, J.D. (1981) Abrupt change in head position and cerebral infarction. *Stroke* **12**: 2–6. (Note: the first three cases were previously reported in Easton and Sherman, 1977.)

Solomon, G.D., Spaccavento, L.J. (1982) Lateral medullary syndrome after basilar migraine. *Headache* **22**: 171–172.

Sorenson, B.F. (1978) Bow hunter's stroke. *Neurosurgery* **2**: 259–261.

Spaccavento, L.J., Solomon, G.D., Mani, S. (1981) An

association between strokes and migraines in young adults. *Headache* **21**: 121.

Stewart, D.Y. (1962) Current concepts of "Barre syndrome" or the posterior cervical sympathetic syndrome. *Clin. Ortho. Rel. Res.* **24**: 40–48.

Sturzenegger, M. (1994) Headache and neck pain: the warning symptoms of vertebral artery dissection. *Headache* **34**: 187–193.

Tatlow, W.F.T, Bammer, H.G. (1957) Syndrome of vertebral artery compression. *Neurology* **7**: 331–340.

Taylor, H.H. (1981) Letter to the editor. *J. Chiropract.* **18**: 11–12.

Terrett, A.G.J. (1983) Importance and interpretation of tests designed to predict susceptibility to neurocirculatory accidents from manipulation. *J. Aust. Chiro. Assoc.* **13**: 29–34.

Terrett, A.G.J. (1984) The neck tongue syndrome. *J. Aust. Chiro. Assoc.* **14**: 100–107.

Terrett, A.G.J. (1987a) Vascular accidents from cervical spine manipulation: report on 107 cases. *J. Aust. Chiro. Assoc.* **17**: 15–24. (Reprinted in: *J. Chiropract.* 1988; **25**: 63–72. Note: case 4 also reported in: Cervical manipulation: anatomy of a disaster. *Med. Pract.* 1986 (July), 26–27.

Terrett, A.G.J. (1987b) Vascular accidents from cervical spine manipulation: the mechanisms. *J. Aust. Chiro. Assoc.* **17**: 131–144.

Terrett, A.G.J. (1988) The neck tongue syndrome and spinal manipulative therapy. In: *Upper Cervical Spine Syndrome: Chiropractic Diagnosis and Treatment* (Vernon, H., ed.). Baltimore: Williams & Wilkins, pp. 223–239.

Terrett, A.G.J. (1989) Tinnitus, the cervical spine, and spinal manipulative therapy. *Chiro. Techn.* **1**: 41–45.

Terrett, A.G.J. (1990a) It is more important to know when not to adjust. *Chiro. Techn.* **2**: 1–9.

Terrett, A.G.J. (1990b) Osteopathic iatrogenics and the need for government regulation. *J. N.Z. Register Osteopaths* **4**: 42–45.

Terrett, A.G.J. (1993) Cerebral dysfunction: a theory to explain some of the effects of chiropractic manipulation. *Chiro. Techn.* **5**: 168–173.

Terrett, A.G.J. (1994) Letter to the editor. *Chiro. Techn.* **6**: 110–112.

Terrett, A.G.J. (1995) The cerebral dysfunction theory. In: *Foundations of Chiropractic: Subluxation* (Gatterman, M.I., ed.). St Louis, Mosby: pp. 340–352.

Terrett, A.G.J. (1996) *Malpractice Avoidance for Chiropractors, Vertebrobasilar Stroke following Manipulation.* 1452–29th Street, West Des Moines, Iowa: National Chiropractic Mutual Insurance Company.

Terrett, A.G.J., Kleynhans, A.M. (1992) Cerebrovascular complications of manipulation. In: *Principles and Practice of Chiropractic,* 2nd edn (Haldeman, S., ed.). Norwalk, CT: Appleton & Lange, pp. 579–598.

Terrett, A.G.J, Webb, M.N. (1982) Vertebrobasilar accidents following cervical spine adjustment/manipulation. *J. Aust. Chiro. Assoc.* **12**: 24–27.

Tettenborn, B., Caplan, L.R., Sloan, M.A. *et al.* (1993) Postoperative brainstem and cerebellar infarcts. *Neurology* **43**: 471–477.

Thiel, H., Wallace, K., Donat, J., Yong-Hing, K. (1994) Effect of various head and neck positions on vertebral artery blood flow. *Clin. Biomech.* **9**: 105–110.

Toole, J.F., Tucker, S.H. (1960) Influence of head position upon cerebral circulation: studies on blood flow in cadavers. *Arch. Neurol.* **2**: 616–623.

Tramo, M.J., Hainline, B., Petito, F. *et al.* (1985) Vertebral artery injury and cerebellar stroke while swimming: a case report. *Stroke* **16**: 1039–1042.

Weiner, H.L. (1981) Transient ischemic attacks, when do they foreshadow a stroke? *Diagnosis* (Jul), 51–57.

Weintraub, M.I. (1992) Beauty parlor stroke syndrome: report of 2 cases. *Neurology* **42** (suppl 3): 340.

Weintraub, M.I. (1993) Beauty parlor stroke syndrome: report of five cases. *J.A.M.A.* **269**: 2085–2086.

White, R.P., Chapleau, C.E., Dugdale, M., Robertson, J.T. (1980) Cerebral arterial contractions induced by human and bovine thrombin. *Stroke* **11**: 363–368.

Wing, L.W., Hargrave-Wilson, W. (1974) Cervical vertigo. *Aust. N.Z. J. Surg.* **44**: 275–277.

Yang, P.J., Latack, J.T., Gabrielson, T.O. *et al.* (1985) Rotational vertebral artery occlusion at C1–2. *A.J.N.R* **6**: 98–100.

Yates, P.O. (1959) Birth trauma to the vertebral arteries. *Arch. Dis. Child.* **34**: 436–441.

Zimmermann, A.W., Kumar, A.J., Gadoth, N., Hodges, F.J. (1978) Traumatic vertebrobasilar occlusive disease in childhood. *Neurology* **28**: 185–188.

Further reading

Anonymous (1991) *A Case of Altered Records.* Back Talk National Mutual Chiropractic Mutual Insurance Company. (Fall), 5–6.

Attali, P. (1957) Accidents graves après une manipulation intempestive par un chiropractor. *Rev. Rheum.* **24**: 652.

Bakewell *v.* Kahle (1952) Medicolegal abstracts. Chiropractors: rupture of brain tumor following adjustment. *J.A.M.A.* **148**: 699. (Note: see Krueger & Okazaki (1980) for discussion of this case 30 years later.)

Bayerl, J.R., Buchmuller, H.R., Pohlmann, B. (1985) Nebenwirkungen und Kontraindikationen der manuellen therapie im bereich der Halswirbelsaule. *Nervenarzt* **56**: 194–199.

Bladin, P.F., Merory, J. (1975) Mechanisms in cerebral lesions in trauma to high cervical portion of the vertebral artery rotation injury. *Proc. Aust. Assoc. Neurol.* **12**: 35–41.

Bolton, S.P. (1987) Vascular accidents. *J. Aust. Chiro. Assoc.* **17**: 75. Case commented on in Terrett (1987b).

Boshes, L.D. (1959) Vascular accidents associated with neck manipulation. *J.A.M.A.* **171**: 1602.

Bouchet, M.M., Pailler, P. (1960) Surdite brutale et chiropractie. *Ann. Otolaryngol. (Par.)* **77**: 951–953.

Boudin, G., Barbizet, J., Pepin, B., Fouet, P. (1957) Syndrome grave du tronc cerebral après manipulations cervicales. *Bull. Mem. Soc. Med. Hop. Paris* **73**: 562–6.

Braun, I.F., Pinto, R.S., DeFilipp, G.J. *et al.* (1983) Brain stem infarction due to chiropractic manipulation of the cervical spine. *South. Med. J.* **76**: 1199–1201.

Bridges, R. (1994) Trial or settlement: circumstances that prompt the decision. *J. Chiropract.* **31**: 44–47.

Carmichael, J.P. (1994) Transient global amnesia following rotational manipulation of the upper cervical spine. Proceedings of the 1994 International Conference On Spinal Manipulation. 1701 Clarendon Boulevard, Arlington, Virginia 22209, Foundation for Chiropractic Education and Research, p. 65.

Cellerier, P., Georget, A.M. (1984) Dissection des artères vertebrales après manipulation du rachis cervical. A propos d'un cas. *J. Radiol.* **65**: 191–196.

Chen, T.W., Chen, S.T. (1987) Brainstem stroke induced by chiropractic neck manipulation – a case report. *Chung Hua I Hsueh Tsa Chih (Chinese Med. J.)* **40**: 557–562.

Cook, J.W., Sanstead, J.K. (1991) Wallenberg syndrome following self induced manipulation. *Neurology* **41**: 1695–1696.

Dahl, A., Bjark, P., Anke, I. (1982) Cerebrovaskulaere kompliskasjoner til manipulasjonsbehandling av nakken. *Tidsskr. Nor. Laegeforen.* **102**: 155–157.

Davidson, K.C., Weiford, E.C., Dixon, G.D. (1975) Traumatic vertebral artery pseudoaneurysm following chiropractic-manipulation. *Radiology* **115**: 651–652.

Dunne, J.W., Conacher, G.N., Khangure, M., Harper, C.G. (1987) Dissecting aneurysms of the vertebral arteries following cervical manipulation: a case report. *J. Neurol. Neurosurg. Psychiatry* **50**: 349–353. (Note: case also reported in Terrett (1987a) and Haynes (1994).)

Fast, A., Zinicola, D.F., Marin, E.L. (1987) Vertebral artery damage complicating cervical manipulation. *Spine* **12**: 8402.

Ford, F.R. (1952) Syncope, vertigo and disturbances of vision resulting from intermittent obstruction of the vertebral arteries due to defect in the odontoid process and excessive mobility of the second cervical vertebra. *Bull. Johns Hopkins Hosp.* **91**: 168–173.

Ford, F.R., Clark, D. (1956) Thrombosis of the basilar artery with softenings in the cerebellum and brain stem due to manipulation of the neck. *Bull. Johns Hopkins Hosp.* **98**: 37–42.

Foster *v.* Thornton (1934) Medicolegal. Malpractice: Death resulting from chiropractic treatment for headache. *J.A.M.A.* **103**: 1260. (1935) Malpractice: Cerebral hemorrhage attributed to chiropractic adjustment. *J.A.M.A.* **105**: 1714. (1937) Malpractice: Death resulting from chiropractic treatment for headache. *J.A.M.A.* **109**: 233–234.

Frisoni, G.B, Anzola, G.P. (1991) Vertebrobasilar ischaemia after neck motion. *Stroke* **22**: 1452–1460.

Fritz, V.U., Maloon, A., Tuch, P. (1984) Neck manipulation causing stroke. *South Afr. Med. J.* **66**: 844–846.

Frumkin, L.R., Baloh, R.W. (1990) Wallenberg's syndrome following neck manipulation. *Neurology* **40**: 611–615.

Gittinger, J.W. (1986) Occipital infarction following chiropractic cervical manipulation. *J. Clin. Neuro Ophthalmol.* **6**: 11–13.

Godlewski, S. (1965) Diagnostic des thromboses vertebro basilaire. *Assises Med.* **23**: 81–92.

Goodbody, R.A. (1976) Fatal post-traumatic vertebro basilar ischaemia. *J. Clin. Pathol.* **29**: 86–87.

Gorman, R.F. (1978) Cardiac arrest after cervical spine mobilization. *Med. J. Aust.* **2**: 169–170.

Green, D., Joynt, R.J. (1959) Vascular accidents to the brain stem associated with neck manipulations. *J.A.M.A.* **170**: 522–524.

Hamaan, G., Felber, S., Haass, A. *et al.* (1993) Cervicocephalic artery dissections due to chiropractic manipulations. *Lancet* **341**: 764–765.

Hardin, C.A., Williamson, P., Steegman, A. (1960) Vertebral artery insufficiency produced by cervical osteoarthritic spurs. *Neurology* **10**: 855–858.

Haynes, M.J. (1994) Stroke following cervical manipulation in Perth. *Chiropract. J. Aust.* **24**: 42–46.

Haynes, M.J. (1995) Cervical rotational effects on vertebral artery flow: a case study. *Chiropract. J. Aust.* **25**: 73–76.

Hensell, V. (1976) Neurologische Schaden nach Repositions massnahmen an der Wirbelsaule. *Med. Welt.* **27**: 656–658.

Heyden, S. (1971) Extra kranier thrombotischer arterienverschlussals folge von kopf-und halsverletzung. *Mat. Med. Nordm.* **23**: 24–32.

Horn, S.W. (1983) The "locked-in" syndrome following chiropractic manipulation of the cervical spine. *Ann. Emerg. Med.* **12**: 648–650.

Janzen-Hamburg, R. (1966) Schleudertrauma der Halswirbelsaule, neurologische probleme. *Langenbecks Arch. Klin. Chir.* **316**: 461–469.

Jentzen, J.M., Amatuzio, J., Peterson, G.F. (1987) Complications of cervical manipulation: a case report of fatal brainstem infarct with review of the mechanisms and predisposing factors. *J. Forensic Sci.* **32**: 1089–1094.

Johnson, D.W. (1993) Cervical self manipulation and stroke. *Med. J. Aust.* **158**: 290.

Jung, A., Kehr, P., Jung, F.M. (1976) Das posttraumatiche zervikal-syndrom. *Man. Med.* **14**: 101–106. (This case is also reported in Vedrine and Spay (1968) and Roche *et al.* (1963).)

Kanshepolsky, J., Danielson, H., Flynn, R.E. (1972) Vertebral artery insufficiency and cerebellar infarct due to manipulation of the neck. *Bull. LA Neurol. Soc.* **37**: 62–66.

Katirji, M.B., Reinmuth, O.M., Latchaw, R.E. (1985) Stroke due to vertebral artery injury. *Arch. Neurol.* **42**: 242–248.

Kipp, W. (1975) *Todlicher Hirnstamminfarkt nach HWS Manipulation* (dissertation). Tubingen, Eberhard Karls Universitaet, p. 39.

Kommerell, G., Hoyt, W.F. (1973) Lateropulsion of saccadic eye movements. *Arch. Neurol.* **28**: 313–318.

Kosoy, J., Glassman, A.L. (1974) Audiovestibular findings with cervical spine trauma. *Tex. Med.* **70**: 66–71.

Kramer, K.H. (1974) Wallenburg Syndrom nach manueller-Behandlung. *Man. Med.* **12**: 88–89.

Krieger, D., Leibold, M., Bruckmann, H. (1990) Dissektionen der arteria vertebralis nach zervikalen chiropraktischen manipulationen. *Dtsch Med. Wochenschr.* **115**: 580–583.

Kunkle, E.C., Muller, J.C., Odom, G.L. (1952) Traumatic brain stem thrombosis: report of a case and analysis of the mechanism of injury. *Ann. Intern. Med.* **36**: 1329–1335.

Lorenz, R., Vogelsang, H.G. (1972) Thrombose der arteria basilaris nach chiropraktischen Manipulationen an der Halswirbelsaule. *Dtsche Med. Wochenschr.* **97**: 36–43.

Malm, J., Olsson, T., Fagerlund, M. (1990) Cervikal manipulation kan ge hjarninfarkt. *Lakartidningen* **87**: 3877–3879.

Martin, H., Guiral, J. (1960) Surdite brusque au cours d'une manipulation vertebrale. *J. Franc. Oto-Rino-Laryngol.* **9**: 177–178.

Mas, J.L., Henin, D., Bousser, M.G. *et al.* (1989) Dissecting aneurysm of the vertebral artery and cervical manipulation: a case report with autopsy. *Neurology* **39**: 512–515.

Mehalic, T., Farhat, S.M. (1974) Vertebral artery injury from chiropractic manipulation of the neck. *Surg. Neurol.* **2**: 125–129.

Meyermann, R. (1982) Moglichkeiten einer schadigung der arteria vertebralis. *Man. Med.* **20**: 105–114.

Miglets, A.S. (1986) Discussion in sudden sensorineural hearing loss following manipulation of the cervical spine. *Laryngoscope* **96**: 166–170.

Miller, R.G., Burton, R. (1974) Stroke following chiropractic manipulation of the spine. *J.A.M.A.* **229**: 189–190.

Murase, S., Ohe, N., Nokura, H. *et al.* (1994) Vertebral artery injury following mild neck trauma: report of two cases. *No Shinkei Geka* 22: 671–676.

Nick, J., Contamin, F., Nicolle, M.H. *et al.* (1967) Incidents et accidents neurologiques dus aux manipulations cervicales: à propos de trois observations. *Bull. Mem. Soc. Med. Hop. Paris.* 118: 435–440.

Nielsen, A.A. (1984, 22 Oct) Cerebrovaskulaere insulter forarsaget af manipulation af columna cervicalis. Ugeskr Lager. 3267–3270. (Note: also reported in: Melhede AIL. Dod hos kiropraktor: Blev behandlet for nakke hold. *Berlingske Tidene* (Denmark) 1984 (23 October): 6. and in: Jensen L. Ga bare til kiropraktoren. *Berlingske Tidene* (Denmark) 1984 (24 October).

Nyberg-Hansen, R., Loken, A.C., Tenstad, O. (1978) Brainstem lesion with coma for five years following manipulation of the cervical spine. *J. Neurol.* 218: 97–105.

Pamela, F., Beaugerie, L., Couturier, M. *et al.* (1983) Syndrome de deefferentiation motrice par thrombose du tronc basilaire apres manipulation vertebrale. *Presse Med.* 12: 1548.

Phillips, S.J., Maloney, W.J., Gray, J. (1989) Pure motor stroke due to vertebral artery dissection. *Can. J. Neurol. Sci.* 16: 348–351.

Ponge, T., Cottin, S., Ponge, A. *et al.* (1989) Accident vasculaire vertebro-basilaire après manipulation du rachis cervical. *Rev. Rhum.* 56: 545–548.

Pratt-Thomas, H.R., Berger, K.E. (1947) Cerebellar and spinal injuries after chiropractic manipulation. *J.A.M.A.* 133: 600–603.

Pribek, R.A. (1963) Brainstem vascular accident following neck manipulation. *Wisc. Med. J.* 62: 141–143.

Raskind, R., North, C.M. (1990) Vertebral artery injuries following chiropractic cervical spine manipulation – case reports. *Angiology* 41: 445–452.

Rothrock, J.F., Hesselink, J.R., Teacher, T.M. (1991) Vertebral artery occlusion and stroke from cervical self manipulation. *Neurology* 41: 1696–1697.

Schellhas, K.P., Latchaw, R.E., Wendling, L.R., Gold, L.H.A. (1980) Vertebrobasilar injuries following cervical manipulation. *J.A.M.A.* 244: 1450–1453.

Schmitt, H.P. (1976) Rupturen und thrombosen der arteria vertebralis nach gedecklen mechanischen insulten. *Schweiz. Arch. Neurol. Neurochir. Psychiatrie* 119: 363–369. (This case was also described by Schmitt, 1978.)

Schmitt, H.P., Tamaska, L. (1973) Disseziierende ruptur der arteria vertebralis mit todlichem vertebralis und basilaris Verschluss. *Z. Rechtsmed.* 73: 301–308. (This case was also described by Schmitt, 1978.)

Schwarz, G.A., Geiger, J.K., Spano, A.V. (1956) Posterior inferior cerebellar artery syndrome of Wallenberg after chiropractic manipulation. *Arch. Intern. Med.* 97: 352–354.

Shekelle, P.G., Brook, R.H. (1991) A community based study of the use of chiropractic services. *Am. J. Public Health* 81: 439–442.

Shekelle, P.G., Adams, A.H. *et al.* (1991) *The Appropriateness of Spinal Manipulation for Low Back Pain: Project Overview and Literature Review.* Monograph no. R-4025/1-CCR/FCER. Santa Monica, California: RAND.

Sherman, M.R., Smialek, J.E., Zane, W.E. (1987) Pathogenesis of vertebral artery occlusion following cervical spine manipulation. *Arch Pathol. Lab. Med.* 111: 851–853.

Simmons, K.C., Soo, Y.S., Walker, G., Harvey, P. (1982) Trauma to the vertebral artery related to neck manipulation. *Med. J. Aust.* 1: 187–188.

Sinel, M., Smith, D. (1993) Thalamic infarction secondary to cervical manipulation. *Arch. Phys. Med. Rehabil.* 74: 543–546.

Smith, R.A., Estridge, M.N. (1962) Neurologic complications of head and neck manipulations. *J.A.M.A.* 182: 528–531.

Sullivan, E.C. (1992) Brain stem stroke syndromes from cervical adjustments: report on five cases. *J. Chiro. Res. Clin. Invest.* 8: 12–16.

Teasell, R.W. (1994) Vertebro-basilar artery stroke as a complication of cervical manipulation. *Crit. Rev. Phys. Rehabil. Med.* 6: 121–129.

Terrett, A.G.J. (1987) Vascular accidents. *J. Aust. Chiro. Assoc.* 17: 117. (Case also reported in Bolton, 1987.)

Terrett, A.G.J. (1995) Misuse of the literature by medical authors in discussing spinal manipulative therapy injury. *J. Manipul. Physiol. Ther.* 18: 203–210.

Terrett, A.G.J (1997) Vertebrobasilar stroke after spinal manipulation therapy. In: *Advances in Chiropractic*, vol. 4 (Lawrence, D.J., ed.). Illinois: Mosby Year Book (in press).

Terrett, A.G.J., Gorman, R.F. (1995) The eye, the cervical spine, and spinal manipulative therapy: a review of the literature. *Chiro. Techn.* 7: 43–54.

Vedrine, J., Spay, G. (1968) Problèmes medico legaux posés par les thromboses consécutives à un traumatisme fere des art'eres vertébrales. *Lyon Med.* 27: 5–21. (This case is also reported in Roche *et al.*, 1963 and Jung *et al.*, 1976.)

Vibert, D., Rohr Le Floch, J., Gauthier, G. (1993) Vertigo as manifestation of vertebral artery dissection after chiropractic neck manipulations. *J. Oto-Rhino-Laryngol.* 55: 140–142.

Weinstein, S.M., Cantu, R.C. (1991) Cerebral stroke in a semi-pro football player: a case report. *Med. Sci. Sports Exerc.* 23: 1119–1121.

Wood, M.J., Lang, E.K., Faludi, H.K., Woolhandler, G.J. (1971) Traumatic vertebral artery thrombosis. *J. Louisiana Med. Soc.* 123: 413–414.

York v. Daniels. (1955) Medicolegal abstracts. Chiropractors: injury to spinal meninges during adjustments. *J.A.M.A.* 159: 809.

Zak, S.M., Carmody, R.F. (1984) Cerebellar infarction from chiropractic neck manipulation: case report and review of the literature. *Ariz Med.* 41: 333–337.

Zauel, D., Carlow, T.J. (1977) Internuclear ophthalmoplegia following cervical manipulation. *Ann. Neurol.* 1: 308.

Index